Velvet Glove, Iron Fist

A History of Anti-Smoking

Christopher Snowdon

First published in Great Britain in 2009
by Little Dice

Copyright 2009 © Christopher Snowdon

ISBN 978-0-9562265-0-1

MayerBenham
55 Athenlay Road
London
SE15 3EN

Little Dice
Trinity Farm, Middleton Quernhow
Ripon, North Yorkshire
HG4 5HX, England

Cover by Devil's Kitchen Design
www.devilskitchendesign.com

www.velvetgloveironfist.com

1. 'Joyful news out of the new found world'

2. 'A smokeless America by 1925'

3. 'Your body belongs to the Fuhrer'

4. 'Some women would prefer having smaller babies'

5. 'Smokers should be eliminated'

6. 'Nonsmokers arise!'

7. 'A smoke-free America by 2000'

8. 'This is a crusade, not a lawsuit'

9. 'I have a comic book mentality'

10. 'Do not let them fool you'

11. 'How do you sleep at night Mr Blair?'

12. 'Developed societies are paternalistic'

13. 'The next logical step'

14. 'The scene is set for the final curtain'

Abbreviations

ACL	Anti-Cigarette League
ACS	American Cancer Society
ACSH	American Council on Science and Health
ALA	American Lung Association
AMA	American Medical Association
ANR	Americans For Nonsmokers' Right
ASH	Action on Smoking and Health
BMA	British Medical Association
BMJ	British Medical Journal
Cal-EPA	Californian Environmental Protection Agency
CDC	Centers for Disease Control
CHD	Coronary Heart Disease
EPA	Environmental Protection Agency
ETS	Environmental Tobacco Smoke
FCC	Federal Communications Commission
FDA	Food and Drug Administration
FTC	Federal Trade Commission
FORCES	Fight Ordinances & Regulations to Curtail & Eliminate Smoking
FOREST	Freedom Organisation for the Right to Enjoy Smoking Tobacco
GASP	Group Against Smoking Pollution
IARC	International Agency for Research on Cancer
JAMA	Journal of the American Medical Association
L & M	Liggett & Myers
MCS	Multiple Chemical Sensitivity
NCI	National Cancer Institute
NSNS	National Society of Non-Smokers
RWJF	Robert Wood Johnson Foundation
SCOTH	Scientific Committee On Tobacco or Health
WCTU	Women's Christian Temperance Union
WHO	World Health Organisation
YMCA	Young Men's Christian Association

Introduction

A unique case?

It is the summer of 2007. A humble council meeting in the Californian town of Belmont has attracted a degree of attention from the world's press to which this quiet suburban community is wholly unaccustomed. Extra security has been ordered after several councillors received death threats. On the internet, a photo of the mayor is being circulated with the image doctored to show her in full Nazi regalia.

Inside the town hall, local politicians debate a bill which, if passed, will ban smoking on every street, park and sidewalk in Belmont, as well as in all apartments and many private homes. Only detached houses will be exempt. Even nonsmokers face possible prosecution; it will be illegal for any citizen to fail to report an infringement to the police.

The debate is heated. The mayor, Coralin Feierbach, raises her voice and waves her arms as she makes her case:

"I'm thinking of the children, that's the most important thing.
Not necessarily the restaurants, not necessarily the condos,
but the children in the community."

Warming to her theme, she bangs her fist on the table three times as she shouts:

"Children! Children! Children!" (1)

This being California, it goes without saying that it is already illegal to smoke in offices, bars and restaurants. For years, the 'Golden State' has built a reputation for being tough on smoking but even ardent nonsmokers are beginning to wonder whether the anti-smoking campaign has crossed the line between protecting public health and intruding on personal freedom. "I don't know where the boundaries of a truly legally defensible ordinance are," concedes Councillor Dave Warden, a keen supporter of the bill, "I really believe that we're so close to the line that no one can really tell."(2)

As the press gathers in Belmont, the town's councillors are contemplating the most far-reaching anti-smoking law of modern times, but it will not be long before a more extreme ordinance is passed in some other part of the world and the media will move on. Smokers and civil libertarians will continue to complain of discrimination and the public health lobby will continue to devise new ways to stamp out the smoking habit.

None of this is new. The English Puritans who settled in Massachusetts and Connecticut banned smoking in the street in the 17th century. In Russia, Turkey, China and elsewhere smokers were punished with mutilation, torture and death. For five centuries tobacco was besieged on the basis of religious conviction, public morality, fire safety, racial superiority, political doctrine and often - but never exclusively - health. The fascists of Germany viewed smoking as a Communist habit just as the socialists regarded it as suspiciously bourgeois. For Christians, it was a pagan custom; for Muslims, it was a Christian invention. The anti-Semites associated it with the Jews, the teetotallers linked it to the drunks and the chaste linked it to the debauched. Wherever there was a popular cause, there were bands of anti-tobacconists ready to attach themselves to it.

Time and again the anti-smokers gathered momentum only to overreach themselves and tumble into obscurity. The political ideologies with which they allied themselves would fall out of favour, their charismatic leaders would die, their followers would come to be seen as cranks and the myriad diseases they blamed on the hated herb - infertility, blindness, hysteria, herpes and insanity, to name but a few - would be exposed as the products of fevered imaginations.

And then, in the mid-20th century, solid evidence finally surfaced which showed that the latest and most popular tobacco product - the cigarette - did indeed cause some serious diseases and all of a sudden the cranks and the moralists disappeared. No longer did anyone oppose tobacco because it led to drink or debauchery. No longer did anyone condemn it as irreligious. No one fretted about cigarettes causing fires and no one insisted - as they had only a few years earlier - that their consumption would infect the gene pool and wipe out the white race. For the first time since Columbus's first encounter with the weed, the zealots and fanatics of the anti-tobacco leagues simply vanished. In their place came a host of new organisations whose agenda was strikingly similar to that of the tobacco-haters of bygone days but whose members declared themselves to be motivated only by concern for the public health.

By now, however, the smoking public had grown used to ignoring the shrill voices that for generations had fed them tall tales about the devilish herb and so there was an urgent need to educate them about this genuine peril. It started with a warning label. In the 1960s, governments around the world ordered the tobacco industry to label each pack of their extraordinarily lucrative product with a cautionary note to its customers. Soon afterwards, the government brought the curtain down on televised cigarette commercials.

The industry complained that its right to free speech was being trampled on. In the United States, where the right to free expression was enshrined in the Constitution, they may have had a case but it was hard to deny that, as a legal product, cigarettes were unusually dangerous. American politicians remained reluctant to over-regulate business, curtail free speech or challenge the public's right to smoke, but they banned broadcast advertising all the same because cigarettes posed a "unique danger" which required unique policies.

Around the world, taxes on tobacco rose, the warnings became stronger, tobacco advertising was banned in all its forms and the number of places in which smokers could engage in their habit dwindled. Some complained that smokers were being persecuted by joyless puritans set on the outright criminalisation of tobacco. Others warned that the anti-smoking endeavour represented the thin end of a wedge that would ultimately lead to the state dictating what people ate, drank, how much they should exercise and what they should spend their money on. "Today it's cigarettes," announced one cigarette company in 1994, "Will high-fat foods be next?"(3) Such warnings fell on deaf ears, particularly when they came from the discredited tobacco industry. Those who warned that society was sliding down a slippery slope of government intrusion were accused of indulging in hyperbole bordering on paranoia. The cigarette, it was said again, was a unique case - a product that could kill when used as the manufacturer intended - and it was ludicrous to compare eating a steak or drinking a glass of wine with smoking a pack of cigarettes.

The educational campaign against smoking inspired millions of smokers to kick their habit but millions more persisted and, much to the surprise of the anti-smoking groups, millions more took up the habit in full knowledge of the hazards. For those who sought tobacco's destruction, the well of government measures that could be deployed to dissuade individuals from risking their own health was running dry and so a new theory emerged.

The evidence that tobacco smoke was still dangerous at vastly diluted levels in the form of secondhand smoke was scant but the idea was invaluable to those who wanted the anti-smoking campaign to shift up a few gears. With it, the hated, stinking smoke became a menace to all and could be prohibited as a threat to the lives of others. Smokers stubbornly continued to puff away in streets, doorways and in their homes but the end, it seemed, was nigh.

By the time the councillors of Belmont were debating the merits of banning smoking in people's own homes, the battlers for public health had long since expanded their horizons beyond cigarettes and were campaigning for legislation against products which were neither unique nor necessarily dangerous. This, too, began with a warning label. Today, the spokesmen and spokeswomen of the health organisations demand warnings be placed on wine bottles, food packaging, cars, gambling machines, aeroplanes, bottled water and large-sized clothes. Activists of all kinds wrestle with one another for the prize of having their cause seen as "the new smoking."

As before, the warnings serve to identify certain products and forms of behaviour as socially undesirable and, also as before, they are merely a prelude to fresh bans and further legislation. Advertising executives now accept that the days of promoting alcoholic drinks on television are numbered. Commercials for hamburgers, chips, cheese and full-fat milk have begun to disappear from the airwaves in Britain and elsewhere. Politicians are regularly advised to slap 'sin taxes' on food and drink, to issue their citizens with pedometers, to limit the number of drinks that can be served in bars, to deny medical treatment to the overweight, to compel restauranteurs to put warnings on their menus, to ban smokers from adopting children and to prohibit perfume, aftershave and other supposed 'toxins' in the workplace.

Are these pragmatic measures to protect the public health or unwarranted intrusions into private behaviour? Do these new laws represent the next logical step or the slippery slope? These are questions that have been asked for generations. We have been here many times before. To give but one example, the American temperance movement of the 19th century began by condemning heavy drinking and hard liquor. Temperance - as its name suggests - meant moderation, not abolition, but within a few decades the anti-saloon activists were calling for the complete criminalisation of the production and consumption of all forms of alcohol.

Prohibition was achieved in 1919 and one newspaper compared the ranks of victorious teetotallers to "a soldier of fortune after the peace is signed."(4) Suddenly redundant, but with no intention of disbanding, it took the moral crusaders only a matter of weeks before they had set their sights on banning tobacco and were rallying round the banner of 'Nicotine Next.' Seventy-five years later, the vice-president of the country's foremost anti-smoking group, Americans for Nonsmokers' Rights, was asked what she would do if tobacco should miraculously disappear. Her candid answer was that she would "simply move on to other causes."(5)

This is the story of just one cause, a cause that for many years seemed doomed but which ultimately set the template for the public health campaigns of the present-day. It is a story populated by characters who had little in common beyond a mutual hatred of tobacco, and it is a story that began long before any of the elements that colour our perception of the smoking issue today existed. When Columbus explored the New World there was no tobacco industry and no advertising industry. The link between smoking and cancer was unknown. There was no concept of passive smoking, let alone 'passive drinking' or 'secondhand obesity.' The battle against smoking began without any of this and yet it began all the same, almost from the moment the Spanish lit their first pipes, and it rarely let up in the five hundred years that followed.

CHAPTER ONE

'Joyful news out of the new found world'

The first European to smoke tobacco was the first to be persecuted for it. In October 1492, after two months at sea, Christopher Columbus reached America. When he landed in Cuba a month later, two of his crew - Rodrigo de Jerez and Luis de Torres - were greeted by Native Americans who presented them with tobacco leaves as an offering of friendship and the two Spaniards were initiated in the art of smoking.

The Indians of North and Central America had been chewing and smoking the plant in religious rituals since around 5000 BC, believing it to be a gift from God with the power to drive out evil spirits. Used in medicine, it was thought that tobacco smoke could cure a variety of physical ailments and, over time, men of higher status began to use it as a mild recreational drug. When used socially, tobacco greased the wheels of social interaction and eased tensions, most famously when the pipe of peace was smoked.

The Native Americans Columbus and his men encountered used a Y-shaped pipe called a 'toboca', from which the Spanish derived the word 'tobacco'. The great explorer later described how they would take the pipe, light it at "one end and at the other chew or suck or take it in their breath that smoke which dulls their flesh and as it were intoxicates and so they say that they do not feel weariness."(1) Both the pipe and the weed were alien to Europeans and, as Columbus's description indicates, they had no verb with which to describe the process. For years it would be known as "drinking smoke."

From the very outset, the people of the Old World were divided between those who swiftly became enamoured of tobacco and those who

ii

found the smell unpleasant and the habit depraved. Whether Columbus himself tried smoking the pipe we do not know for sure. Certainly he did not like the look of it. Sent on a mission to find gold, he must have been deflated to find that the natives considered these dried leaves to be amongst the New World's greatest treasures. Not seeing any worth in it for himself, Columbus was bewildered and appalled when Rodrigo de Jerez and other members of his crew readily embraced the herb and he berated them for descending to the level of 'savages'. Tellingly, and in spite of his remonstrations, he observed that "it was not within their power to refrain from indulging in the habit."(2)

Within days of first laying eyes on it, Columbus had identified some of the key characteristics of tobacco smoking; that it relieved tiredness and hunger, aided relaxation and that it was a habit which, once started, was not always easy to give up. Assuming this curious plant to be of no financial value, Columbus did not include it in the cargo for the return journey and it was left to other crew members to introduce it to his homeland.

Since tobacco was uniquely associated with the godless 'Red Indians', the Catholic Church considered it suspect, if not outright heretical, and was immediately hostile to those who indulged in it. The Spain of Ferdinand and Isabella was not a good place to ally oneself with devilry and pagan savagery. Our man Rodrigo de Jerez was interrogated by the Spanish Inquisition and imprisoned for seven years for the crime of being an unrepentant smoker.

With such violent opposition to its use, tobacco remained an arcane curiosity for many years. Grown on the other side of a wide ocean it was, in any case, unavailable to the public in abundance. Even when seeds, rather than leaves, were brought to European shores, tobacco was a difficult and needy plant to cultivate. It was not until the middle of the 16th century, after many more transatlantic voyages and the appearance of the first tobacco crops at home, that tobacco generated any real interest.

In the New World, however, tobacco was in plentiful supply and many European settlers smoked habitually, often whilst enjoying another new discovery: the hammock. But for every convert to the weed there was someone else who found it disagreeable. Gonzalo Fernadez de Oviedo y Valdes went to the West Indies in 1514 and was shocked to find that tobacco use had taken hold even amongst "some Christians." He called smoking a "bad and pernicious custom" and wrote that "the man who acts thus merely passes while still alive into a deathly stupor."(3) Another observer, writing in 1527, noted that Indians who smoked tobacco were consumed by "a species of intoxication" and called it, not for the first or last time, "a disgusting habit."(4)

Despite those who complained of the "diabolical stench,"(5) tobacco began to find pockets of support, first in Portugal, then in Spain and France, on the back of its supposed curative effects. The Portuguese explorer Magellan introduced it to India and China via the Phillipines in the 1560s and physicians found themselves intrigued by the plant wherever they came across it. Andre Thevet, observing Native Americans in 1557, wrote: "They say it is very good to drive forth and consume the superfluous moisture in the head. Besides, when taken this way, it makes it possible to endure hunger and thirst for some time."(6) In 1571, the Seville physician Nicholas Monardes wrote what amounted to a love letter to tobacco - *Joyfull Newes out of the Newe Founde Worlde* - in which he identified more than twenty medical ailments which could, he claimed, be cured by tobacco. Like Columbus, Monardes remarked on its peculiar capacity to stimulate at one time and sedate at another.

Jean Nicot, a French diplomat who spent much time in Portugal, was instrumental in bringing tobacco to the courts of northern Europe. The practice of snuffing had been first witnessed in Mexico by early explorers and tobacco users in this period were as likely to put it up their nose as they were to stuff it in a pipe. In 1560, Nicot advised the ageing Catherine de Medici - by this time France's Queen Mother - to take snuff for the good of her health. She and her circle soon became enthusiastic snuffers and Catherine decreed that tobacco be known as *Herba Regina*. So influential and persuasive was Nicot in popularising tobacco that his surname was used when its active ingredient - nicotine - was discovered, isolated and named in 1828.

The actual *smoking* of tobacco was largely confined to sailors and settlers until the mid-1560s, when the practice was introduced to

England by Sir John Hawkins and Sir Francis Drake. In the 1580s, Drake recommended it to Sir Walter Raleigh who, in turn, became a great advocate of the weed. In 1585, smoking was still rare enough for Raleigh to be doused in water by a servant who walked in and assumed him to be on fire (although this story may be apocryphal), but England was entering an era in which it would become uniquely identified with smoking. The upper echelons of Elizabethan society, perhaps including the Queen herself, smoked tobacco recreationally, and the lower orders duly imitated them. By the end of the century, smoking - usually through a long-stem pipe - was common throughout all sections of English society and was beginning to spread through mainland Europe and parts of Asia.

As it did so, tobacco's reputation as a medical panacea continued to grow. Anthony Chute's *Tobacco*, published in 1595, was the first book on the subject to be written in the English language. In it, Chute echoed Monardes' bold claims on behalf of the herb, recommending its use as a "sovereign remedy against coughs, rheum in the stomach, head and eyes." There was nothing, he wrote, "from the girdle upward, [that cannot] be taken away with a moderate use of tobacco."(7)

Four years later, Henry Buttes, in *Dyets Dry Dinner*, wrote that tobacco smoking benefited the throat, lungs and stomach and was particularly good for the head and chest. Others endorsed it as a cure for gonorrhoea and plague, and as a disinfectant and tooth-whitener. Rather less absurdly, some claimed it could be used to treat depression, as well as that much discussed malady of the age, melancholy.

That such extravagant and wrongheaded claims were ever made for smoking, even in early modern Europe, is difficult to fathom. One is tempted to suggest that the effects of nicotine were addling its devotees' brains to the point of wide-eyed delusion. And yet, physicians did have a crude idea that germs were carried through the air and there was a belief that smoke, any kind of smoke, could cleanse the atmosphere.

A mystical belief in smoke, if not *smoking*, had been part of European culture since Classical times. Hippocrates had recommended the use of smoke around the genitals to treat hysteria in women, the Catholic Church had long used candles and incense to represent purification and, like the native Americans, Christians used smoke to ward off evil spirits. When an outbreak of plague hit a community - as happened with devastating regularity throughout the medieval period - it was common to find townsfolk lighting bonfires so that, through a combination of smoke and heat, the pestilence would be banished. In this context, the notion that the body could be cleansed and fumigated by inhaling smoke was not so extraordinary.

As the 16th century wore on, the Catholic Church's opposition to tobacco began to wane. In 1575, smoking was prohibited in every church in the Spanish empire and Pope Urban VIII issued a papal bull against tobacco use in church, but these moves were more practical than theological. The papal bull was issued as a direct response to the widespread smoking and chewing of tobacco in the church in Seville; the floor of which had become "filthy with tobacco juice spittings during Mass."(8) By 1600, neither the Catholic Church nor the growing Protestant movement were any longer doctrinally opposed to tobacco.

The counter-blaste

The dizzying rise of tobacco use in Elizabethan England was as unregulated as it was unrestrained. When King James VI of Scotland became King James I of England in 1603, smoking, much to his disgust, had never been more popular. One can only speculate as to what lay at the root of James I's hatred of smoking, although we do know he loathed Sir Walter Raleigh with an equal passion. Judging from the prolific use of the word 'stinking' in his anti-tobacco tracts, the king found the smell of tobacco smoke obnoxious and was bewildered by his new subjects' eagerness to embrace it. Scornful of the perceived medicinal benefits that tobacco's advocates claimed for the weed, he put its popularity down to a mindless fad. "And so from hand to hand," he wrote, "it spreads till it be practised by all, not for any commodity that is in it, but only because it is come to be in fashion."(9)

In 1604, he wrote the first great anti-smoking treatise, *A Counter-Blaste to Tobacco*, in which he famously described smoking as a habit "loathsome to the eye, hateful to the nose, harmful to the brain, dangerous to the lungs." He claimed that autopsies of smokers revealed their organs to be infected "with an unctuous oily kind of soot" and added - several hundred years before the term 'passive smoking' entered the vocabulary - that smokers infected others with this "soot" by "soiling and infecting" the air around them.

The term "soot" was one for which anti-smokers of this era had a great fondness. Another anti-smoking tract, pointedly entitled *Work For Chimney Sweeps*, claimed that tobacco made smokers sterile and their brains 'sooty'. Witnessing smoking for the first time was always a shock to the uninitiated and, lacking any frame of reference, observers could only compare the smoker's head to a chimney. 'Soot' therefore became the favoured word to describe the black residue they assumed must remain in the smoker's brain. An examination of the residue left in the smoker's pipe appeared to bear out their analysis.

Health concerns were not James I's only reason for despising smoking. Tobacco's origins amongst "those beastly Indians" continued to be held against it. Smoking - or "the Indian vice," as he called it - was "barbarous" and "savage" as well as being ungodly and idolatrous. Worse still, it had been brought to England by "a father so generally hated" (a reference to Raleigh, who he would later have beheaded). King James was evidently little impressed with the New World. He considered its main gifts to Europeans to have been first tobacco, then syphilis. Needless to say, tobacco's blinkered supporters believed that it cured syphilis too.

Although *Counter-blaste* was published anonymously, it was not long before the author's regal identity became public knowledge and, when it did, something of a national debate ensued, culminating with an actual debate at Oxford University which was attended by the king himself. Both students and faculty were obliged to put away their pipes until he left.

Counter-blaste inspired a spate of anti-smoking articles and poems in England. These were often penned by palace favourites and cronies and had a relentlessly sycophantic tone. Smoking was variously attacked as immoral, heretical, a fire hazard, a waste of farmland and a gateway to drunkenness and decadence. Court poet Joshua Sylvester wrote the lengthy diatribe *Tobacco Battered* in which tobacco was described as "a weed; which to their idols, pagans sacrifice." In 1626, Orpheus Junior wrote *The Golden Fleece* in which it was suggested that smoking damaged a man's lungs, throat, circulation and sperm:

> "It breeds a wheezing in a narrow breast,
> The hectic fever or thick phlegm at least,
> A bastard heat within the veins it leaves,
> Which spoils the infant if the wife conceives"(10)

It was health too, which concerned Samuel Rowlands when he returned to the concept of 'soot' in his *Epigram 18*: "In head, heart, lungs, doth soot and cobwebs breed," he wrote (11). George Wither, in *On Vanity: Satire 1*, reiterated James I's contention that those who smoked did so only to fit in with others:

> "So they have seen some do: and therefore they forsooth must use it to."

William Shakespeare never once mentioned tobacco in his plays, despite smoking being widespread in the Globe theatre. Possibly he did not wish to displease James I but, if so, the bard cannot personally have had anything against smoking, otherwise he would surely have tried to further curry favour with the king by attacking it on stage (12).

The other great playwright of the age had much stronger views on smoking and was happy to advertise them. Ben Johnson mercilessly satirised the outlandish claims made on tobacco's behalf and, in 1621, lamented that "the scent of the vapour before and behind hath foully perfumed most part of the isle."(13) Tobacco, said Johnson, was "good for nothing but to choke a man and fill him full of smoke and embers." Even Anthony Chute, who had glorified tobacco in 1595, was condemning those who smoked it recreationally by the time his *Tobacco* reached its sixth edition in 1626. In a shameless about-turn, he now called it "a vicious habit."

England's legion of smokers did not take this criticism lying down. *A Defence of Tobacco* was soon published as a counter-blast to *Counterblaste* and was as genial and light-hearted as James I's essay had been po-faced and humourless. Sensibly choosing to publish anonymously - men had lost their heads for less - the author suggested that rather than viewing tobacco as the work of the devil, it would be "a more charitable notion to think that it came from God."(14) He questioned the king's assertion that smokers were full of soot, saying that there was no comparison between a man and a pipe, and challenged him to examine the throats and noses of smokers. If he did, the author promised, James would find them "as clean mouthed and throated as any man alive."(15)

Edmund Gardiner went further in 1610, making tobacco sound more like a psychedelic drug that opened the doors of perception when he asserted that through tobacco "we may see the wonderful works of God, how that he can make things strange, great, and incomprehensible and wonderful to man's judgment." This was precisely the kind of hyperbole that Ben Johnson delighted in lampooning, but the anti-smokers' claims about the dangers of smoking, while occasionally stumbling upon a medical truth, had no more basis in science than the pro-smokers' claims to the contrary. Cancer was barely recognised and even less well understood. Before the arrival of the cigarette, tobacco was not deeply inhaled into the lungs. Nicotine was primarily absorbed through the gums and the health effects of pipe-smoking were far from clear (nor are they now). The death from nose cancer of renowned smoking advocate and scientist Thomas Hariot in 1586 attracted little comment from either side.

If you can't beat them, tax them

There was nothing to prevent James I from making tobacco illegal in 1604. If he believed everything he said about the terrible dangers of tobacco smoking then criminalisation was the most obvious course of action. Doubtless he would have relished any opportunity to stamp the habit out by force but he was faced with a dilemma that has dogged many men and women of like mind ever since. In the space of twenty years, smoking had spread throughout every corner of his kingdom and banning it would be wildly unpopular, wholly impractical and utterly unenforceable.

In spite of the dull English climate, coarse tobacco was being grown domestically and superior American varieties could be smuggled into the country with relative ease. England was a major exporter of tobacco and all Virginian tobacco had, by law, to be distributed via English ports. This made it doubly difficult to keep tobacco imports away from an English population that had developed a substantial appetite for them.

Faced with the practical failure and political unpopularity of prohibition, James I became the first to do what many have done since: he turned to taxation. In 1604, he increased the duty on tobacco by an eye-watering 4,000%. This, he anticipated, would reduce consumption while increasing government revenue. He then limited the amount of tobacco that could be imported from Virginia in a bid to raise the market price further still.

This proved to be too much for England's smokers. Smuggling rose and English farmers grew tobacco in prodigious quantities. So heavy was the trade in contraband that, despite the massive tax rise, the treasury found itself receiving less revenue from tobacco duty than it had before. Not too proud to turn pragmatist, James I reversed his decision and lowered the tax while banning tobacco farming at home. In 1624, he made the tobacco industry a royal monopoly (16).

Events abroad mirrored the English experience. Philip III of Spain was no friend of the Indian vice and, in 1606, he restricted tobacco farming in his South American colonies. When, eight years later, it became apparent that the treasury was forgoing a fortune in lost taxation, he repealed the ordinance but ordered - under penalty of death - that all tobacco be channelled through Seville. At a stroke, Seville became the world capital of tobacco and would remain so for the rest of the century.

Louis XIII of France saw smokers as a bountiful source of revenue and placed a duty of 30 sols on every pound of tobacco imported. His son and heir Louis XIV was a more vocal opponent of smoking and would have liked to prohibit it entirely but he could not afford to sacrifice the money that tobacco added to his coffers. Napoleon Bonaparte could not bear the taste of tobacco but Napoleon III became a great consumer of it, reputedly smoking fifty cigarettes a day. On being asked to ban the "vice" of smoking, the younger Napoleon replied he would happily do so "as soon as you can name a virtue that brings in as much revenue."(17)

The cruel and the unusual

If smokers felt aggrieved at having to pay a little more tax to support their habit, they might have consoled themselves that they lived in northern Europe. There were plenty of countries elsewhere in the world where smokers faced far tougher anti-smoking measures than mere punitive taxes.

The first half of the 17th century saw draconian laws brought in to eliminate tobacco use from Sicily to China. The czar of Russia banned the sale and consumption of tobacco completely in 1634 after a series of fires were blamed on smokers. He complained that the Russian people were spending their last pennies on tobacco instead of food and filling the churches with smoke. First offenders were flogged and had their nostrils slit; those caught a second time were executed.

In 1644, the Chinese emperor Chongzhen banned smoking and ordered that tobacco importers be beheaded. In Japan, tobacco was banned virtually as soon as the English introduced it at the dawn of the 17th century. Again, the penalty for disobedience was death.

Feeling against tobacco was particularly strong in the Muslim world. Just as some in Europe regarded smoking as a pagan activity, many Muslims viewed it as a pernicious Christian custom. Successive rulers were ferocious in their zeal to nip the tobacco threat in the bud. In Hindustan, the Mogul emperor Jahangir decided that since "the smoking of tobacco has taken a very bad effect upon the health and mind of many persons, I order that no one should practice the habit."(18) Offenders had their lips slit. His brother Shah Abbas, the ruler of Persia, punished both smokers and tobacco merchants with death, saying: "Cursed be that drug that cannot be discerned from the dung of horses."(19)

After Shah Abbas's death, his son continued to wage war on smokers, sentencing them to be executed by having molten lead poured down their throats. In Turkey, the fanatical Murad IV (1623-40) banned smoking after a fire in Constantinople and had offenders gruesomely executed, on one occasion having twenty army officers tortured to death for flouting the law.

In those days of absolute monarchy, laws on smoking were dictated according to the whims of emperors and kings. Where despots, overlords and princes were absent, it was left to reforming groups to act against tobacco collectively. In Switzerland, early anti-smoking activists petitioned a number of town councils to "take steps against the 'epidemic of smoking.'"(20) A Chambre de Tabac was established and those caught smoking in public were fined, pilloried or imprisoned.

In North America, the clamp down on tobacco began when the Puritan element came to dominate the politics of New England in the 1620s. Those settlers who tried growing tobacco for a living were quickly restrained and, in 1632, Massachusetts banned smoking in public. Connecticut only allowed its residents to smoke in their own home and, even then, just once a day. Smokers had to be at least 20 years old, be alone and be in possession of a smoking license. The Governor of New Amsterdam (now known as New York) banned smoking entirely in 1639 and, in 1676, it became a crime for residents of New France (now known as Canada) to smoke or carry tobacco in the streets.

Considering the brutality of the punishments dished out to smokers in large parts of the world it is remarkable that the habit not only survived but thrived during the 17th century. Even in the Muslim world people continued to light up because, as the contemporary Turkish writer Katib Chelebi put it: "Men desire what is forbidden."(21) The Turkish ban was lifted in 1647.

When Sicily criminalized smoking, the law was ignored to such a degree that the government was reduced to spreading a rumour that the Turks had poisoned Sicily's tobacco imports in a desperate bid to get its citizens to stop. Even in Switzerland, where anti-smoking laws came about democratically rather than despotically, tobacco use flourished; Swiss authorities admitted that they faced "a spirit of opposition which is not easy to suppress."(22)

The unintended consequence of China's ban on tobacco was an upsurge in the smoking of opium and few observers regarded this as a step forward. Anger at the tobacco ban is thought to have been a factor when the peasantry stormed the Imperial palace two years later and the law was subsequently repealed. The dissident anti-smoking scholar Fang Yizhi described the triumph of smoking in the years that followed:

> "It gradually spread within all our borders, so that everyone now carries a
> long pipe and swallows the smoke after lighting it with fire;
> some have become drunken addicts." (23)

The Chinese writer Quan Zuwang, on the other hand, wrote that smoking provided "pure pleasure and spiritual sublimity" and could "dispel boredom and preoccupation, a necessity for daily life."(24)

Tobacco's unstoppable ascent in the 17th century was helped along by war and pestilence. Soldiers fighting in the Thirty Years War (1618-48) found smoking a pipe the perfect way to alleviate stress, boredom and hunger and when the Great Plague swept through Europe in the 1660s, people again put their faith in the power of smoke. Charles II's physician announced that tobacco offered effective protection from the disease and pupils at Eton were given a pipe to smoke each morning. The great diarist Samuel Pepys instinctively bought a pouch of tobacco upon hearing that the plague had reached his district of London. Tobacco would continue to be prescribed by doctors in Europe for everything from bronchitis to smallpox until the late 19th century.

Every attempt to bring the smoking craze to a halt ended in dismal failure and by 1700 most countries had abandoned criminalisation in favour of taxation. As anti-smoking laws fell apart so too did the anti-smoking movement, insofar as a scattering of individuals speaking out against smoking could be described as a movement.

For those who still objected to tobacco, it was the pervasive smell that most riled them. Smokers, wrote one 17th century German, "stink just like pigs and goats." Another wrote that "they always stink so horribly - like a smouldering heap of ruins - that no-one can bear to be in their company." Another writer with a great fondness for the adjective 'stinking' was Jakob Balde, a Jesuit priest, who in 1658 wrote an anti-smoking treatise which described smoking as 'dry drunkenness' and asked: "What difference is there between a smoker and a suicide except that the one takes longer to kill him than the other?"(25) By this time, judging by the dearth of anti-smoking literature from the period, such sentiments were the preserve of a small group of die-hard anti-tobacconists living on the fringes of a smoky mainstream society. Tobacco had triumphed.

The fall and rise of smoking

The ubiquity of pipe smoking amongst the lower classes drove the English aristocracy to seek out new and exclusive methods of enjoying tobacco. In the 1700s, this elite turned its back on smoking and, inspired by the French, adopted snuff. Charles II had picked up the snuff habit when he was exiled in Paris during the English Civil War and it became popular with his courtiers. In 1702, the English navy plundered thousands of barrels of snuff and this plentiful supply, combined with the aristocracy's Francophilia, led to an upsurge in its use.

Working men continued to smoke their clay pipes throughout the 18th century but for the upper and middle classes snuffing was all the fashion and Samuel Johnson was perplexed to find that in the circles in which he mixed, smoking had all but died out. "I cannot account," he said, "why a thing that requires so little exertion, and yet preserves the mind from total vacuity, should have gone out."(26)

Snuff's supporters credited the powder with fantastic qualities on a par with those claimed by tobacco's earliest fans. They claimed it cured, amongst many other things, bronchitis, consumption and apoplexy. One formerly blind man was quoted as saying:

"On taking one small pinch...my eyes opened.
I am now 96, can read the smallest type without glasses by moonlight, and drink barrels of the most potent beverages without a dream of a headache."(27)

Since snuff was smokeless it did not pose a fire risk and, perhaps more importantly, was less liable to cause offence to those who did not have a nose for tobacco. It thereby escaped much of the criticism that had been laid at the door of pipe and cigar smoking. In America, the phenomenal popularity of chewing tobacco pacified anti-smokers in much the same way.

Praise for snuff was more common than vilification, but it was still tobacco and so it still had its detractors. As a sign of debauchery and immorality, snuff use was considered little better than smoking. The allegations made against the habit had a familiar ring to them. It was variously described as a cause of dyspepsia, nausea and apoplexy, it was said to ruin the vocal cords and, once again, to fill the brain with 'soot'.

In any case, the love affair with snuff did not survive the turn of the century. The English gentry's emulation of Gallic behaviour came to an abrupt halt when the French began sending their own aristocracy to the guillotine in 1789. Snuff's decline was even more sudden in France itself, where its use was viewed as a gesture of solidarity with the royal family.

And so it was that smoking made a rapid resurgence in respectable society at the end of the 18th century, with the English adopting the cigar and the French turning to the hand-rolled cigarette. Matches were invented in 1827, helpfully ushering in an era of trouble-free smoking.

British soldiers fighting the Spanish in the Peninsula War (1808-14) found that clay pipes broke too easily and adopted cigars, which they brought back home when peace broke out. Cigar imports into Britain rose at a startling rate; from just 26 pounds a year in 1800 to 250,000 pounds in 1830 (28). In the United States, cigars had for years been too closely associated with British imperialism for them to gain popularity and it took a war with Mexico (1846-48) for them to gain a foothold in the market, again due to provincial soldiers being introduced to foreign smoking habits.

Of greatest lasting significance was the Crimean War (1854-56) for it was in the Crimea that British soldiers encountered cigarettes for the first time, courtesy of their Turkish allies. The British had always viewed cigarettes as a foreign and unmanly mode of smoking but they were practical on the front-line and soldiers sought them out when they returned home. But cigarettes were little more than a novelty in Britain and were not always easy to find. Spotting a gap in the market, a Bond

Street tobacconist began hiring girls to hand roll cigarettes for the soldiers and students who were asking for them. The tobacconist's name was Philip Morris.

The Victorian anti-tobacco movement

The 19th century saw the emergence of campaigns for such diverse causes as vegetarianism, Sunday observance, healthy living and animal rights (29). Public health crusaders worked to clean up the water supply and end the epidemics of cholera which plagued Britain's towns and cities. Temperance and teetotalism became the dominant reforming movements of the age, underscored by the religious convictions of the Methodist Church and a genuine desire to save the working classes from impoverished lives and early deaths.

In England, the holiday industry pioneer Thomas Cook became the first well-known anti-smoker of the Victorian era when he published a journal by the name of *Anti-Smoker and Progressive Temperance Reformer* in 1841, the world's first anti-smoking newsletter (30).

In Australia, and in the same decade, Dr Robert Welch spoke out against tobacco in a speech to the Total Abstinence Society and, in an article in *The Temperance Advocate*, endorsed the view that smoking went hand-in-hand with drinking. He was followed by the self-styled 'Professor' James Rennie, a fifty-three year old Scottish school master, who arrived in Sydney and gave a speech denouncing smoking as "one of the most extensively diffused evils with which the new world has infected the old."(31) It proved not to be a popular cause and Rennie was roundly ridiculed in the Australian press.

There was very little in the way of organised opposition to tobacco in Britain until April 1853 when the Anti-Tobacco Society was formed by Canon Stowell and Thomas Reynolds. The newspapers were unsupportive, with *The Saturday Review* reporting on one of their meetings thus:

"Tobacco does not agree with them.
There are a good many people with whom the Indian herb does not agree...

> But we have a right to hint to them that their dislike of tobacco
> should not teach them to violate truth and charity...
> There are - we own that we are of that party - many to whom pride and ignorance,
> bad logic and cant, are as insufferable as tobacco is to Mr Stowell." (32)

The Anti-Tobacco Society did not have anything original to add regarding the effects of smoking on the human body and their claims that it caused deafness, blindness, hysteria, dyspepsia, impotence and paralysis had all been heard before. Coming from a temperance background, its members' principle concern was that smoking would lead to drinking, vice, breach of Sunday observance and idleness. Tobacco was, as its secretary Thomas Reynolds proclaimed, "the stepping-stone to other evils."(33)

It was Reynolds who would become the movement's guiding light and its best known character, a result of his tireless public speaking and a inclination towards self-mythology that bordered on the histrionic. When he lectured in churches, boys' clubs and temperance halls he was received with cautious enthusiasm but when he presented his fearless views to the less sympathetic audiences of the British Association for the Advancement of Science or Cambridge University he received some frosty receptions; the latter meeting concluded with the police escorting him from the room for his own protection.

Faced with an unhelpful combination of apathy and contempt, the Anti-Tobacco Society was largely ignored in its early years and had achieved virtually nothing by 1857, when the esteemed medical journal, *The Lancet*, published an article by Samuel Solly, himself a member of the Society and an ex-smoker. Solly wrote that he knew of "no *single* vice which does so much harm as smoking" (emphasis in the original), and asserted that it caused paralysis and various other terrible ailments. As a retort to those who celebrated tobacco's psychologically calming effects, he added that those who were "troubled in mind" should not be smoking but should instead take the quintessentially Victorian remedy of "submitting to the rod, and rising strengthened by chastisement."(34)

Solly's views were contentious. The medical establishment had for years considered smoking to be largely benign, if not downright beneficial. As a "single vice," most doctors agreed that drinking was much the greater peril. For the next twelve months, the pages of *The Lancet* became home to an international debate on the 'tobacco controversy'. Although the arguments were unsophisticated from a modern perspective, a calm assessment of the views of the world's doctors was overdue: it helped move the debate on from the cycle of unfounded claim and counter-claim between the pro and anti-smokers that had barely matured since the 16th century.

Only three years earlier John Lizars, an Edinburgh surgeon and another member of the Anti-Tobacco Society, had revived the memory of James I with a report stating that smoking caused "giddiness, sickness, vomiting, dyspepsia, viticated taste of the mouth, loose bowels, diseased liver, congestion of the brain, apoplexy, mania, loss of memory, [blindness], deafness, nervousness, palsy, emasculation and cowardice."(35) The esteemed surgeon also believed that syphilis was spread by the sharing of a pipe.

In reality, scientific evidence that smoking could be lethal was very thin on the ground. John Hill had reported an association with cancer of the nasal passages in 1761, citing Thomas Hariot's death from this disease in 1586 as (rather anecdotal) evidence. In Germany, Samuel T. von Soemmerring associated smoking with cancer of the lip and, in the 1850s, the Frenchman Etienne-Frederic Bouisson reported that of the 68 lip cancer patients he had studied, 63 smoked a pipe. Since all but two of these cancer cases had smoked a short pipe, Bouisson put this down to the heat rather than the tobacco. These slender findings represented the sum total of four hundred years of medical research into tobacco.

The Lancet debate exhibited prejudice, special pleading, common sense, peculiarity and perception in equal measure. Some doctors regurgitated the argument that smoking turned good boys bad and led to debauchery. One correspondent countered Solly's claims that smoking caused sterility and lunacy by noting that the nation's birth rate was rising and that most lunatics were women. Dr Pidduck wrote in to report that fleas did not attack smokers because their blood was so foul that it could kill leeches (it was not clear if this was a good or a bad thing for smokers).

More presciently, Dr J.B. Neil wondered whether insurance companies should ask their customers whether they smoked and another correspondent speculated that if a time ever came when tobacco smoke came into contact with the lungs or bronchial tubes, men would soon stop smoking. A German correspondent said that his own country had become "the great tobacco furnace of the age" and suggested that "the tendency of Germans to disease of the lungs may be traced to their incredible passion for smoking."

The Lancet debate did not result in any firm conclusions being reached about smoking and health, largely because neither side could substantiate their claims. In general, the medical community felt that although there might be some cause for concern it was of little consequence as a public health threat, especially when compared to the great tuberculosis and cholera epidemics of the day.

The Anti-Tobacco Society attempted to harness *The Lancet* controversy as a means of spring-boarding their cause into the public's consciousness. They launched *The Anti-Tobacco Journal* in 1858 and published a number of pamphlets condemning tobacco but interest in the subject, which at one point had reached the pages of *The Times*, was already waning. After a brief period of failure the Anti-Tobacco Society went into decline, trundling along with a few hundred members until the end of the century. All the while it was mocked for its extremism, unpopularity and penury by *The Times*, *Punch* and, most relentlessly, *Cope's Tobacco Plant*. The latter was the journal of the eponymous Liverpool tobacco company which, dominant to the point of arrogance, suggested Reynolds form an Anti-Teapot Society. For all the impact Reynolds had on changing attitudes towards smoking, he might as well have taken their advice.

In 1877, Emile Decroix founded France's first anti-smoking society, The Society Against the Abuse of Tobacco. Decroix had been fighting a two-pronged war against tobacco and horse meat since the 1850s and he assembled a group of around one hundred opponents of tobacco, including Louis Pasteur, to campaign against the weed. Decroix's society owed less to the temperance movement than that of Britain and instead rode the wave of France's *fin-de-siecle* healthy living movement. This did not make them any less prone to hyperbole; one of their spokesmen blamed smoking for France's defeat in the Franco-Prussian War, saying it had robbed their soldiers of their intellect, emaciated their limbs and made them physically unable to move towards the enemy. Emile Decroix's death in 1901 coincided with the end of the great Gallic health reform movement in general and the Society Against the Abuse of Tobacco in particular.

Across the Atlantic, 1857 saw the publication of the first issue of America's own *Anti-Tobacco Journal*, the brainchild of the Reverend George Trask who appointed himself the 'Anti-Tobacco Apostle'. Trask had formed his own Anti-Tobacco Society in 1850 as an adjunct to the American anti-liquor movement. He lived in the old Puritan stronghold of Massachussetts where it remained illegal to have a lit pipe out of doors (36), and he called tobacco "Satan's fuel for the drinking appetites."(37) A teetotalling ex-smoker, Trask published his journal for 15 years and was, quite literally, a one-man movement; as well as writing the newsletter, he was the society's vice-president, secretary, treasurer and spokesman.

Since chewing tobacco had long been the most popular way of consuming tobacco in America, it was on this that Trask focused his attention. The health implications were particularly murky with regard to chewing tobacco (although Trask hazarded a wild guess that 20,000 Americans died each year from tobacco related diseases) and so the same old arguments about tobacco leading to alcohol were rehashed. A few individuals lent their names to the cause, including P.T. Barnum, and while they were not without an audience in 19th century America, statements like "tobacco eating and devilry are both one" were unlikely to make many new converts, particularly in a country that owed so much of its wealth to tobacco. *The Anti-Tobacco Journal* did not appear again after 1873 and the Society struggled on for only a little while longer.

The failure of anti-tobacconism

It would be very easy to exaggerate the influence of the anti-smoking leagues prior to the era of the cigarette. The anti-tobacconists were never more than a slim minority who were invariably viewed as poor cousins of the temperance movement. Both Thomas Reynolds and George Trask died in 1875. A friend gave the former a fitting epitaph:

> "Here lies a man who in his great regard for things spiritual
> well-nigh forgot things temporal." (38)

On his death, Reynolds' daughter took over the reins of the Anti-Tobacco Society but its influence became, as the historian Matthew Hilton put it, "minimal to the point of obscurity."(39) Smoking was now so rife that it was senseless to legislate against it and with taxation from tobacco exports making up an eighth of the UK's total revenue there was no political will to curb it.

This was, after all, the golden age of liberalism and smoking was viewed as a fairly harmless practice which adult males were free to indulge in. Even Reynold's Anti-Tobacco Society never called for tobacco to be made illegal but he, and the other anti-smoking activists of the time, were still widely viewed as fanatical kill-joys.

For every dedicated anti-smoker there were any number of passionate smokers to scoff at them and their rhetoric. One such fellow wrote the following verse - taken from one of several late 19th century anthologies of tobacco poetry. Although the poem is scathing towards the enemies of tobacco, it indicates that smokers were at least aware of their existence:

> "I will smoke, and, I will praise you
> My cigar, and I will light you
> With tobacco-phobic pamphlets
> By the learned prigs who fight you." (40)

The idea of sparking up tobacco with anti-smoking literature was one that also appealed to Mark Twain, writing at length, and with some anger, about the health reform movement of America:

> "I don't want any of your statistics; I took your whole batch and lit my pipe with it.
> I hate your kind of people. You are always ciphering out how much a man's health

is injured, and how much his intellect is impaired, and how many pitiful dollars and
cents he wastes in the course of ninety-two years' indulgence in the fatal practice
of smoking; and in the equally fatal practice of drinking coffee; and in playing billiards
occasionally; and in taking a glass of wine at dinner, etc. etc...
And you never try to find out how much solid comfort, relaxation, and enjoyment
a man derives from smoking in the course of a lifetime (which is worth ten times the
money he would save by letting it alone), nor the appalling aggregate of happiness lost in
a lifetime by your kind of people from not smoking.
Of course you can save money by denying yourself all those little vicious enjoyments
for fifty years; but then what can you do with it? What use can you put it to?
Money can't save your infinitesimal soul...
Now you know all these things yourself, don't you? Very well, then, what is the use of
your stringing out your miserable lives to a lean and withered old age?
What is the use of your saving money that is so utterly worthless to you?
In a word, why don't you go off somewhere and die,
and not be always trying to seduce people into becoming as ornery and unlovable as
you are yourselves, by your villainous 'moral statistics'?"(41)

None of the European anti-smoking societies of this period
survived the death of their founders who were, for the most part,
energetic and charismatic individuals. While the campaigners against
alcohol scored several successes, the anti-tobacco societies achieved none.
The anti-smokers relied too much on exaggeration, xenophobia and
religious zealotry, all of which were treated with scepticism by the
political mainstream and ultimately led to their failure to garner much
support outside of temperance and Methodist circles. The major
exception to this was the United States where, as we shall see in the next
chapter, a popular campaign against cigarettes flourished in the last years
of the century.

CHAPTER TWO

'A Smokeless America by 1925'

James Buchanan Duke made for an unlikely villain. A soft-spoken Methodist from North Carolina, 'Buck' Duke - as he was known to all - was a pioneer of hydroelectricity and one of the most generous philanthropists of his time. His name lives on in the American South where the reservoir which provides electricity to residents in the west of North Carolina, owned by the still-thriving Duke Energy, was named Lake James in his honour. The Duke Endowment trust fund, which he set up with $105 million of his own money (the equivalent of $1.2 billion today), continues to support hospitals, orphanages and churches in the two Carolinas. Duke University, once known as Trinity College, was renamed in 1924 as a tribute to the lavish endowments it was given by the Duke family, who asked for nothing in return but that it "open its doors to women, placing them on an equal footing with men."(1)

Had he done all this and nothing more, Buck Duke would still be fondly remembered today in the Deep South. As it is, his achievements in the fields of renewable energy and charitable giving are mere footnotes in the story of the man who first mass-produced cigarettes and almost single-handedly created the modern tobacco industry.

Buck Duke

In 1881, at the age of just twenty-four, Buck Duke was the proprietor of W. Duke & Sons, a tobacco company which was struggling to compete with its local rival Bull Durham. Both firms were based in Durham, North Carolina but while Bull Durham made the world's best-selling brand of loose tobacco, Duke's operation was an also-ran. Unable to keep pace with his competitor in the sale of chewing tobacco, pipe tobacco or cigars, Buck took the gamble of investing in the only product it had neglected: the ready-rolled cigarette.

Bull Durham executives would have years to regret this oversight but it cannot have seemed such a mistake at the time. Manufacturing cigarettes was an extremely labour intensive process. Every one of the 500 million cigarettes sold in the United States had to be hand-rolled by factory workers. The market for them was on the rise - five years earlier a mere 42 million had been sold - but even 500 million cigarettes equated to just 50,000 people smoking 20 a day; less than one percent of the population. For Americans, chewing tobacco (or 'plug') remained by far the most popular tobacco product and the national appetite for cigarettes would have to grow dramatically for Buck Duke to justify directing his entire business towards them.

Cigarettes and cigarillos had been smoked by the Spaniards for centuries and by the French since the revolution. Even the English had taken to them with sufficient enthusiasm for tobacconists like Philip Morris to make a tidy sideline out of manufacturing them. Americans, on the other hand, had no history of smoking cigarettes and most of those sold in the US went to European immigrants working in cities like New York where F. S. Kinney had launched the first ready-rolled cigarettes just twelve years earlier.

Cigarettes had for years been considered effeminate, foreign and possibly narcotic. Although they had been adopted by some soldiers, the predominant view was that they were unmanly. Worse than that, they were associated with the Spanish at a time when Spaniards were held up as a symbol of national decline in much the same way as the British regarded that other great cigarette smoking nation, Turkey.

With Bull Durham out of the running, Duke's main competitor in the cigarette market was Allen & Ginter, the makers of *Pet* and *Richmond Straight Cut No. 1* and the inventors of the cigarette card. In 1881, Duke launched the *Duke of Durham* brand of cigarettes and hired 125 Russian immigrants to hand-roll them. For the young entrepreneur, this was a temporary measure. He knew the only way to make real money out of cigarettes was to find a machine to do the work and, to that end, experimented with an automatic rolling machine that had recently been patented by a twenty-two year old Virginian named James Bonsack. The machine was not yet reliable enough to be used for commercial production but, aware that Allen & Ginter had been eyeing up the contraption, Duke took a chance and bought two of them at a preferential rate.

Sure enough, the Bonsack machines proved to be awkward and prone to faults. It was not until 1884, after three years of tireless experimentation, that Duke had them working well enough to begin production on a grand scale. By the mid-1880s the Bonsack machines were producing 300 cigarettes a minute and, for the first time, ready rolled cigarettes became widely available at an affordable price.

Having secured the supply end, Duke devoted his attention to creating demand. Circumstances were beginning to work in the young man's favour. In 1883, the federal government slashed the rate of tax on a thousand cigarettes from $1.75 to 50 cents and, starting around 1880, a huge wave of immigration brought Europeans into the cities of the United States. These new arrivals did not share their hosts' penchant for chewing tobacco, and pipe smoking was too sluggish and elaborate for the fast pace of urban life. Cigarettes, however, could be lit and stubbed out with ease, could be carried in one's pocket, did not require any paraphernalia and took only a few minutes to smoke. They were ideal for city living.

No city took as many immigrants as New York and no city adopted the cigarette with such unabashed relish. As late as 1910, New Yorkers were smoking a quarter of all the cigarettes consumed in the United States and Buck Duke ruthlessly marketed his products to the young, metropolitan working-class. He hired the canny Edward F. Small to head up the firm's marketing operations and initiated an advertising campaign on a scale never before attempted by a tobacco company; one that swallowed a fifth of his annual profits.

Never too proud to borrow ideas from his competitors, Duke gave away collectable cigarette cards in packs just as Allen & Ginter had been doing and endowed his new brands with catchier, trendier names like

Cameo and *Cross Cuts.* He gave tobacconists financial incentives to promote his brands to the exclusion of all others, he was the first to package cigarettes in cardboard boxes and he pioneered the giving away of free samples. It all worked extraordinarily well. Cigarettes, specifically those made by W. Duke and Sons, sold at a phenomenal rate. In 1884, the company produced 744 million cigarettes, and production rose rapidly thereafter as Duke acquired more Bonsack machines.

Buck Duke was never accused of thinking small. "I had confidence in myself," he would later remark, "I said to myself 'If John D. Rockefeller can do what he is doing in oil, why should I not do it in tobacco?'"(2) With this ambitious upstart in the mix, much of the initial reaction against cigarettes came not from anti-smoking activists but from his rivals in the tobacco industry. Pipe and plug manufacturers had the most to lose from a switch to cigarettes and they fought a rearguard action by playing on dormant fears and prejudices. One frequent claim - repeated for years - was that cigarettes were laced with opium and morphine. This, it was supposed, explained the markedly more addictive nature of cigarettes as compared to other forms of smoking.

Disgruntled cigar manufacturers threw anything they could at the new product alleging, amongst other things, that cigarette papers were "bleached with arsenic and white lead, that the contents were tobacco scraps from the gutter, and that the cigarette paper came from Chinese leper colonies."(3) The *New York Times* went along with the hysteria when it declared, in 1884, that "the decadence of Spain began when the Spaniards adopted cigarettes, and if this pernicious practice obtains among adult Americans the ruin of the Republic is close at hand."(4)

But it would take more than silly scare stories and knee-jerk xenophobia to hold back the rise of the cigarette and sales continued to spiral upwards. Just five years after getting his Bonsack machines up to scratch, Duke controlled 40% of the US cigarette market and was able to dictate terms to his dwindling rivals - or at least those he had not yet bought out. On April 23 1889 he met with the directors of Allen & Ginter, F. S. Kinney and the two other major cigarette companies to form a consortium of which he was president.

Duke called his new company American Tobacco.

Lucy Page Gaston

While Duke was busy carving up the cigarette market, Lucy Page Gaston, three years his junior, was teaching school children in Illinois. Born in Delaware, Ohio, Gaston was the daughter of a teetotalling, nonsmoking father who had been involved in many of the great reforming movements of the day, including the battle against slavery. Lucy inherited his fighting spirit. She grew up to be an enthusiastic and active member of the Women's Christian Temperance Union (WCTU) and the Anti-Saloon League. As a student at Illinois State Normal School, she led raids on saloons and gambling halls, smashed bottles of liquor and shouted temperance slogans at startled customers.

It was while working as a school teacher that Gaston first noticed what she called the 'cigarette face' - the insolent and apathetic expression on the faces of the boys at the back of her school-room whom she assumed to be smokers. Convinced that these boys were heading for a life of failure, alcoholism, crime and immorality she became increasingly concerned about the effects of cigarettes on the nation's youth. As the 1880s wore on, Gaston's focus shifted from the elimination of drinking towards tackling what she viewed as the cigarette menace.

Anti-tobacco sentiment was not uncommon in the temperance circles in which Lucy Page Gaston moved. The WCTU had been formed in 1874 by teetotal members of the Presbyterian church and was fervently opposed to tobacco in all its forms. Believing that only women had the strength of character to resist drink and bring about prohibition, the WCTU swiftly became one of the major reforming organisations of late 19th century. Its members were resolute in their opposition to smoking and a Mrs. M. B. Reese of Ohio was appointed superintendent of the Department of Narcotics and put in charge of the 'Effort to Overthrow the Tobacco Habit'.

The WCTU lobbied politicians for restrictions on cigarette sales, urged businessmen not to employ those who smoked 'coffin nails' and distributed copious anti-smoking literature. In 1882, the WCTU successfully petitioned the Senate Committee on Epidemic Diseases to classify cigarettes as a public health hazard. By the 1890s, under pressure from the WCTU, four states had completely banned cigarettes from sale.

By that time, Gaston had singled out the cigarette as uniquely dangerous and viewed it as more harmful than even the demon whiskey. She felt sure the lethal ingredient in cigarettes was not, as some had suggested, nicotine, but a substance called 'furfural' which, she insisted, was fifty times more toxic than alcohol. In 1893, feeling unfulfilled in her teaching career, she resigned and moved to the teetotal town of Harvey, Illinois where she set up a local newspaper, *The Harvey Citizen*, and wrote anti-smoking and anti-saloon articles which eventually attracted the attention of WCTU president Frances Willard.

Willard was an unusual and striking individual. A vegetarian, teetotal, nonsmoking spinster, this ex-University professor had a tendency to dress in a masculine fashion and had "wild crushes on girls" in her youth (5). Fiercely opposed to both alcohol and meat, she was one of a small number of public figures to consistently - and loudly - denounce tobacco. Willard always blamed tobacco for her brother Oliver's death (aged 43) but it was the assumed link with alcohol that most raised her ire. Under her presidency the WCTU adopted the striking slogan 'Smoking leads to drinking and drinking leads to the devil'.

Willard died in 1898, lamenting that a "world free of meat-eaters, drinkers and smokers" was "utterly crazy for the nineteenth century."(6) The following year Lucy Page Gaston founded the Anti-Cigarette League of Chicago with herself as president. Gaston, like Willard, was the archetypal 19th century reformer. Though not completely without humour, she presented a stern, unsmiling face to the world - a face that even she admitted resembled a beardless Abraham Lincoln. Well educated and unmarried, she would dedicate the rest of her life to the anti-smoking cause.

The Anti-Cigarette League (ACL) took its cue - and much of its name - from the Consolidated Anti-Cigarette League founded in New York six years earlier by the educationalist Charles Hubbell. But while the pipe-smoking Hubbell was almost exclusively interested in preventing teenagers from smoking cigarettes, the ACL, from the very outset, stated that its goal was to bring about the complete prohibition of what they called the 'little white slavers'.

Cigarette smoking suddenly became less popular in the last years of the 1890s and it appeared to some that the fad had finally come to an end. Quite why cigarette sales fell at the tail-end of the 19th century has never been fully explained. The Anti-Cigarette League naturally attributed the downturn to their own efforts but some contemporary commentators put it down to the surge of interest in cycling. In fact, mundane economic factors are more likely to have been responsible. Federal tax on cigarettes trebled between 1896 and 1898 and such was the resulting drop in sales that the US government collected just $2.3 billion from cigarette taxes in 1901 compared with some $4.2 billion five years earlier (7). Cigarettes had previously been the cheaper smoking option but the tax hike, coupled with a revival of the wider economy, enabled more people to buy cigars.

Whatever its cause, the sudden decline in the fortunes of the cigarette convinced the anti-smokers that the little white slavers could be defeated entirely. If a world without alcohol was, as Frances Willard had reluctantly conceded, "crazy for the nineteenth century," a world without cigarettes suddenly seemed a realistic proposition. Members of temperance groups who had viewed earlier anti-tobacco campaigns as a lost cause jumped at the chance of supporting a movement whose time, it seemed, had come. In 1900 the superintendent of the WCTU's Anti-Narcotic Department said that "work against other narcotics has gone steadily on, but the cigarette habit is of such great importance that other things seem to sink almost into insignificance."(8)

The Anti-Cigarette League of Chicago now claimed to have a membership of 300,000 - mostly children - and, in 1901, Gaston renamed it the National Anti-Cigarette League. This was an exciting time for Gaston and her followers. They visited schools, churches and town halls across middle America giving speeches and handing out anti-smoking pamphlets featuring slogans like 'Don't tobacco-spit your life away.'(9)

On at least one occasion the ACL hired a private police force to arrest children who were caught smoking, but its grass-roots activity tended to favour the velvet glove of persuasion over the iron fist of force. The ACL ran stop-smoking clinics around the country and one of its members, Dr D.H. Kress, discovered the use of silver nitrate as a solution to cigarette addiction and many a boy had his mouth swabbed with this chemical. Having been thus treated, he would become sick if he smoked tobacco within the next few days.

The ACL concentrated on children and teenagers (its newsletter was called *The Boy*) but its stated intention was to wipe out tobacco use amongst all sections of society. As important as the grass-roots crusade was, the Anti-Cigarette League had its greatest influence as a political lobby group. Between 1901 and 1908 their efforts were instrumental in persuading the states of Oklahoma, Indiana, Wisconsin, Arkansas and Illinois to ban the sale, manufacture and possession of cigarettes.

Gaston worked tirelessly and obsessively, signing letters with "Yours, for the extermination of the cigarette, Lucy Page Gaston." Having given up her teaching career to work full-time for the ACL she relied on charity and reputedly lived on milk and graham crackers for much of her life (10). By the turn of the 20th century, she had become one of the most famous reformers in America, eclipsed only by the formidable anti-saloon activist Carry Nation.

Born Carry Amelia Moore in 1846, Carry A. Nation's story is perhaps the oddest in the history of the temperance movement. Her mother was insane and believed herself to be Queen Victoria. Her father was little better; he responded to his wife's regal fantasies by building her a golden carriage. Carry was a keen and active member of the WCTU and the Anti-Saloon League but her first husband, it later transpired, was not only an alcoholic but a smoker and a Freemason. She left him and went on to marry David Nation from whom she acquired the memorable moniker of which she was immensely proud and which she regarded as a symbol of her destiny as the saviour of America. Standing over six feet tall and convinced that she had conversations with Jesus, Nation had an awesome propensity for violence which included, but was not confined to, thwacking courting couples with her umbrella and laying waste to saloons.

At the age of 53, she felt compelled to charge into a drugstore that was (illegally) selling liquor and, accompanied by another WCTU member, smashed a barrel of whisky with her sledgehammer. With the wind in her sails, she moved on to a nearby town where she attacked three saloons with hammers, rocks and billiard balls all the while shouting "Smash! Smash! For Jesus' sake, smash!" Swapping the sledgehammer for the large hatchet that became her trademark, these spates of anti-saloon violence soon became regular events all over Kansas. She waged a continuous, raging campaign against smokers, drinkers and Freemasons through her publication *The Smasher's Mail* and offered a policy of direct action she called 'hatchetization' as the solution.

Nation rivalled even Gaston in her hatred of cigarettes. When the two great reformers met in Gaston's office in 1904, the hatcheteer spotted a picture of Theodore Roosevelt on the wall and exclaimed: "My dear Miss Lucy, why do you have that picture in here? Don't you know he's a cigarette smoker? Let me tear it up!"(11) Mixing several centuries of ideas about tobacco with Gaston's belief in a distinctive 'cigarette face' she once said:

"I believe that, on the whole, tobacco has done more harm than intoxicating drinks.
The tobacco habit is followed by thirst for drink.
The face of the smoker has lost the scintillations of intellect and soul.
The odour of his person is vile, his blood is poisoned...
The tobacco user can never be the father of a healthy child." (12)

Such was her fame that, in her later years, Nation would appear on stage before packed houses re-enacting her days as a 'smasher,' although a lecture tour had to be cancelled when she expressed sympathy with the assassin of the well known smoker President McKinley. She died in a mental institution at the age of 65, not living to see her dream of Prohibition become reality.

In the early years of the 20th century the United States saw the anti-cigarette cause generate a great degree of public sympathy. There was genuine concern about the number of children smoking, some apparently as young as five (13). By 1890, twenty-one states had enacted laws restricting the purchase or consumption of tobacco by children but they were rarely enforced with any vigour. In 1894 the Brooklyn School Board admonished the police for not doing more to halt the widespread use of cigarettes by local children. Duly chastised, one of the officers on the beat could only complain that the culprits were "very sly."(14)

Cigarettes were still popularly assumed to be laced with drugs and it was believed that people, especially children, could literally drop dead while smoking, a belief that seemed to be confirmed by newspaper headlines like 'Cigarette Fiend Dies' and 'Cigarettes Killed Him'. Anti-smokers insisted that "many an infant" had been killed by fathers smoking in their room as they slept (15). One such account of passive smoking was recounted by a French journalist:

"A farmer, with two companions, smoked one evening in a chamber where
a young man was asleep. When, at midnight, the visitors withdrew,
the farmer found the youth insensible.
A doctor was summoned, but all efforts for his restoration were fruitless.
At the post mortem it was pronounced that he had died of congestion of the brain,
caused by the respiration of tobacco-smoke during sleep."(16)

In 1907 the Reverend J.Q.A. Henry of the Christian Temperance Campaign described the story of a nineteen year old who dropped dead in this fashion. It was said that the lad was found shrivelled "like an old man" and that he had no blood left in his veins. No doubt born of Chinese whispers and regurgitated by credulous journalists, such reports seem preposterous today, but with 'coffin nails' so new and misunderstood these urban legends gained a foothold in the public consciousness. It must be remembered that many people in America, particularly in rural areas, would never have seen a cigarette, let alone tried one. By concentrating its attention on the cigarette and turning a blind eye to other tobacco products, the Anti-Cigarette League was able to marshal not only its own natural supporters but also smokers of pipes and cigars, chewers and even drinkers against this suspect newcomer.

One did not have to be anti-smoking to be anti-cigarette, nor did it do any harm to be a little xenophobic, like the former heavyweight boxing champion who advised in 1906:

"It isn't natural to smoke cigarettes. An American ought to smoke a cigar, an Englishman a briar, a Harp a clay pipe and a Dutchy a Meerschaum. It's the Dutchmen, Italians, Russians, Turks and Egyptians who smoke cigarettes and they're no good anyhow."(17)

Dr John Kellogg, of the eponymous cornflake company, formed the International Health and Temperance Association in 1879 and called for tobacco to be banned altogether in his book *The Living Temple* (1903). Kellogg called smoking "a savage practice, without a single redeeming feature [introduced by] the American savage"(18), and while he found the smell of tobacco very unpleasant to his own nose, his objections went well beyond personal distaste and casual racism. A temperance man who had been friendly with Frances Willard, Kellogg had instinctive moral objections to smoking and believed that cigarettes posed any number of hazards to the human body. He reputedly sold several hundred thousand copies of his various anti-tobacco tracts and signed up 20,000 children to his anti-tobacco pledge in the 1880s. He also spoke out against tea and coffee and would drink neither because, he said, they contained "from three to six percent of a deadly poison."(19)

Unlike Kellogg, who would not smoke tobacco in any form, other industrialists saw no irony in puffing on a cigar or a pipe while they denounced the evils of cigarettes. Thomas Edison was a prolific smoker of cigars and credited them as a great aid to inspiration but he refused to employ cigarette smokers because he believed that acrolein in cigarette paper caused brain damage. Henry Ford considered smokers of cigarettes to be less productive employees and he, too, would not hire them.

Ford expanded on his anti-cigarette theme in four volumes of his book *The Case Against the Little White Slaver* which, among other things, explained how cigarette smoking bred criminality. With no employment laws to prevent them from being discriminated against, cigarette smokers were sacked even if they did not smoke at work. John Wannamaker would not even allow pictures of people smoking to be hung in his department stores.

For all of Lucy Page Gaston's efforts, journalists of the time gave these prominent industrialists much of the credit for the wave of anti-smoking legislation passed in the early part of the 20th century. In 1907, the *New York Times* wrote that "Business...is doing what all the...anti-cigarette specialists could not do."(20) Three years later *Harpers Weekly* noted that: "Legislation against the cigarette has not been brought about directly by the agitation of those reformers who crusaded against it."(21) By this time no fewer than thirteen US states had outlawed the sale and consumption of cigarettes.

The cigarette around the world

In Europe, the cigarette rose faster and with fewer impediments than in the United States. In 1900, when the US was smoking just 1% of its tobacco in cigarettes, the figure for the UK was closer to 13%. Several European countries had temperance and moral reform movements which were as strong as those of America and yet the idea that cigarettes posed a unique threat to the nation never took hold.

England's first popular machine-made cigarettes were the *Woodbine* and *Cinderella* brands made by Bristol tobacconists W.D and H.O. Wills. The Wills brothers were impressed by James Bonsack's contraption when the inventor exhibited it at the 1883 Paris Exhibition and bought the exclusive British rights. As a result, they were able to dominate the cigarette market in Britain for the rest of the century at the expense of the Bond Street tobacconists Philip Morris and Benson & Hedges*.

There was something of a national public outcry when, during the Boer War, the chief recruiting inspector revealed that of the 12,235 men who applied to join the army, 8,223 were turned down as being unfit to serve and a third of those rejected were said to be suffering from 'tobacco heart'. The army inspector did not, however, identify the

---

* Benson & Hedges were given the first royal warrant by the Prince of Wales - later Edward VII. The Prince was widely known to be an aficionado of cigarettes and his patronage helped remove some of the remaining prejudice against them.

cigarette as being any more likely to cause this wheeziness than other forms of smoking and few guessed at any such connection. Some proud pipe and cigar smokers disapproved of the cigarette because they viewed it as a faddish, unsophisticated and disposable product that was conducive neither to contemplation nor conviviality. But even this somewhat snobbish line of reasoning did not presuppose that cigarettes were any more harmful to the body than cigars, unless, as was often observed, they led to immoderate consumption.

The British Anti-Tobacco & Anti-Narcotic League was the only anti-smoking organisation of any stature in Europe at the close of the 19th century. With a membership of around 600 souls it was hardly a mass movement. Formed in Manchester in 1867 by nonconformists and moral reformers, the league went through several name changes before adding the reference to narcotics in 1872 to signal its opposition to opium, chlorodyne and laudanum. Their pleas for abstinence fell on deaf ears. Politicians had little to no interest in discouraging smoking and actually lowered tobacco duty in 1887, thereby enabling the budget brand *Woodbine* to retail at five for a penny.

With the cigarette in the ascendancy and smoking more popular than ever, the Anti-Tobacco League ceased trying to stop adults smoking and focused on children instead. In this they were not alone. Winston Churchill and Baden Powell both lent their support to the International Anti-Cigarette League's campaign to limit access to cigarettes to those over 16 years old but neither man had the faintest objection to adult consumption. The growing concern about juvenile smoking was not a reflection of a general belief that tobacco was any more harmful to minors than to adults. Rather, it was a result of the Victorian glorification of childhood and the recent invention of the concept of adolescence which dictated that children be kept children for as long as possible and that adult pleasures/vices be kept from them until they reached maturity. Smoking was, in the words of one historian, "socially incompatible with idealised notions of adolescent behaviour"(22) and the late 19th century saw a popular campaign to prevent minors from having access to any form of tobacco.

This crusade found allies in the emerging Social Darwinist

movement which feared for the future of the nation's stock and claimed that children were constitutionally ill-equipped to handle tobacco. By 1907, this view had become so widely accepted that Britain had no fewer than 14 societies dedicated to tackling the issue (23).

A ban on juvenile smoking had gone before Parliament before and been rejected but in 1908, with the Liberal party moving away from the doctrine of *laissez-faire*, a proposal to ban the sale of tobacco to the under 16s was tacked onto the Children's Act and passed into law. At a stroke, the wind went out of the anti-smokers' sails. The groups dedicated to outlawing juvenile smoking disbanded and the British Anti-Tobacco League was deprived of the only part of its agenda that had ever garnered it any real public support.

Unlike the American anti-tobacconists, neither the League nor Reynolds' earlier Anti-Tobacco Society campaigned to have tobacco criminalised. British anti-smoking groups never questioned the right of adults to lead their lives as they chose and they favoured persuasion over coercion. But the British Anti-Tobacco League conspicuously failed to persuade the nation to curb its tobacco use and although it continued to publish its journal *Beacon Light* into the 1920s it, like the Anti-Tobacco Society, withered and died.

Australia was home to a number of notable anti-smoking reformers in the late 19th century and they, too, did not find a campaign of persuasion particularly fruitful. Instead, the Australian WCTU campaigned (unsuccessfully) for a total ban on cigarettes in South Australia and its membership rose as high as 10,000. The WCTU continued to campaign against smoking until the 1950s but the high watermark of its crusade against vice came with the 6pm pub closing law that it petitioned for during the First World War.

The Children's Protection Bill of 1898 would have prohibited the sale of tobacco to juveniles throughout Australia but it was defeated. Somewhat farcically, it would anyway have allowed children to buy cigarettes if they claimed them to be for their parents. It did nothing to allay public fears about cigarettes and their supposed role in juvenile delinquency or, as it was known, the 'larrikin problem'. It was therefore left to individual states to make their own laws and by 1906 they had all banned tobacco sales to the under 16s with the exception of Western Australia which would finally follow suit in 1917.

Cigarettes under threat of prohibition

With cigarettes banned in thirteen US states and countless other anti-smoking bills under review, Lucy Page Gaston and the Anti-Cigarette League had developed a seemingly unstoppable momentum but all was not as it appeared. Their successes were coming almost exclusively in the mid-west, where cigarettes had never been popular to begin with. On the East coast, in the tobacco growing states and in the biggest cities, anti-smoking sentiment was weak and it was in these places that cigarette consumption rocketed.

In 1900, 2 billion cigarettes were sold. By 1913 it was 14 billion. The *New York Times*, which had in 1884 issued its overwrought warning about cigarettes signalling the "end of the Republic," reversed its opposition and took a more libertarian stance during the ACL's golden years when it consistently spoke out against statewide cigarette bans. When the first such law was passed it said:

"The smoking of cigarettes may be objectionable, as are many other foolish practices,
and it may be more injurious than other modes of smoking tobacco,
but it is an evil which cannot be remedied by law." (24)

The *New York Times* blamed resentment at Buck Duke's domination of the tobacco industry when Washington State banned cigarette sales in 1895 and when, ten years later, Indiana enacted its own cigarette ban, the newspaper called it "as scandalous an interference as can be conceived with constitutional freedom." (25) *Outlook* magazine concurred, describing the ban as "a foolish piece of legislation."(26)

Those states which did ban cigarettes found it nigh-on impossible to enforce the prohibition. Like many a 17th century despot, American politicians soon learnt that banning a product was no guarantee of eliminating it. Cigarette trafficking over state-lines took place on a large enough scale to keep those who wanted cigarettes supplied with them.

Only criminal gangs and black marketeers benefitted. The police had neither the funds nor the manpower to stem the flow of contraband and they could do even less about those who chose to smoke in their own homes.

As the drawbacks of cigarette prohibition became apparent, lawmakers elsewhere began to think twice before enacting similar bans in their own states. It did no one any favours to bring in unpopular and unenforceable legislation. As Senator Josiah Collins said: "When you pass a law you know is going to be violated...you are merely bringing all law into contempt."

Meanwhile, Lucy Page Gaston spent her time arguing with politicians in her adopted state of Illinois where a statewide ban on cigarette sales was passed in 1907 before being ruled unconstitutional by Illinois's Supreme Court. This, in turn, contradicted the decision of the national Supreme Court which, in 1901, had allowed states to ban cigarettes and it was an indication of how chaotic the rules on the issue had become. For Gaston, success in Illinois had obvious symbolic significance and she fought the decision for years. She succeeded in preventing the law from being officially repealed (technically this did not happen until 1967) but no new anti-smoking laws were passed in the state, including her suggestion that smokers be compelled to walk in the middle of the street.

Buck Duke's American Tobacco Company did not take the Anti-Cigarette League's activities lying down. Showing himself to be the true father of the modern tobacco industry, Duke issued writs, launched lawsuits, appealed decisions and pointed to the damage the bans would do to the economy. By the turn of the century, he had expanded into Canada and signalled his intention to dominate the British tobacco industry by buying up Liverpool's British Ogden Tobacco. In an effort to fend him off, the British tobacco companies joined forces and formed the Imperial Tobacco Company.

For the first time in his career, Duke found himself outnumbered and outgunned. In 1902, he sold his British acquisitions to Imperial and agreed to leave the British market to his rivals on the proviso that they merge with American Tobacco to corner the market outside of Britain and the US. The result was the mighty British American Tobacco, an international behemoth which still thrives today.

Back in America, antipathy towards Duke's dominance of the tobacco industry - not least from disgruntled tobacco farmers whose prices Duke pushed ever downwards - resulted in an anti-trust suit being filed against American Tobacco in 1908. The Justice Department accused the company of using its position to charge excessive prices and eliminate competition. Duke was astounded. He freely admitted to undercutting the competition, buying out rival firms, making special agreements with suppliers and arranging exclusive distribution deals with retailers. He saw all of this as good business practice and said so in court.

In truth, it was hard to see how Duke had broken the law. It was true that he had closed down most of the 32 tobacco companies he had bought, but he still had no shortage of competition and it was difficult to see how the man who had given America the five cent pack of cigarettes could be accused of charging excessive prices. Nonetheless, Duke was found guilty of restraining trade to form a monopoly and, in 1911, the Supreme Court ordered American Tobacco to be splintered into a number of independent companies of which the largest were Lorillard, Liggett & Myers, RJ Reynolds and a much diminished American Tobacco. Duke retired from the industry a bitter man and turned his attention to generating hydro-electric power for the factories of North and South Carolina.

The break-up of American Tobacco created the tobacco industry as we know it today. Suddenly free to operate autonomously, Dick Reynolds of RJ Reynolds Tobacco reputedly said "Now watch me give Buck Duke hell." His company launched its *Camel* brand in 1913 with a phenomenally successful advertising campaign and within five years found itself with 40% of the US cigarette market. Other enduring brands were introduced in the years immediately preceding America's involvement in World War One, notably Liggett & Myers' *Chesterfield* ('They satisfy') and American Tobacco's *Lucky Strikes* ('It's toasted').

Philip Morris, the man, was long gone - he died in 1873 - but his company crossed the Atlantic and opened for business in the US in 1902. The firm had never been part of American Tobacco, nor had it ever been more than a minnow compared to the likes of American Tobacco or RJ Reynolds. It sold a mere seven million cigarettes in 1903 but the company announced its arrival with a brand of cigarettes aimed at the upper end of the market called *Marlborough* which, when shorn of three letters, would end the century as the world's best selling cigarette.

The Nonsmokers' Protective League

Undeterred by a seven-fold increase in cigarette sales in the first decade of the 20th century, Lucy Page Gaston had her eyes firmly fixed on the complete prohibition of tobacco and, by 1911, was campaigning under the banner: "A Smokeless America by 1925." Her new emphasis on eliminating all smoke rather than mere *cigarette* smoke alarmed some previously supportive pipe and cigar men but the ACL marched on, changing its name to the Anti-Cigarette League of America in recognition of its growing number of Canadian branches.

The major American cities remained largely untouched by the anti-smoking crusade, with the notable exception of New York where, in 1911, Dr Charles G. Pease founded the Nonsmokers' Protective League (NPL). Pease was a fifty-six year old dentist and homeopathic physician who spent his long life fighting the 'poisons' which he believed were leading Americans towards racial degeneracy. A New Yorker by birth, he took against coffee at the age of twelve and went on to add tea, chocolate, alcohol, vinegar, cocoa, meat, "artificially flavoured lollipops" and - above all - tobacco to his long list of genetic toxins.

Gaston's crusade against cigarettes was explicitly a war of extermination and she made no secret of her abolitionist intentions. The agenda of the Nonsmokers' Protective League was different in so far as it fought against what is today known as 'secondhand smoke' and confined its ambitions to restricting smoking in public. Announcing itself in the pages of the *New York Times*, NPL secretary Milton Willis insisted that:

> "The league does not seek to abridge the personal rights of any one, but it seeks to awaken the sense of fairness in those who use tobacco and to impress upon them the fact that they have not the right to inflict discomfort and harm upon others." (27)

A crowded city with more than its fair share of smokers, New York was a fertile breeding ground for a nonsmokers' rights movement. Unrestrained smoking on public transport, in particular, was bothersome to many. *Harper's Weekly* bemoaned "the men who bring lighted cigars into street-cars and smoke in the face of every passenger who crowds past them to get on or off, clearly and scandalously disregarding the rights of others."(28) In an editorial marking the league's formation, the *New York Times* commented:

> "Anything that may be done to restrict the general and indiscriminate use of tobacco in public places, hotels, restaurants, and railroad cars, will receive the approval of everybody whose approval is worth having."

But the newspaper struck a note of caution with regard to Pease himself who had already gained some notoriety:

> "But we also note the name of a somewhat rabid and aggressive anti-tobacco agitator, Dr Charles G. Pease, who may turn out to be the originator of the movement. Dr Pease, if our memory serves, is a wildly emotional hater of tobacco. His associates must bear in mind that pipes and cigarettes cannot be suppressed. Mankind cannot be made over the Pease model." (29)

Pease was indeed the "originator of the movement" and if his associates had sought to hide this fact from the press, they could not do so for long since the controversial doctor was a prolific letter writer and a tireless public speaker. But despite the misgivings of the *New York Times*, Pease's campaign was successful. In 1913, two years after the formation of the NPL, smoking was banned in subways, street-cars and ferries.

Thereafter, Pease became something of an anti-smoking vigilante, making dozens of citizen's arrests on the New York subway as smokers continued to flout the law. He called for smoking restrictions in the city's parks and announced that he had received a letter from a "pure young woman" called Annette Hazelton who agreed with all he said about the evils of tobacco and who would do all she could to help his cause. Pressed further about this mysterious admirer, Pease produced the letter in question but it was quite obviously written in his own hand and he never fully recovered from this minor scandal.

That he felt compelled to fabricate evidence of having just one loyal supporter is indicative of how low Pease's stock had sunk in New York City. In August 1913, the Central Federated Union, which represented 300,000 workers, appealed to politicians not to be used by Pease in "his endeavours to prohibit smoking by those who wish to smoke." Calling him a "meddler, who is contriving schemes to abridge personal liberty," the union said:

> "We strongly advise Dr Pease, if he is sincere in his motive and not a charlatan or
> notoriety seeker, to use his energies in the direction of doing something for
> the general public and forming plans to reduce the high cost of living and make
> life less of a burden than it is." (30)

In the months after the ban on public transport, city councillors were repeatedly asked to make exemptions to the law and 72,000 people signed a petition to demand that one in five carriages allow smoking. Pease attended a council meeting to fend off this latter suggestion, only to be sat next to a doctor who launched a scathing attack on those "who do not like tobacco themselves and protest against others using it, either under their own or another name"; a comment that was met with laughter and cries of "Annette Hazelton!"(31) At another meeting, a smoker eloquently complained:

> "Spare a little for our vices. We shall be a long time dead. They have a constitutional right
> to breathe fresh air; haven't we got a constitutional right to the pursuit of happiness?"(32)

The ban was not amended but, faced with a spirited opposition and a discredited leader, the Nonsmokers' Protective League failed to have any further anti-smoking legislation passed when the First World War intervened and changed everything.

The triumph of the cigarette

Every war since the 17th century led to an upsurge in tobacco use in one way or another but none had so dramatic an effect as that which was fought in the fields of Europe between 1914 and 1918. America's involvement lasted little over eighteen months but it was long enough for any remaining prejudices against cigarettes to be comprehensively overturned. Cigarette use by the nation's heroes in the trenches was so widespread that anti-smoking sentiment came to be seen as something close to treason. General John J. Pershing famously announced to the nation: "You ask me what we need to win this war. I answer tobacco as much as bullets"(33) and, in an urgent cable to Washington, wrote "we must have thousands of tons of it without delay."(34)

The War Industries Board identified tobacco as an essential industry and the US government swiftly took control of it, bringing the sixty-year old Buck Duke in from the cold to advise them on how they could maximise production. US cigarette production trebled between April 1917 and November 1918. The War Department bought everything Bull Durham produced. To the delight of RJ Reynolds, whose *Camel* brand was the best-selling cigarette in the country, the make up of cigarette rations was based on pre-war market share and the company promoted itself at home with the patriotic line: "When our boys light up, the Huns will light out."

Responding to requests for cigarettes, the public contributed to campaigns to supply their soldiers with as many as possible. The widow of the American war hero - and committed smoker - Admiral George Dewey set up a fund to send cigarettes to Europe in 1917 and The *New York Sun* ran a hugely popular 'smokes for soldiers' campaign which was personally supported by President Wilson. (A similar drive in Britain provided over 230,000,000 cigarettes during the course of the war and inspired the popular song 'Don't forget the cigarettes for Tommy.')

The anti-smoking movement crumbled almost overnight. As the US prepared to go to war in 1917 the Democratic Senator George E. Chamberlain had drawn up a bill to outlaw tobacco in and around military bases. It had already been passed in the House and was awaiting

Senate approval when the country declared war on Germany, at which point public opinion shifted dramatically. Newspapers called Chamberlain a "small souled zealot" peddling "perverse and hateful puritanism." *The Cleveland Leader* said that "even a fanatic could hardly have proposed such a thing seriously." So popular were cigarettes becoming with young men that the *New York Times* speculated that the bill was a deliberate peace-nik ploy to discourage them from joining the army (35).

The charitable and Christian organisations which had preached against tobacco before the war changed their tune when they experienced the horrors of the Western Front first-hand. The YMCA had been sermonising against cigarettes for years before becoming one of the world's largest distributors of them during the war, selling them in over 1,500 canteens on military bases as well as giving them away for free as part of aid. Daniel Poling, YMCA member and editor of The *Christian Herald* talked about 'nicotine bondage' back home in the USA but became more sympathetic to cigarette use after working on the Western front, saying:

> "There are hundreds of thousands of men in the trenches who would go mad, or at least
> become so nervously inefficient as to be useless, if tobacco were denied him...
> The argument that tobacco may shorten life by five or ten years,
> and that it dulls the brain in the meantime, seems a little out of place in a trench
> where men stand in frozen blood and water and wait for death." (36)

The YMCA was not the only Christian organisation to make an abrupt U-turn on the cigarette issue with the onset of war. Before hostilities began the Salvation Army had portrayed cigarettes as the work of Satan; a drug that led young men down the road to drunkenness, degeneracy and death. But by late 1918 they had given away 15 tons of tobacco to soldiers on the front line and had become much loved by the troops as a result. Anti-smoking articles in the Salvation Army's *The War Cry* and the YMCA's *Association Men* made way for photos of smiling soldiers being handed cigarettes by the charities' workers.

A few voices were raised to suggest that cigarette use was a factor in the number of recruits failing fitness tests through bronchial infections, lung damage and 'tobacco heart' but even they conceded that these ailments only affected 'immoderate smokers'. The hardcore anti-smoking organisations continued to speak out against the cigarette but their audience was now confined to those in the prohibitionist heartland where true believers pointedly sent soldiers Bibles instead of smokes. Lucy Page Gaston was making herself unpopular with her anti-cigarette pronouncements; at one point accusing the army of 'doping up' soldiers. She could no longer claim to represent mainstream public opinion. By 1918, the *New York Times* was publicly asking whether anti-smokers should be prosecuted under the Espionage Act as an "alien enemy."

In the face of this sea-change, previously supportive temperance reformers began to distance themselves from the anti-smoking brigade. The anti-cigarette campaign had originated in the fringes of a broader reform movement and had only become more dominant when those within it saw it as a winnable fight. When the public became less sympathetic to the cause it began to retreat to the fringes again.

It was no coincidence that this occurred as the anti-saloon crusade sensed victory against alcohol. The WCTU was as opposed to tobacco as it had ever been but it could not fight more than one vice at a time and soldiers were exposed to all of them. In a bid to keep the troops away from alcohol and prostitutes, the reformers turned a blind eye to tobacco while they geared up for a nationwide ban on alcohol when the war was over.

The Chamberlain bill had failed in banning cigarette use in the army but its other provision - that alcohol be banned on US military bases - was passed into law in August 1917. This was a major coup for the anti-saloon activists, even though it was ostensibly made on the basis that farmland would be more efficiently used to produce food than hops. The Anti-Cigarette League argued, quite reasonably, that if that was the case why could tobacco farms not be converted for food production as well but their support was ebbing away. The reform movement had not finished with tobacco but its reluctant, tactical decision to ease off it while the world was at war allowed the cigarette to flourish like never before.

A memorable piece of popular poetry appeared in the 1910s which read:

> Tobacco is a dirty weed. I like it,
> It satisfies no normal need. I like it,
> It makes you thin, it makes you lean,
> It takes the hair right off your bean,
> It's the worst damn stuff I've ever seen,
> I like it. (37)

During the First World War a grimmer piece of 'tobacco verse' was written. It succinctly explains the rise of the cigarette in these years:

> 'Coffin Nails' is what we said,
> But the war has changed the name,
> The cigarette is now first aid,
> In this hellish, killing game. (38)

Handed out free of charge to all who wanted them, cigarettes were regarded as essential rations for anxious, bored, cold and tired troops. A month after the war broke out *The Lancet* said it was "time to brush aside much prejudice against the use of tobacco" particularly for soldiers and sailors for whom it was "a real solace and joy" in a "nerve-racking campaign."(39) After the war, the calming effect of cigarettes on the mind was viewed as no less valuable in alleviating the stresses of modernity. Britain's *Morning Post*, while mourning the decline of the pipe, noted that without the "soothing influence" of the cigarette, lives of city-dwellers would be "unendurable."(40)

The cigarette age had truly begun.

CHAPTER THREE

'Your body belongs to the Fuhrer'

"Prohibition is won, now for tobacco," proclaimed the great anti-saloon preacher Billy Sunday in 1919 (1). Within months of the war in Europe coming to an end, the US federal government passed the 18th Amendment and the sale of alcohol was banned across the nation. The temperance dream was now a reality and, for those who had spent years campaigning for it, prohibition was the first step towards the moral regeneration of the country. The next step was to stamp out tobacco.

In 1919, Frederich W. Roman published a book with the ominous title *Nicotine Next* and its author confirmed smokers' fears in an interview with The *New York Tribune*, saying: "We have been holding back our agitation during the war for patriotic reasons, but now that the war is over we intend to push it vigorously."(2) 'Nicotine Next' was soon adopted by the WCTU as its pithy, post-war slogan and Clarence True Wilson, leader of the Anti-Saloon League, urged anti-tobacconists to "strike while the iron is hot."(3)

For a time a total nationwide ban on tobacco seemed within reach. Gaston's Anti-Cigarette League set up eight new chapters and in 1919 changed its name once again, this time to the Anti-Cigarette League of the World. Gaston petitioned the Food and Drug Administration to reclassify cigarettes as a 'habit forming drug'. The federal government increased tax on cigarettes by 50%, a policy the tobacco industry blamed on "professional reformers and honest lunatics."(4) Across the country companies refused to employ smokers, the YMCA resumed its anti-smoking stance, and Charles Pease of the Nonsmokers' Protective League announced that "we shall launch our campaign for legislation that will prohibit the growth, importation and sale of tobacco." (5)

Anti-smoking groups believed they could start from where they had left off before the war but they failed to appreciate how much the public's attitude to cigarettes had softened in the intervening years. The reformers had banished alcohol and they expected to banish tobacco. But alcohol had never been described as "indispensable" by the supreme commander of the US armed forces. Tobacco had.

While the federal government was busy outlawing booze, Nebraska, Tennessee and Oklahoma were quietly repealing their bans on cigarette sales. Wisconsin and South Dakota had already done likewise. Of the thirteen states that had banned cigarettes in their entirety only four had their bans in place by the end of 1919. At least 22 other states contemplated legislation but decided against it. In 1921 alone, no fewer than 92 anti-smoking measures were being considered in 28 states but very few of them ever made it into law and those which did focused on the relatively uncontroversial issue of juvenile smoking.

The tobacco industry set up the Tobacco Merchants Association to fight the anti-smoking lobby and it was joined by grass-roots organisations, for the anti-smokers did not have a monopoly on lobbying groups. Anti-Prohibitionists set up the Allied Tobacco League of America in 1919 and New Yorkers formed Smokers Against Tobacco Prohibition. In Utah, the Freeman's League argued that the state's tobacco ban was illiberal, ill conceived and bad for the economy; the law was overturned in 1923.

The sheer number of people smoking cigarettes after the war made the anti-smokers' task a difficult one. By the reckoning of the Assistant Secretary of War, 95% of the military used tobacco in some form during the First World War. Previously, cigarette smoking had been largely confined to the nation's cities. Many in middle America would not have known a cigarette smoker personally and it was easy for them to believe the worst of what was said about 'coffin nails'. The return of the troops to American shores shattered those prejudices. The *Camel* smoking heroes of the Western front bore little resemblance to the weak-bodied, brain-damaged, degenerate cigarette fiends of popular imagination.

With solid medical evidence against smoking thin on the ground and with many physicians stoutly defending the habit, the public began to scrutinise the anti-smokers' claims against the cigarette. The likes of Lucy Page Gaston and Henry Ford, it was pointed out, had no medical qualifications and there was little or no scientific evidence behind the multitude of allegations made against tobacco. By what authority did the WCTU label cigarettes, tea, aspirin and ginger as narcotics?

Stories of boys dropping dead after one cigarette and tobacco being spiked with opium were treated with greater scepticism once the cigarette began to transcend class boundaries. Having donated to the war-time Smoke Funds it would have been somewhat incongruous for the public to demonise tobacco and the anti-smokers could not persuade them to perform such a U-turn.

The prohibition of alcohol was proving to be as unworkable as it was unpopular. Billy Sunday had welcomed in the Prohibition era, saying:

> "The reign of tears is over. The slums will soon be a memory.
> We will turn our prisons into factories and our jails into storehouses."(6)

This was as woeful a prediction as any in history. Alcohol consumption soon returned to 60-70% of pre-1919 levels, tens of thousands were killed by bad moonshine, half a million people were prosecuted for alcohol violations, respect for the law was undermined and large sections of the public became resentful of authority. Fuelled by the trade in illicit liquor, organised crime reared its head in the early 1920s and the murder rate began a steady rise (which peaked in 1933, the year the law was finally overturned).

The unpopularity of Prohibition only served to stiffen opposition to further anti-cigarette measures. Many feared for the future of the country if its leaders continued to pander to the illiberal and puritanical element that appeared to be holding the whip hand. When it became clear that the reform movement would not be appeased by outlawing drink, the nation's libertarian spirit reasserted itself. Where would it stop?

The New York World cautioned its readers:

> "The unprotesting generation that lost its right to drink may yet lose its
> right to smoke, and also, if it submits gracefully,
> its right to walk under a full moon or sit on the grass." (7)

Reformers, police and politicians were finding that removing alcohol from the country was not as simple as getting a bill signed into law. The WCTU, anxious to protect the 18th Amendment at all costs, spent more time monitoring speak-easies than it did campaigning for further legislation. Ageing and increasingly directionless, the WCTU and the Anti-Saloon League were prepared to keep their own counsel on the smoking issue for the sake of public relations. Both groups issued statements distancing themselves from the Anti-Cigarette League and assured the public that Prohibition was not the thin end of a hefty wedge. The WCTU continued to publish F. W. Roman's *Nicotine Next* but diplomatically dropped the word 'next' from its title. By 1921, even Billy Sunday was assuring the public: "I have never been a crank about tobacco."

As the inherent problems of Prohibition came to the surface, the wisdom of criminalising another hugely popular vice came under question. There was also a financial aspect, and not just for tobacco farmers and their supporters on Capitol Hill. Not only was there the issue of how much a ban would cost to enforce but states were faced with a deficit if they had to operate without tobacco tax revenue. This was doubly important now that alcohol could no longer be taxed. Rather than banning tobacco, politicians were increasingly inclined to raise the duty on it to make up the tax shortfall caused by alcohol prohibition.

In 1921, Iowa set the tone for the years ahead by repealing its ban on cigarettes and adding a tax of two cents a pack instead. Other states took notice and followed the centuries old practice of justifying tax rises on health or moral grounds while boosting their own finances. The WCTU came to reluctantly support this approach and in the process abandoned its pre-war stance that taxing cigarettes was a recognition of their status as a legitimate product. In the 1920s the anti-smoking movement, aside from a scattering of Gastonites, focussed on raising the price of cigarettes and limiting advertising. The movement gradually dropped moral arguments and instead talked up the rights of nonsmokers.

With the anti-tobacconists now emphasising the comfort of nonsmokers, public smoking bans were proposed in South Carolina and Minnesota in the early 1920s. The latter went the furthest, covering theatres, streetcars, railway coaches, train stations, buses, taxis, barber shops and all state-owned buildings. Although neither made it into law, Minnesota revived the bill in all its essentials half a century later when it became the first US state to impose restrictions on smoking in public places.

The early 1920s saw Idaho and Utah bring in bans on the sale of cigarettes but, at the same time, two other states repealed their laws and the Idaho law was reversed during the same session of legislature, leaving just two states with laws prohibiting the product.

The decline of the Anti-Cigarette League

Lucy Page Gaston, meanwhile, was not for turning. In 1920, she announced her intention to run for the presidency of the United States against the 'cigarette face' William G. Harding and she wasted what little money she had left on this futile endeavour. Harding was elected to the White House and soon became the first sitting president to be photographed smoking a cigarette.

Gaston's unkind remarks about cigarette smokers became so vociferous, and fell so far out-of-step with mainstream opinion, that she suffered the indignity of being fired by her own organisation in 1921. In a measured statement to the press, the ACL announced that it "contented itself with spreading scientific and other information to protect the youth from forming the cigarette habit" and that its decision would "leave Miss Gaston free to carry out her more drastic and prohibitory methods."(8)

Still adored by a small retinue of dedicated abolitionists, Gaston left for the tobacco-free haven of Kansas where she joined the local Anti-Cigarette League. She lasted just two months, during which time she compared herself to Jesus Christ, before her comments were found to be too rich for Kansas and she was fired again. She retreated to her adopted city of Chicago to form the all new National Anti-Cigarette League but after six months she was, again, shown the door.

Gaston's failure to compromise in her later years left her an isolated figure, considered by the press and even some of her erstwhile supporters to be a dogmatic zealot. Whatever else might have been said about her, she was consistent. She was calling for cigarettes to be criminalised long after others had reduced their ambitions to clamping down on underage smoking. She wrote strongly worded letters to such well-known smokers as Queen Mary and President Harding and was virtually penniless in January 1924 when she was run over by a street-car after attending an anti-smoking meeting. Aged 64, she was sufficiently robust to survive this ordeal only to succumb - somewhat ironically for someone who never drank or smoked - to throat cancer, from which she died in August.

The year Gaston died, 73 billion cigarettes were sold in the US, five times more than had been sold a decade earlier and twenty times more than had been sold when Gaston began her campaign. Three years later, Kansas became the last state to repeal its ban on cigarettes. In 1930, *Outlook* published an article reviewing Lucy Page Gaston's life and work. It was simply titled 'Lost Cause'.

Women smokers

The anti-smoking crusade would have collapsed entirely in the 1920s had it not been for the controversy over women smoking. It was a curious paradox that while cigarettes were branded effeminate, no respectable woman would want to be seen smoking one. In the late 19th century some feminists took up smoking as a statement of equality and, by the 1890s, women who smoked were generally assumed to be anarchists, Suffragettes or prostitutes. Cigarettes were considered bad enough for men and boys. For women, with all their perceived emotional instability, delicate nervous systems and weak bodies, they were assumed to be disastrous.

That anti-tobacconists continued to garner popular support on the issue of women smoking was due, in part, to the widely held belief in the weaker constitution of the fairer sex. In 1920 the Surgeon General advised women not to smoke because, as he delicately put it, "a woman's nervous system is more highly organised than a man's."(9) The *Journal of the Indiana State Medical Association* said women should avoid tobacco because of "the generally recognised emotional instability of the female sex."(10)

These notions of feminine fragility were allied with more odious beliefs in Social Darwinism and eugenics. The US minister Josiah Strong made the bond between progressive reform and white supremacy explicit in his book *Our Country* (1885) and such theories had already inspired a programme of sterilisation in California in the 1890s. These ideas did not come from an obscure corner of political thought nor were they espoused by a small group of racist ideologues. They were a largely uncontested part of mainstream thinking, informing debate about the future of mankind in the first half of the 20th century and only came to a halt with the discovery of the death camps of Auschwitz and Belsen.

If smoking was injurious to women, the argument went, physical degradation would be passed onto their children and drag down the Anglo-Saxon race. Mrs John B. Henderson, the widow of a US Senator, campaigned vigorously against the cigarette and recommended US colleges expel female smokers in 1925 on the basis that they would "inevitably lead, sooner or later, to physical bankruptcy and race degeneracy."(11)

Dr Charles G. Pease preached a similar message in New York and it was in that city that women's fight for the right to smoke came to a head*. Female New Yorkers took to cigarettes in growing numbers and there was a concerted attempt by conservatives and anti-tobacconists to nip this unwelcome trend in the bud. In 1908, women were banned

---

*New York City continued to be as notable for its anti-smokers as for its huge number of smokers. Vida Milholland, one of the city's best-known social reformers, described cigarettes as the "enemy of American progress" and, pre-empting the city's public smoking ban by eighty years, said that if smokers had to indulge their "mind-destroying habit" they should so do in private.

from smoking in public buildings in New York City. The Non-Smokers Protective League applauded the ban but called for a fresh law making it an offence to smoke in the presence of women. Two attempts were made, in 1908 and 1911, to outlaw women smoking in the street. Both failed, as did similar proposals in Washington DC and Massachusetts, but the police made arrests anyway.

In 1908, a 29 year old woman was jailed for a day after being caught smoking in public and, in the same year, a woman was jailed for 30 days for 'endangering her children's morals' by smoking in front of them (12). In 1922, an 18 year old Brooklyn woman was charged with disorderly conduct for smoking a cigarette while with her 15 year old friend. She was acquitted on appeal but was immediately rearrested for the same incident on a charge of 'corrupting the morals of a minor.'(13) In 1912, a court acquitted a man of assaulting his wife after he smacked her in the face while trying to knock a cigarette out of her mouth. The judge recommended he spank his wife for smoking (14).

Marketing cigarettes at women was unheard of. Buck Duke was fiercely opposed to women smoking and never contemplated breaking this taboo, but his successors began to wonder if it might be worth the risk. Although the anti-smoking movement dwindled after the war, the threat of a nationwide ban on cigarettes was, for a time, real enough to put the tobacco industry on its best behaviour. When the threat receded in the mid-1920s - and with the prospect of doubling its business if cigarette use amongst women became acceptable - the tobacco companies began to aim their advertising towards this emerging market.

In 1919, Lorillard launched two brands aimed at women including *Murad*, a cigarette cheekily named after the brutal anti-smoking ruler of 17th century Turkey, Murad IV. Both failed to make an impact and the industry did not make another attempt to cross the gender divide until 1927 when Philip Morris re-branded *Marlborough* as *Marlboro* and gave it the slogan 'Mild as May.' One *Marlboro* advert from 1927 read:

"Women quickly develop discerning tastes. That is why *Marlboros* now ride in so many limousines, attend so many bridge parties, and repose in so many handbags."

Liggett & Myers came closest to breaking the taboo on showing women smoking in their advertisement of 1926 for *Chesterfield* which showed a young lady requesting her smoking gentleman friend "Blow some my way." The following year, American Tobacco went beyond invitations to be exposed to passive smoke with a *Lucky Strikes* campaign which showed an emancipated woman enjoying a cigarette.

By this time, cigarette use amongst women had become common enough for the tobacco industry to dare to exploit it and no company did so more effectively than American Tobacco. In 1928 it appealed to women on diets by suggesting they 'Reach for a *Lucky* instead of a sweet' if they wanted to 'Avoid that future shadow.' The company had its gamble repaid with a trebling in sales in just one year. The following year, American Tobacco pulled off a marketing masterstroke with a 'Freedom March' in New York City in which women dressed as the Statue of Liberty walked down Fifth Avenue holding cigarettes aloft as 'torches of freedom'. By the end of the decade, a tobacco industry insider estimated that half the women in New York were smoking cigarettes and *Lucky Strikes* had overtaken *Camel* as the nation's favourite brand.

In Britain, where the tobacco industry faced little opposition and had no reason to fear a popular backlash, gold tipped cigarettes and scented cigars had been marketed towards women since the 1890s. Tobacco use was not uncommon amongst female factory workers and their numbers rose sharply during the war. Working for the war effort gave women a level of independence they could not have enjoyed as domestic servants and an income they would not have received as housewives. Newly liberated, female munitions workers took to cigarettes in sufficient quantities for several groups, including the Young Women's Christian Association, to register their disapproval but to little avail.

Although prejudice against women who smoked was less pronounced in Europe than in the US, it was not until the late 1920s that smoking began to lose its down-market reputation in respectable society. Thereafter, female smoking rates soared. By the time the next world war had come to an end, around 40% of women were regular, usually light, smokers.

Certain rules continued to apply to middle and upper class ladies.

An etiquette book from 1933 titled *No Nice Woman Swears* considered it perfectly acceptable for a lady to smoke in a car or taxi but noted that "it's still not the thing for a woman to smoke on the street."(15) A guide to good hospitality, also from 1933, indicated the dominance of the cigarette in the inter-war years, instructing that a good hostess always keeps cigarettes "to hand in every reception room whether you smoke yourself or not."(16) For many years the description of Agatha Christie, as written on the back of her hugely popular detective novels, mentioned that she was a reluctant nonsmoker. She had tried "many times" to smoke but could not enjoy it. She described this with no pride and just a little shame.

A new British organisation, the National Society of Nonsmokers spoke out against this new threat to the nation's womenfolk from its inception in 1926. Echoing the arguments about racial degeneration that were being heard in America and Germany at the time, its newsletter *Clean Air* asserted that tobacco damaged the reproductive system and that even if it did not, smoking had such a negative effect on a woman's appearance that no man would want to marry her. Similar rhetoric was being spouted by Charles Pease and his Nonsmokers' Protective League but neither they, nor the National Society of Nonsmokers, had more than a negligible influence on public opinion.

Cigarette smoking had become an unstoppable phenomenon among both sexes and anti-smoking as a movement was at its lowest ebb, all but completely disappearing for the next thirty years. By the time Count Corti published his *History of Smoking* in 1931, he was in no doubt that the anti-tobacconists were now an irrelevance, concluding that: "Although the fight between smokers and nonsmokers still drags on, a glance at the statistics proves convincingly that the latter are but a feeble and ever-dwindling minority."(17)

Health fears begin to emerge

Few were aware of it, but a growing body of evidence on the dangers cigarettes posed to health was coming to light in the 1930s. Lung cancer deaths in the US rose from 0.6 per 100,000 in 1914 to 1.7 in 1925. In the UK, the rate rose from 1.0 per 100,000 in 1910 to 2.33 in 1926. Although the increase was observable to doctors who dealt with the disease, few suspected a connection with cigarettes. Little was known about lung cancer and the numbers dying of it were still small when compared to other cancers, tuberculosis or epidemics like the recent and devastating Spanish 'flu that famously killed more people than the First World War.

An indication of the disease's lowly status amongst health professionals was provided by Isaac Adler, who wrote the first medical guide on lung cancer in 1911, a book that began with an apology for writing about such an obscure ailment. In 1919, a Washington University student, Alton Ochsner, was offered the rare chance to witness lung cancer surgery. He was told he would probably never get such an opportunity again and yet in 1937, in the space of 8 months, he saw another six cases. All were men and all were heavy smokers of cigarettes.

The Lancet noted in 1927 that nearly every case of lung cancer studied involved smokers. A 1928 study of 217 cancer cases in Massachussetts found that of the 35 site-specific cancer cases (e.g. lung, lips, tongue, etc.), 34 were heavy smokers. Still, after the First World War, most men *were* smokers and the authors found little difference in overall cancer risk between smokers and nonsmokers. The following year, The *American Review of Tuberculosis* said there was "no definite evidence" that smoking contributed to lung cancer. But in Argentina, A.H. Roffo of the Buenos Aires Cancer Institute conducted experiments on animals and by the end of the 1930s had concluded that cigarette tar caused tumours of the lung.

The most compelling evidence came from Germany. In 1929, Fritz Lickint showed a link between smoking and lung cancer and by 1935 was saying that there was "no doubt" of causation. Another German doctor, Franz Muller, wrote the pioneering 'Tobacco misuse and lung carcinoma' in 1939 and reported that 83 of the 86 lung cancer patients he studied had been smokers. Muller also found that lung cancer victims were six times more likely to be "extremely heavy smokers."

Had they been taken together, these studies would have made a strong case against the cigarette, but these researchers were scattered throughout the world and their reports appeared without fanfare over two decades. Since the most thorough research was carried out in Nazi Germany it was largely ignored by the rest of the world at the time and was disregarded after the Second World War*. Franz Muller disappeared during the war, possibly killed in combat, and Fritz Lickint's work on lung cancer faded into obscurity even in his homeland. Those who warned of a growing public health problem were treated with scepticism thanks, in part, to their warnings being so reminiscent of discredited scare stories peddled by abolitionists in recent memory and by other fanatics in preceding centuries.

To the disgust of the temperance movement and the delight of drinkers, the 18th Amendment was repealed in 1933 (as if making a concession to prohibitionism, the US government chose the same year to outlaw marijuana). Post-Prohibition America was not a fertile breeding ground for reformers wanting to dictate to people how to live their lives. Even if cigarettes posed a threat, went the popular argument, it was not of epidemic proportions, it did not outweigh the perceived benefits of smoking and it was, in any case, a calculated risk.

In 1938, *Scientific American* told its readers that smoking damaged the body "to some extent, usually not great" but added that it was also dangerous "to climb mountains and stepladders, play football, cross the street, or merely to exist, but the risk is so small that we willingly accept it."(18) As late as 1948 the *Journal of the American Medical Association* was saying that "more can be said on behalf of smoking as a form of escape from tension than against it."(19)

---

* Despite Muller's study being published in the prestigious *Journal of the American Medical Association* in 1939.

Just as it had in the 1920s, cigarette consumption doubled in the 1930s. By 1940, the US had 7,121 cases of lung cancer, up from 2,357 in 1930 and dramatically up from 1914 when the recorded figure was just 371. Few were exclusively blaming smoking for the rise and, as the tobacco industry pointed out, there was no causal relationship. Smokers were dying of lung cancer but so were nonsmokers and the vast majority of both groups remained unaffected. Perhaps the blame lay elsewhere. This was the age of the cigarette but it was also the age of X-Rays, asphalt, diesel, urban living, motor cars and better diagnosis of disease. All were considered possible culprits. In Europe, some blamed the rise in lung cancer on the influenza pandemic or the use of chemical weapons during the war.

One perfectly valid partial explanation for the rise of lung cancer - and all other forms of cancer - was that people were simply living longer. In 1900, average life expectancy was 47. The average age of lung cancer death is 71. With more people making it into their sixties, seventies and beyond, it was inevitable that rates of lung cancer would increase, but this hardly explained why smokers were dying of lung cancer at a faster rate than nonsmokers. For the time being, however, there was sufficient confusion for the public to give cigarettes the benefit of the doubt.

'Just what the doctor ordered'

The tobacco companies were aware of the murmurings that cigarettes might be deleterious to health and they began to subtly market their products towards the more health-conscious smoker. Reluctant in the extreme to concede that cigarettes had any seriously unpleasant side-effects - and lacking any evidence to show their brands were safer than their rivals' - they resorted to pseudo-science, suggestion and euphemism.

The most famous example was Liggett & Myers' unforgettable 'Just what the doctor ordered' slogan but Lorillard set the ball rolling with their 'Not a cough in carload' campaign for *Old Gold* in 1925 and by 1933 *Chesterfield* was being marketed as 'Just as pure as the water you drink.' *Lucky Strikes'* long-running but ambiguous 'It's toasted' slogan referred to the way the tobacco was heated and treated before being put in the cigarette, but the unspoken message was that *Luckies* benefited from some unique process which effectively removed irritating and harmful elements. In reality, the process was neither unique nor effective and the Federal Trade Commission rapped American Tobacco on the wrists for misleading consumers when it investigated industry marketing practices in 1942. The commission also criticised RJ Reynolds for its claim that *Camels* "renew and restore bodily energy."

Philip Morris and American Tobacco brought in doctors - many of whom were themselves prolific smokers and were given cartons of smokes for their support - to back up their spurious health claims. American Tobacco told the public that '20,679 physicians say *Luckies* are less irritating' while Philip Morris placed an advertisement in the *National Medical Journal* claiming that three out of four smokers found their cough "cleared up" after switching to their brands. Philip Morris advertised their eponymous brand on the basis that it "takes the FEAR out of smoking" and lined up scientists to support the company's claim that, by substituting glycol for glycerine, their smokes caused less 'irritation' than its rivals. Neither the FTC nor the magazine *Consumer Reports* found any evidence that this procedure made any difference in clinical trials. *Consumer Reports* found that, once blindfolded, smokers could find little difference between competing brands and it was particularly dismissive of "the 'scientists' whom they [Philip Morris] directly or indirectly subsidise."

In a further bid to diminish and deflect growing health fears, the tobacco industry introduced filter tips. *Parliament* was the first brand to carry a filter in 1931 and in 1936, Brown & Williamson introduced *Viceroy*, with the claim that its cellulose acetate filter removed half the particles from the smoke. This counter-offensive by the tobacco industry was more than enough to quell what little public concern there was about smoking in the 1930s. Smoking became the norm and anti-smokers were viewed as, at best, eccentric throw-backs and, at worst, deranged obsessives. Even uncomplaining nonsmokers were eyed with suspicion. Discussing the effect of tobacco on the mind, the *International Journal of Psychoanalysis* concluded that it caused neither psychosis nor neurosis and added: "One is more justified in looking with suspicion at the abstainer...most of the fanatic opponents of tobacco I have known were all bad neurotics."(20)

The Nazi war on smoking

By the mid-1930s, anti-smoking was a spent force as a social movement in the US and Europe. The lone exception was Nazi Germany. The German anti-smoking tradition was stronger than most. Germans had not taken to tobacco until the Thirty Years War (1618-48) and its introduction was swiftly followed by laws restricting its use. In some parts of the country, smoking was punishable by death as late as 1691. Tobacco was banned in Bavaria, Berlin, Saxony, much of Prussia and parts of Austria until the mid-19th century, whereupon it was condemned as a scourge on society, a debilitator of public health and a destroyer of families.

Germany's first modern anti-smoking organisation was the short-lived German Anti-Smoking Association for the Protection for Non-Smokers, formed in 1904, which was succeeded in 1910 by the Federation of German Tobacco Opponents. Both groups had affiliations with the temperance movement and opposed tobacco on the by-now familiar grounds that it led to drug use, infertility, degeneracy and a whole host of medical ailments both real and imagined. In 1919, while the anti-smoking movement in the rest of the world was sliding towards obscurity, Germany saw the formation of its most successful anti-smoking group. Founded in the cigarette producing capital of Dresden, the German Anti-Tobacco League flew the flag for anti-smoking in the 1920s, before National Socialism adopted it in government.

Under the Nazis, Germany embarked on an unprecedented campaign against smoking. Age-old prejudices against tobacco were wedded to theories of racial hygiene, eugenics, public health and Social Darwinism to become a potent political force. All these ideas had surfaced in other parts of the world in the preceding century but only in the Third Reich were they able to flourish unhindered by compassion, logic or restraint.

Lavishly funded by the state, German scientists soon forged ahead of the pack in the field of smoking and health. In 1939, Franz Muller identified tobacco use as the "single most important cause of the rising incidence of lung cancer," a view that would not be shared by the worldwide scientific community for another twenty years (21). In the same year, Fritz Lickint published *Tobacco and the Organism*, a book that ran to 1,100 pages and that has been described by the historian Robert Proctor as "the most comprehensive scholarly indictment of tobacco ever published."(22) Lickint is also remembered for coining the term 'passive smoking' (*Passivrauchen*) in 1936, a phrase with far-reaching consequences for Germany and, many years later, the rest of the world.

No profession was better represented in the Nazi party than doctors (closely followed by lawyers) and it was they who pushed the policies of preventive medicine and social engineering, with smoking an obvious target. The Reich Health Office viewed tobacco as the chief threat to public health and its leader Leonardo Conti led the crusade. Blind to irony, the Nazis branded tobacco "the enemy of world peace."

Beginning in 1938, laws were passed to ban smoking in public places, including air raid shelters, post offices, theatres and government buildings. Himmler banned policemen and SS officers from smoking on duty and Goering banned soldiers from smoking in the street. Smoking was banned in cars and trams in all the major cities. Schools were ordered to educate schoolchildren against smoking and the boys of the Hitler Youth were obliged to make a smoke-free pledge in the name of the Fuhrer. Tobacco taxes were raised, ostensibly to protect public health but in reality to fund the war effort and as the war escalated so too did cigarette prices. By 1941, 80% of the price of a pack of cigarettes went in tax, a rate not matched in Britain until the 1990s.

The onset of war did not slow down the anti-smoking campaign. German troops were given no more than six cigarettes a day and those who refused them were rewarded with extra food. Women serving as part of military operations were denied a tobacco ration of any kind.

In 1941, advertising restrictions were brought in. Cigarette companies had their marketing strategies closely monitored by the authorities and were banned from portraying their product as sexy, healthy or harmless. Women could not be shown in advertisements nor could the tobacco industry be seen to direct their campaigns at them. The male models who did appear could not be portrayed as manly or sexually attractive. The law also made it clear that "advocates of tobacco abstinence or temperance must not be mocked."(23)

Thus shielded from mockery, the German Anti-Tobacco League demanded still tougher measures through the pages of its journal *Pure Air*. Although complete abstinence was the Aryan ideal, lower yield cigarettes were recommended for those who could not or would not give up. With nicotine wrongly considered to be the carcinogenic agent in cigarettes, the Reich Institute for Tobacco Research set about developing cigarettes with low nicotine and zero nicotine levels. In 1939, a law was passed to regulate nicotine levels. The German Anti-Tobacco League sneered at these measures and responded by saying that no cigarette was safe and that smokers would adjust their smoking habits when smoking lower yield cigarettes to draw out maximum nicotine. Instead they called for tobacco advertising to be banned entirely and for still higher taxes on cigarettes. These abolitionists had no cause to worry about half-measures from the Nazi party. Hitler talked about banning tobacco completely in Europe once the war was over and more far-reaching legislation was only prevented by the destruction of the Reich.

It is tempting to view the Nazi war on smoking as a natural consequence of the pioneering work that German scientists had conducted into lung cancer, abetted by a regime which put little value on the freedom of the individual. This ignores that fact that Nazi anti-smoking ideology predated the work of Muller and Lickint and it was only because Hitler was prepared to fund them so generously that they were able to reach their conclusions (24). However prescient their research into smoking and health may have been, it cannot adequately explain the scale of the Nazi anti-tobacco endeavour. The tail did not wag the dog. Other countries would later amass a body of evidence against tobacco which dwarfed that of the Third Reich without launching an anti-smoking campaign of the type seen in Hitler's Germany.

Many of those within the Nazi party did not share Hitler's hatred of smoking and some, including top officers like Goering, were prolific smokers themselves. Germany had a tradition of opposition to tobacco but there was nothing inevitable about National Socialism embracing anti-smoking policies and, like the party's fanatical anti-semitism, the Nazi war on smoking was largely a reflection of its leader's own obsessive prejudices.

Adolf Hitler smoked two packs a day as a young and aspiring artist but he was forced to give up when he ran short of money. Thereafter, he became a vehement, life-long anti-smoker. He strongly encouraged his close acquaintances to quit and rewarded those who did so with a gold watch (Goering was never able to summon enough willpower to earn his, and Hitler's girlfriend Eva Braun smoked until the end).

In some speeches Hitler even attributed his success, and therefore the success of National Socialism, to the moment he threw his cigarettes in a river. One of these, from May 1942, suggested that the world would never have heard of him had he continued smoking:

> "I am convinced that if I had been a smoker, I never would have been able
> to bear the cares and anxieties which have been a burden to me for so long.
> Perhaps the German people owe their salvation to that fact."

Hitler was the driving force behind the creation of the Reich's anti-smoking institutions, including the Bureau Against the Hazards of Alcohol and Tobacco and the Bureau for the Struggle against Addictive Drugs. The grandest of these was the Jena Institute for Tobacco Hazards Research. The centre cost 100,000 Recihmarks and, in 1941, while waging total war on several fronts, Hitler found time to send a telegram to those attending its opening ceremony, saying: "Best of luck in your work to free humanity from one of its most dangerous poisons."(25) At the same opening ceremony Professor Otto Graf proposed banning smoking from all workplaces because of the risks of passive smoking.

The Jena Institute was run by Karl Astel, a brutal anti-Semite and eugenicist who had been actively involved with the Nazi party since its earliest days. When not plotting tobacco's downfall, he toured mental hospitals selecting patients for extermination. He sacked Jews and smokers from academic posts at the University of Jena and compiled lists of Jews to be sent to concentration camps. Under his directorship, all smokers and non-Aryans were refused employment and, like Hitler, he made plans to completely eliminate smoking once the war was concluded.

In the Nazi world-view smoking was an insidious habit that crept under the skin of the Aryan race, enslaving their minds and debilitating their bodies. In the paranoid fantasy of Nazi propaganda this could only be the work of the countless perceived enemies who lined up to undermine the German people, above all the Jews. The German Seventh-Day Adventists openly called smoking an 'un-German' habit propagated by Jews and the Nazi party shared this peculiar belief. Grinning, devilish Jewish caricatures were portrayed on posters and on the cover of *Pure Air*, showering cigarettes and pipes on helpless Germans.

Neither truth nor sanity were prerequisites for Nazi smear campaigns and the anti-tobacconists cast their net far and wide. Tobacco was viewed as fit only for blacks, gypsies and communists. One Nazi poster declared that smoking was the habit of "Jews, Africans, Indians, loose women and decadent intellectuals." The 1939 peace treaty with the USSR and the heavy-smoking Stalin posed a public relations problem that was overcome by airbrushing the pipe from his mouth in billboards celebrating the accord. When Operation Barbarossa abruptly ended the rapprochement in June 1941, anti-smokers were again free to publicise the fact that Stalin - like Churchill and Roosevelt - was a 'nicotine addict.' Hitler was always proud that his allies Mussolini and Franco were both nonsmokers.

The Nazi anti-smoking effort was part of a broader 'clean life' crusade which also attacked caffeine, meat-eating, alcohol and drugs. Organic food and high-fibre diets earned government approval. Foods containing fat or preservatives did not. Nor did anything containing stimulants. The Bureau for the Struggle Against Addictive Drugs spent much of its time attacking tobacco but it also denounced *Coca-Cola*, sleeping pills and morphine. This healthy living campaign was not without public support - a 1939 rally in Frankfurt held to oppose tobacco and alcohol was attended by no fewer than 15,000 people. Accompanying this obsession with health, country living and racial purity was the assault on liberal decadence, American degeneracy, jazz music, abstract art and swing-dancing. Even white bread fell under suspicion after the Nazis accused it of being a 'French revolutionary invention'.

The belief that individuals were free to do what they wanted with their bodies was considered a Marxist invention; one that undermined a strong and disciplined society. The doctrine of 'public health' disputed the notion that health was an essentially private matter and was fully embraced by a totalitarian regime which viewed it as a suitable target for state regulation. The individual could not make decisions without considering his or her part in the Reich. Citizens had a 'duty to be healthy' (*Gesundheitspflicht*) - to be fit for war and to be fit to breed - a concept epitomised by the contemporary slogan: "Your body belongs to the Fuhrer!"

As future mothers of the master race, women were targeted above all. Tobacco was "a genetic poison" which caused infertility and corrupted the all-important German "germ plasm." At best, it would undermine and debase future generations and, at worst, leave women unable to conceive at all. Fritz Lickint had already established that nicotine was not a carcinogen but the Nazis used the fact that the substance was present at trace levels in breast milk to support their bizarre rhetoric about 'racial poisoning'(26). After a campaign by the Federation of German Women, restaurants and cafes were prohibited from selling cigarettes to women and tobacco rations were not given to women who were under 25, over 55, or pregnant. The German Anti-Tobacco League went further, demanding a ban on all sales of tobacco to women of all ages.

Hitler remained closely involved with the crusade against tobacco to the very end. He banned smoking at his Austrian base, the Wolf's Lair, and in the Fuhrerbunker in Berlin. In 1942, he voiced regret that he had ever allowed his troops a tobacco ration; a ration he would soon be forced to increase to boost morale when the war went from bad to worse. In 1943 he made it illegal for persons under the age of 18 to smoke in public places. A year later, with the Third Reich crumbling around him, Hitler personally ordered smoking to be banned on city trains and buses to protect female staff from secondhand smoke.

Throughout all this, per capita cigarette consumption continued to rise, nearly doubling between 1935 and 1940; overtaking that of heavy-smoking France in the process. Like Germany's military success, cigarette consumption peaked in 1942 and only fell when the economy collapsed in the last months of the war. By that time, conditions for German troops had become so desperate that even avowed anti-smokers were sympathising with soldiers who wanted to smoke.

Hitler committed suicide in April 1945 and, after burning his body, SS troops lit cigarettes in the Fuhrerbunker for the first time. Within weeks, cigarettes became the unofficial currency of Germany, with a value of fifty US cents each. Hitler ultimately, if inadvertently, succeeded in reducing smoking in Germany but only by bringing the country to its knees. With the post-war German economy in meltdown, per capita cigarette consumption in 1950 was lower than it had been in 1935; a reflection of nothing more than the perilous state of the nation's finances. As the country rebuilt itself, Germans were again able to buy cigarettes and, by 1963, consumption had more than trebled (27).

My lady nicotine

At the height of the Nazi war on tobacco, the only major anti-smoking voice in the United States was the far milder and notably less totalitarian *Readers Digest*. The onset of war had a familiar effect on the smoking habits of Americans. Cigarette consumption doubled again in the 1940s and by the time the peace was concluded more than half of all men and a third of women were regular smokers. In Britain, four out of five men were smokers.

War had once again been a boon to the cigarette companies but tobacco industry insiders were becoming increasingly uncomfortable about the effect their products were having on health. Research from Johns Hopkins University added to the small but growing body of evidence against cigarettes when it showed that smokers were simply not living as long as nonsmokers. This news was brought to the American public's attention to great effect by former heavy-weight champion Gene Tunney. Published in *Readers Digest* in 1941, his article - *Nicotine*

Knockout - was a full-blooded condemnation of tobacco as something that makes you unfit while alive and makes you die before your time. He promised he would beat current champion Joe Lewis if only Joe would start smoking.

And yet, tobacco - and specifically cigarettes - had become more popular than ever before. What was it about cigarettes that made them almost universally popular by the mid-twentieth century? The question of why people smoke is one for which the modern world has an easy, ready-made answer: They begin to smoke because of peer pressure (and advertising) when they are young and continue smoking because they become hooked. In this analysis, nicotine does nothing for the body except keep it wanting more. By smoking cigarettes, the smoker gets back to a state of normality akin to that enjoyed every moment by the nonsmoker. Why else would smokers claim that cigarettes both give them energy and help them relax? Or help them both concentrate and unwind? Surely these contradictory claims indicate that smokers are engaging in self-delusion; they are merely satisfying a craving.

This tidy answer, beloved of anti-smokers and often used to strengthen the resolve of those trying to quit, does not tell the whole story. Physical dependence cannot explain the number of people who return to tobacco weeks, months or years after giving it up. The physical withdrawal symptoms last only a few days and most quitters are able to abstain for this period. Most of those who 'relapse' do so when there is no longer any physical reason to do so. The idea that these full-grown men and women are drawn back into the habit purely because of peer pressure or advertising will not do. Like every drug from coffee to cocaine, nicotine provides tangible pharmacological benefits which provide pleasure whether one is trying it for the first time or is a long-term user.

That cigarette addiction has a psychological element is widely known. Smoking provides a channel for 'divergent activities'. When others might doodle, touch their hair or fiddle with coins, the smoker smokes. This is of greatest use when uncomfortable or bored; smoking is often merely a way of killing time. Doodling, however, is not a worldwide phenomenon engaged in by a billion people twenty times a day and the displacement theory can hardly explain the full appeal of nicotine. The pharmacological effects of nicotine have been described superbly in David Krogh's *The Artificial Passion* (1991) in which he shows that, although its benefits may not outweigh its hazards, it is an extraordinary drug.

Nicotine behaves like acetylcholine, a neurotransmitter which acts on a number of 'nicotinic sites' in the body. It will, for example, prompt the adrenal glands to release epinephrine, also known as adrenaline. It will prompt the blood vessels to release norepinephrinen and increase dopamine in the brain's 'reward centres'(28). These stimulants cause the heart rate to rise and blood pressure to go up, making the smoker feel more alert. But at higher doses nicotine impedes transmission at the synapses and causes the nerve signals to become temporarily blocked, providing a feeling of relaxation. The downside comes when the nicotine is suddenly withdrawn and the nerve cells that were shut down become hyperactive, creating tension and craving. A 19th century anti-tobacco tract described the drug's pharmacologically addictive nature well, saying it "produces, for the time, a calm feeling of mind and body, a state of mild stupor and repose. This condition changes to one of nervous restlessness and a general feeling of muscular weakness when its habitual use is temporarily interrupted."(29)

This is the remarkable thing about nicotine. It *can* sedate as well as stimulate. Furthermore, smokers can easily, and often unconsciously, 'self-medicate,' giving themselves the appropriate dosage for their mood and environment. Mangan and Golding carried out experiments with smokers, putting them in situations of extreme boredom and extreme tension to study their smoking habits. Those put in sensory isolation took sharper and shorter drags on their cigarettes and took fewer drags in order to achieve a stimulating effect on mind and body. Those put in rooms filled with loud white noise took bigger and more frequent drags to calm themselves (30). It has also been well-documented that not only do psychiatric patients smoke more, they draw harder on their cigarettes, literally self-medicating themselves into a state of sedation.

Dozens of studies have shown that nicotine makes smokers less aggressive than nonsmokers. Norma Heimstra, for example, took 20 smokers who weren't allowed to smoke, 20 who were, and 20 nonsmokers, and had them drive a car for six hours straight. In all cases concentration levels fell and tiredness increased but it was nonsmokers who became most aggressive and their levels of 'social warmth' fell more quickly than that of the smokers. Somewhat surprisingly, the smokers who were not allowed to smoke did not become any more aggressive or irritable than the other smokers (31).

Another experiment showed the calming effect of nicotine. In 1984, D. R. Cherek performed an experiment in which volunteers were given three buttons to press. One button accumulated money from the bank, one took money from other volunteers and the third assaulted fellow volunteers with white noise. Those who smoked during the sessions were less likely to take money from others and more likely to accumulate money from the bank. Those smoking high nicotine cigarettes took even less money from the other volunteers.

In the pantheon of drugs, nicotine is unusual because, unlike other sedatives and tranquillisers, it induces neither docility nor slow-wittedness. It does not create a 'high' like opium or marijuana. Because of the subconscious self-medication, even heavy smokers will not 'overdose' or become overwhelmed by its effects. Nicotine use does not lead to hallucinations, paranoia, apathy, violence, hangovers or insanity. As Bismarck once said of his cigar: "It acts as a mild sedative without in any way impairing our mental faculties."(32)

Like coffee, it is a mild drug that can be used throughout the day without intoxicating. This is a point often overlooked by those who argue that since psychedelic and narcotic drugs are banned, then tobacco - which is more harmful to health and more addictive - should also be made illegal. This ignores the fact that illegal narcotics are banned not because they kill those who take them (they rarely do) but because their mind-bending properties make it difficult for their users to lead a productive and organised life and can lead to mental illness.

Far from unbalancing the mind, nicotine can help it focus. It causes electroencephalograph arousal; that is, it arouses and stimulates the brain. Experiments have shown that it is especially useful in maintaining concentration and alleviating boredom during tedious and repetitive tasks. As Dr Johnson noted: "It preserves the mind from total vacuity."(33) Nicotine helps filter out external stimuli and allows the smoker to focus on a single task better than a nonsmoker and for longer. This does not mean that nicotine gives a smoker superior concentration skills over a nonsmoker initially, but after several hours the smoker will remain focussed while the nonsmoker's mind will begin to wander or become tired (34). But when deprived of nicotine for over eight hours, brainwaves will slow (35) and performance levels and reaction times will fall (36) (37).

The writer Richard Kluger regarded these benefits of smoking as being proof only that "smokers remain attentive during the performance of long, boringly repetitive tasks." This may be true, but such tasks became the work of millions in the age of Henry Ford and it may explain why smoking remains far more popular with the working class than with those with more cerebrally challenging jobs, even though such workers are least able to afford it.

Just as nicotine contrarily provides energy and slumber, it offers concentration and dreaminess. While it does not have sufficient psychoactive power to be called mind-altering in the 1960s sense of the word, it can provide a five minute respite from reality without sacrificing lucidity. As one woman said, when asked why she smoked:

> "Do you want the honest answer? I smoke because it provides a sort of stop-gap between myself and life. While I smoke I am not quite in the moment...
> It's a subtle, constant, consistent, reliable break from life."(38)

When an anti-tobacco reformer appealed to a professor to give up his tobacco-chewing habit in the 19th century he was told "I chew a little, if I did not, I should be as fat as a pig"(39) and nicotine's role in aiding weight-loss is no illusion. On average, smokers weigh seven pounds less than nonsmokers and, as Krogh says, the "weight disparity between smokers and nonsmokers increases with age."(40) Despite smokers tending to have a poorer diet than nonsmokers, they are significantly less likely to become obese (41). Contrary to popular belief, this is not because cigarettes are an appetite suppressant or because ex-smokers overeat to compensate when they give up. Smokers and nonsmokers eat roughly the same amount but tobacco reduces the desire for sweet foods and increases the metabolic rate, particularly during exercise (42).

Why do some people smoke when others do not? "Why," as Tolstoy once asked, "do gamblers almost all smoke? Why among women do those who lead a regular life smoke least? Why do prostitutes and madmen all smoke?"(43) Unsurprisingly, smokers tend to be risk-takers and they are more likely to believe in fate and luck. Studies show they are more impulsive, more rebellious, have a higher sex drive and are less concerned about what people think of them. With the exception of pipe-smokers, who are generally quieter, they tend to be outgoing and are much more likely to be extroverts. A very high number of high achievers, artists and geniuses have smoked.

Before smokers get too smug, let us also remember that smokers are also statistically more likely to be poor, badly educated, drinkers and jailbirds. Smokers are more likely to have suffered depression and are twice as likely to commit suicide. One study showed that 60% of heavy smokers have a history of depression (44). The vast majority of schizophrenics smoke and more than half of psychiatric patients and homeless people smoke. Above all, if you smoke cigarettes you will die, on average, seven years before your nonsmoking friends.

The key difference between cigarettes and other forms of smoking is that the tobacco in cigarettes is cured in a way that makes it acidic while pipe and cigar smoke are alkaline. And because the mouth is acidic, the alkaline cigar smoke allows nicotine to be absorbed through the gums while being too harsh to be readily inhaled. The lungs, however, are alkaline and the (acidic) cigarette smoke is able to be absorbed by them, allowing nicotine to go almost instantly into the blood stream and to reach the brain within seconds. This provides all the pleasures and benefits of smoking listed above at a heightened level and accelerated pace and explains the phenomenal popularity of cigarettes by the 1940s. But, as scientists of the time were beginning to suspect, this process poses a serious risk to health. It allows carcinogenic components in the smoke to make contact with the delicate lining of the lungs and bronchial tubes and makes the development of cancer in these areas more likely.

In 1914, America's lung cancer rate was 0.6 per 100,000 people. By 1950 it was 13 per 100,000 and had risen fivefold since 1938; only stomach cancer was more common. Privately, the tobacco industry was coming to terms with the fact that its products were killing people.

CHAPTER FOUR

'Some women would prefer having smaller babies'

Dr Lennox Johnston had been injecting himself with pure nicotine for years before his wife found him lying on the floor and close to death. Suddenly aware of her husband's unusual secret habit, she implored him to put an end to it and, for a time, he did.

Johnston, a Glaswegian GP who lived and worked in Merseyside, had given up smoking with little difficulty in 1928 before joining the National Society of Non-Smokers (NSNS), the organisation that emerged from the ashes of the recently dissolved British Anti-Tobacco Society. The NSNS sacrificed the dream of a nonsmoking world in favour of the more attainable goal of securing smoke-free places for the country's dwindling number of abstainers. Temperance activists were amply represented in the organisation but religious fervour did not dominate the society as it had its predecessors. In Lennox Johnston, however, it had a member as fanatical as any who had ever lived.

Johnston was an extraordinary character by any standard. Fascinated to the point of obsession with the addictive properties of nicotine, his clinical experiments into its effects largely consisted of giving himself injections of small but unadulterated doses of the drug. After being chastised by his wife, he abandoned this line of research but, in 1940, the onset of bombing and the evacuation of his family allowed him to recommence his work.

Thereafter, he gave himself hundreds of nicotine shots before deciding, for the purposes of comparative analysis, to experiment with cocaine but he found himself disappointed with the drug. By 1941, his risky, self-funded research had cost him £10,000 of his own money and had nearly killed him on several occasions. It did, however, yield a scientific paper - 'Tobacco Smoking and Respiratory Disease' - in which Johnston argued that nicotine was addictive and that cigarette smoking was responsible for four out of five of lung cancer deaths.

Johnston then found 35 volunteers and, after repeatedly injecting them with nicotine, observed that the smokers in the group "invariably" found the sensation pleasant. After 80 injections, many, like the doctor himself, preferred the needle to the cigarette and when injections were withheld, cravings became evident. This pioneering research appeared to confirm nicotine's role in both providing pleasure and creating addiction, and demonstrated that this addiction was physiological as well as psychological. Furthermore, it provided hope that nicotine replacement therapy could wean smokers off cigarettes. It was this last discovery that most excited Johnston.

In many ways Lennox Johnston was ahead of his time. Virtually forgotten today, he recognised that smoking was addictive 44 years before the Royal College of Physicians came to the same conclusion, and he correctly identified smoking as a major risk factor in respiratory disease and lung cancer, pointing to the death rate in British men - 80% of whom smoked - which was double that of women. He was aware that while nicotine was the active ingredient in cigarettes, it was not present at high enough levels to be toxic and, therefore, the carcinogenic element must lie elsewhere.

But he went further. In terminology that would not reappear for another fifty years, he referred to tobacco addiction itself as a disease, a psychological "infection" passed from one person to another with every smoker acting as a "living advertisement for tobacco."[1] Johnston's objection was that this addiction inevitably led to "vice" and "moral degeneracy" which, he said, manifested itself in lying about how much one smoked, persuading others to take up the habit and defacing and ignoring no-smoking notices. He hoped that the NSNS and other societies like it would become "pockets of resistance dedicated to the extermination of this death-dealing drug addiction."[2]

Unfortunately for Johnston, few in the medical community were inclined to accept that tobacco was either clinically addictive or dangerous to health and his missionary zeal, notoriously short temper and tendency to assume that anyone who disagreed with him was a deluded smoker was not conducive for winning further support.

In 1940, he wrote to the Medical Research Council to request funding for research to demonstrate that nonsmokers took less time off work than smokers. It was his earnest belief that working men would be more productive if they were made to give up drinking and smoking, and with Britain entering the darkest days of the war, he pitched abstinence as a necessity for the survival of the nation. Not only would the country win the war, he said, but abolishing tobacco would bring about a "gigantic national renaissance." Alas, he was alone, even amongst his friends in the NSNS, in believing tobacco control to be a priority in time of war. Johnston received no reply from the Medical Research Council. Nor did he receive a reply to the two letters that followed it, in which he felt obliged to emphasise that he was not a crank.

Johnston's chief objective in the first years of the Second World War was to have his paper on smoking and health published as soon as possible. Believing that tobacco unconsciously disturbed the mind, he felt there was little hope of it being published by any editor who smoked but, going to London to deliver it to the editor of the *British Medical Journal* in person, found to his dismay that he was indeed a pipe man. As he feared, the editor refused to publish it (on the basis that it was badly written and too long) and in the months that followed Johnston made the trip from Liverpool twice more to remonstrate with the staff of the magazine, on the final occasion crying "Addict! Addict! Addict!" as he stormed out.

Disgusted by the medical establishment, Lennox Johnston resolved to burn down the offices of the British Medical Association. By his own account, he "examined the building several times, and planned the operation in detail many hundreds of times in bed at night," confessing that "the idea comforted me enormously."(3) He also devised a plan to pull Churchill's cigar from his mouth in the street as a publicity stunt and, although he never went through with either scheme, he admitted to committing several unspecified crimes and at one point visited the suffragette Sylvia Pankhurst for tips on how to get arrested.

The fruits of Johnston's fourteen year investigation into tobacco did not see the light of day until December 1942 when *The Lancet* published half of his study. Missing what Johnston regarded as the most important passages and tucked away at the back of the journal, it was ignored by the mainstream media and singularly failed to bring about the nationwide revolt against cigarettes he craved. When the Medical Research Council informed him that they were turning down another of his requests for funding, he flew into such a rage that the organisation refused to have anything more to do with him.

And so it was that the eccentric doctor found himself ostracised from the medical establishment when, after the war, the Medical Research Council began to look more closely at the smoking issue. In 1948, he again asked for funding to conduct official research into lung cancer but was told that two epidemiologists, Richard Doll and Bradford Hill, had already been assigned to a similar project. True to form, Johnston wrote to the MRC's assistant secretary accusing him of being a tobacco addict.

The evidence mounts

On May 27 1950, the *Journal of the American Medical Association* published two epidemiological studies of sufficient size and scope to convincingly implicate cigarette smoking as a major cause of lung cancer. From his study of 236 cancer patients, Dr Morton Levin found a tenfold increase in lung cancer risk for those smoking 20 or more cigarettes a day. In the second study, Ernst Wynder and Evarts Graham studied 684 cancer patients and found that 96.5% of lung cancer cases were moderate or heavy smokers. Evarts Graham was sufficiently disturbed by the findings to quit smoking but it was too late. He died of the disease in 1957, aged 74.

In September 1950, Richard Doll and Bradford Hill published preliminary findings from their study of 1,732 cancer patients in the *British Medical Journal.* They found lung cancer to be fifty times more likely to affect heavy smokers than nonsmokers and Doll, too, gave up smoking during the course of the research.

These papers made for alarming reading but could not, in themselves, be considered conclusive and the tobacco industry was quick to doubt their veracity. The main criticism, which would become an industry mantra in the years to come, was that while there appeared to be a statistical correlation between smoking and lung cancer, there was no proven cause-and-effect and there was no demonstrable biological mechanism to explain how these cancers came about.

The tobacco companies were not alone in casting doubt on the new findings. Doctors, most of whom smoked, remained sceptical. Clarence Little, former director of the American Society for the Control of Cancer, was one of the world's foremost proponents of the theory that cancer was primarily genetic in origin. He was particularly dismissive of environmental factors and in his book *Civilisation Against Cancer* (1933) argued that cancer was caused by the derangement of a single cell and that no one external factor could bring this about.

Little's old organisation became the American Cancer Society (ACS) in 1944 and Alton Ochsner was appointed president. Ochsner had been a young student when he was told, in 1919, that he may never see another lung cancer case again in his lifetime (see Chapter 3). Despite the proliferation of cases coming to light in subsequent years, Oshsner had not been hasty in making a connection with the contemporary rise in cigarette use and the ACS, too, was not about to jump to any conclusions. Eager to get to the bottom of the controversy, the ACS commissioned E. Cuyler Hammond, a smoker who had his own doubts about the studies, to supervise a nationwide survey of 200,000 Americans, their health and their smoking habits. When, three years later, Hammond presented the preliminary results of the survey (Hammond & Horn, 1953) he, too, showed an overwhelming link between smoking and lung cancer.

By this time, Ernst Wynder, a young German scientist who had moved to America during the war, began clinical trials to show that there was not just an association with cancer but a clear cause-and-effect. By painting cigarette tar on the backs of mice he induced tumours at a far higher rate than would otherwise be expected. This was the first time a biological link between tobacco and cancer had been shown but the tobacco industry dismissed the experiments on the basis that the doses of tar were far higher than would come from cigarettes, that the tar had been applied to the skin rather than being smoked and that, ultimately, human beings were not mice.

In response to this mounting weight of evidence the American Cancer Society's spokesman, Dr Charles Cameron, told the press that:

> "It is reasonable that some would want to shuck off this mortal coil
> a few years ahead of schedule as the price for a carefree,
> full-blooded - some would say undisciplined - life."(4)

These are words so far removed from what one would expect to hear from the head of a cancer charity today that it is hard to credit that they were ever spoken at all. Cameron added, perhaps lighting a cigarette as he did so, that the risks from smoking "do not appear to differ significantly in degree from lots of other calculated risks to which modern man exposes himself."(5) A few months later, suddenly mindful that his devil-may-care attitude might seem out of step with the cancer-fighting agenda of his organisation, Cameron issued a statement reminding the public that a link between smoking and lung cancer had indeed been found and that this was not a good thing.

And yet, Cameron's initial reaction - that smoking was a calculated risk and a matter of personal choice - was not uncommon even in medical circles. Around the same time, a correspondent to *The Lancet* wrote that:

> "Even if smoking increases the chance of a man developing lung cancer from 1
> in 10,000 to 1 in 1,000, it remains questionable whether community or individual
> have anything to gain from the abolition of smoking." (6)

Professor Sidney Ross, in 'Smoking and its Effects: With special reference to lung cancer' wrote:

> "It is on the whole a beneficent weed; it helps suffering humanity at many a crisis;
> it relieves the monotony of many humble, uneventful lives;

it staves off hunger and releases the tension in overstrung lives;
it is one of nature's gentlest stimulants." (7)

It was left to the *Readers Digest* to do the job of warning the American public about the dangers of smoking. Under the ownership of the principled DeWitt Wallace, the magazine did not take any advertising at all until 1953 and thereafter refused to advertise tobacco or alcohol; this at a time when cigarette companies spent more money on advertising than any other industry. The millions spent by the tobacco industry on print advertising and their sponsorship of television shows like *I Love Lucy* and *Your Hit Parade* protected it from criticism from large swathes of the media. Throughout the 1950s the tobacco industry was ruthless in withdrawing multi-million dollar advertising accounts from magazines which cast aspersions on its products.

Never reliant on industry dollars, the *Readers Digest* had taken a virtually lone stand against smoking since the 1920s and published more anti-smoking articles than any other organ. In 1952, it published the groundbreaking 'Cancer by the Carton' by Isroy Norr. Norr had previously circulated this summary of the evidence against cigarettes through the pages of *The Christian Herald* under the apt title 'Smokers are getting scared.' Norr was one of the few dedicated anti-smokers of the immediate post-war era, publishing his *Norr Newsletter about Smoking and Health* between 1955 and 1963; his platform for railing against "tobacco propagandists" and "cigarette pushers." He was one of the last notable anti-smokers to come from a temperance background and he worked closely with the Seventh Day Adventists and the American Temperance Society.

'Cancer by the Carton' became the most influential anti-smoking article to have appeared in the country for years and along with newspaper articles reporting the Wynder, Doll, Levin and Hammond studies, helped cigarette sales in the US fall by 2.8% in 1953. This drop did not go unnoticed by the tobacco industry.

The tobacco industry's campaign of confusion

Seeing its profits going into a rare decline, and faced with the prospect of paying huge damages in liability suits, the tobacco industry sprung into action. On December 15 1953, the heads of the largest cigarette companies in the USA (with the exception of Liggett & Myers, who felt it was beneath them) held a rare meeting in which they discussed a unified response to the growing body of evidence against their products. This secret meeting defined the policy of cigarette companies for the next forty years.

Their approach was legalistic and pedantic, as if they were on trial. Everything they said would be true within the letter of the law. They would not promise that their products did not cause disease, only that they could not say for sure. Their spokesmen would always say that they did not "believe" cigarettes to be hazardous. They would blank their critics and, as far as possible, stonewall the government. They would employ scientists to disparage all research that implicated cigarettes as carcinogenic. They would propose alternative theories for the rise in lung cancer deaths and explore every avenue of doubt in the public's mind. Finally, they set up and co-funded the Tobacco Industry Research Committee (TIRC) which would accept that while there were questions to be answered, the case against the cigarette was far from conclusive.

For the makers of cigarettes, it was imperative that the 'tobacco controversy' - as they called it - continue in an atmosphere of claim and counter-claim indefinitely. Above all, they agreed, they had to forget their differences and close ranks against the medical experts and lawyers who were bearing down on them. No tobacco company could accept any liability in or out of court. If just one case was lost, a precedent would be set that would decimate the industry. Every case brought against the industry must be fought, no matter what the financial cost and no matter how long it took. The industry would use its vast profits to outspend plaintiffs, and its lawyers would use every technicality to drag legal proceedings on for years.

This ruthless approach worked spectacularly well. The next 45 years saw the industry face over a thousand liability suits brought by lung cancer victims or their families. Just 24 of them made it before a jury and not one resulted in the industry paying a penny in damages.

The first public manifestation of the industry's counter-attack came in January 1954 when the TIRC published a two page advertisement in hundreds of American newspapers. Under the disingenuous headline 'A Frank Statement to Cigarette Smokers', the industry declared itself deeply concerned about the allegations made against its best selling product while implicitly dismissing them as being without substance:

> "Although conducted by doctors of professional standing,
> these experiments are not regarded as conclusive in the field of cancer research.
> However we do not believe the results are inconclusive, should be disregarded
> or lightly dismissed. At the same time, we feel it is in the public interest to
> call attention to the fact that eminent doctors and research scientists have publicly
> questioned the claimed significance of these experiments...
> For more than 300 years, tobacco has given solace, relaxation and enjoyment to
> mankind. At one time or another during those years, critics have held it responsible
> for practically every disease of the human body.
> One by one these charges have been abandoned for lack of evidence." (8)

Nothing, they assured the public, was more important than the health of their customers and, through the aegis of the TIRC, they vowed to leave no stone unturned in their efforts to unravel the mystery of the lung cancer epidemic. Clarence Little, the experienced, pipe-smoking cancer expert, was appointed scientific director of the TIRC and in April 1954 published *A Scientific Perspective on the Cigarette Controversy*. This booklet, sent out to the media and to 176,800 doctors free of charge, quoted 36 scientists who cast doubt on the 'smoking theory.'

Unconvinced by such assurances, smokers gave up their habit in growing numbers. In the year of the industry's "frank statement," per capita consumption fell by a further 6.1% and the first lawsuits were filed against the cigarette companies. Immediately applying the new code of contesting and prolonging every case, Liggett & Myers fought the first suit full-bloodedly and the plaintiff was forced to drop the action twelve years later. Philip Morris was then required to defend itself against a Missouri smoker who had lost his larynx. This case did at least make it to court, albeit eight years later, but the jury deliberated for just one hour before finding in Philip Morris's favour. RJ Reynolds was sued by Eva Cooper for the death of her *Camel* smoking husband but the court found no evidence that cigarettes had caused his cancer. These early precedents persuaded other would-be litigants that taking the tobacco industry to court would only result in expensive failure and the first wave of tobacco litigation soon subsided.

By 1957, 77% of Americans had heard or read about the results of the ACS's Hammond and Horn study and 50% believed that smoking caused lung cancer. Smokers who were unwilling or unable to give up the habit began to seek safer methods of smoking. It did not seem beyond the realms of possibility for scientists to be able to identify and remove the carcinogenic element from cigarettes, nor was it crazy to believe the tobacco companies capable of minimising or eliminating the risk to health. While publicly denying that such hazards existed, the industry began to alter their cigarettes to allay the public's fears. Unfortunately, they had no better idea than anyone else what the carcinogen was, only that it lay somewhere in the ill-defined part of the smoke known, all too vaguely, as 'tar.'

Dr Oscar Auerbach's research into cell mutation suggested that smoke disabled the body's defence mechanisms and allowed environmental irritants to contaminate the body for longer than would be the case with nonsmokers. Auerbach suggested that this left them more susceptible to all kinds of disease. In a private memo dated 1958, a senior Philip Morris scientist identified benzo(a)pyrene as the harmful agent and instructed his scientists to have it removed. This proved to be impossible but his analysis may have been correct. Nearly forty years later, in 1996, *Science* published a paper that demonstrated that benzo(a)pyrene damages the mechanisms in healthy lungs that suppress cancer.

With no easy way of removing the damaging particles without also removing the nicotine and destroying the flavour, the industry put its faith in filter-tip cigarettes, sales of which had been sluggish since they first appeared in the early 1930s. In 1952, the Lorillard tobacco company began experimenting with a substance called crocidolite and used it in the filters of its *Kent* brand. Secretly developed by the US military in the Second World War, crocidolite was declassified, renamed and marketed by Lorillard as 'micronite.' The company launched the brand with great fanfare at a press conference in New York's Waldorf-Astoria hotel and advertised the micronite filter as "the greatest health protection in cigarette history." *Kent* did not prove to be a big seller and the filter was discontinued in 1956. Its failure in the marketplace would turn out to be a blessing for smokers since crocidolite, as was soon discovered, is the most deadly form of asbestos.

Liggett and Myers were somewhat more successful. They had been head and shoulders above their rivals in the field of scientific research for years and their alpha cellulose filter-tip was described as a "miracle product" when advertised in the pages of *Life* magazine. They went on to develop a charcoal filter that removed 60% of 'cilatoxic materials' and their efforts were rewarded with the emergence of the *Lark* brand, a cigarette that was selling ten billion units in the US by 1964 before fading into obscurity everywhere outside Japan.

RJ Reynolds introduced *Winston* as a filter-tipped brand in the early 1950s and by the end of the next decade it was America's best selling cigarette. In 1956, the company launched its first filter-tipped menthol brand, *Salem*, to challenge the dominance of Brown & Williamson's *Kools*. The only thorny issue was how to market them. It was inherently difficult for the tobacco industry to advertise filtered cigarettes as safer while maintaining that their conventional brands were harmless. One of the earliest filtered cigarettes, *Viceroy*, was marketed as having a filter that meant that tar "cannot reach the throat and lungs." This claim - along with Liggett & Myers' insistence that *Chesterfields* had "no adverse effects on the throat, sinuses or affected organs" - was as close as the tobacco industry was prepared to go in acknowledging the kind of illnesses filter tips might protect smokers from.

In 1950, just 2% of cigarettes had a filter tip. By the end of the decade, with unease about the health implications of smoking hanging heavy in the air, this had rocketed to 50%. The trend continued throughout the 1960s and the decline of *Lucky Strikes* and *Pall Mall* can be put down, in part, to American Tobacco's decision to keep the brands unfiltered long after the trend towards filters had become evident (9).

In 1956, the US lung cancer rate rose to 31 in 100,000 and 29,000 people died of the disease. The following year saw the full publication of the Hammond and Horn study which, once again, showed a clear association between smoking and cancer; of the 448 lung cancer cases recorded, only 15 had never smoked. Hammond and Horn also found a statistical correlation, for the first time, between smoking and increased risk of coronary heart disease. In the same year, the Surgeon General stated that cigarette smoking was a "causative factor" in the development of lung cancer.

The tobacco industry spent millions conducting its own research behind closed doors and was all too aware of the true hazards of smoking. As far back as 1946, a Lorillard scientist had tentatively informed his employers that:

> "Certain scientists and medical authorities have claimed for many years
> that the use of tobacco contributes to cancer development in susceptible people.
> Just enough evidence has been presented to justify
> the possibility of a such a presumption."(10)

Industry funded research in Harrogate, England, confirmed these fears. Worried that their work might be leaked to the outside world, industry scientists were ordered not to use the word 'cancer' and instead use the code-name 'zephyr.' For those who knew the code, this 1957 internal memo was unequivocal: "There is a causal relation between zephyr and tobacco smoking, particularly cigarette smoking." (11)

None of this was ever relayed to the public. In 1958, the industry set up the Tobacco Institute to lobby on its behalf and, speaking on behalf of American Tobacco, Robert Barney Walker told *The New Yorker*, "There is not a weight of evidence. There is a mounting wave of propaganda."(12) Clarence Little of the TIRC, in 1960, insisted that "the tobacco theory is rapidly losing much of the unique importance claimed by its adherents at its original announcement,"(13) a perverse assessment of a decade's worth of research which had almost exclusively supported the 'tobacco theory.'

Not all dissenting voices came from the tobacco industry. Hans Jurgen Eysenck, one of the best known and most respected psychologists in Britain, proposed the 'constitutional theory' which suggested that those who contracted cancer did so because they were genetically predisposed to do so. They were, he said, also predisposed to suffer from stress and it was this stress that led them to smoke. Consequently, any group of smokers was bound to contain a larger than average number of cancer patients. A neat theory, perhaps, but one with an obvious flaw. It failed to explain why so many more people had become 'predisposed' to lung cancer since the coming of the cigarette age.

A similar hypothesis came from one of the fathers of modern epidemiology, Sir Ronald A. Fisher, who believed that lung cancer began in adolescence and developed gradually. According to Fisher, individuals smoked tobacco to bring relief from the - presumably subtle - pain that this embryonic disease caused. Others suggested that lung cancer was more likely to be diagnosed in known smokers because doctors had been led to expect them to contract the disease. This was barely more believable. Doctors were often heavy smokers themselves and even if some were misdiagnosing patients, it could not be enough to explain 85% of lung cancer cases being smokers.

Legislation against cigarettes

By the end of the 1950s, Richard Doll and Austin Bradford Hill had become internationally lauded as scientific pioneers while Lennox Johnston remained practically unknown. The two English epidemiologists, rather than the Scottish doctor, took the credit for associating smoking with lung cancer and Johnston admitted that this resulted in his "mental equilibrium" being "disturbed for months."(14)

Johnston never disguised the bitterness he felt towards Doll and Hill and dismissed them as mere "statisticians" who were not brave enough to compromise their popularity by pushing for what Johnston considered the only logical outcome of their findings - "the abolition of smoking."(15)

"Only true pioneers," wrote Johnston, "are prepared to endure extreme unpopularity," and it was in this spirit that he called for higher taxes on cigarettes and the banning of smoking everywhere from factories to restaurants. In 1952, with his theories in the ascendancy, he succeeded in having a second paper on nicotine and addiction published in *The Lancet* and was interviewed by *Time* magazine. "Anti-smokers must do all they can," he said, "besides speaking up, they should write untiringly to the newspapers and to Management Boards and committees."(16) Believing that he could persuade 75% of smokers to give up if given access to television, he petitioned the BBC on four occasions to allow him to address the nation but to no avail.

Johnston's call for tax hikes, smoking bans in virtually all public places, a total ban on tobacco advertising and a state-funded anti-smoking campaign foreshadowed the agenda of every anti-smoking group that would follow by several decades. Once again, the Liverpool doctor was ahead of the pack but his militancy left him very much on the fringes of the debate. Unappreciated in his own day, his achievements have been buried with the passing of time and few today know his name. His only book - *The Disease of Tobacco Smoking and its Cure* - was published in 1957 and has been out of print ever since. He was writing letters to the *British Medical Journal* as late as 1979 (17), still insisting that smoking and drinking were the Western world's most serious preventable diseases, but he then disappears from record and this author has been unable to even ascertain when or where he died.

Few in Britain fell over themselves to embrace 'the smoking theory.' In 1957, the *British Medical Journal* was still accepting cigarette advertising and the nation's health minister declared that: "We cannot interfere with what is a matter for the individual."(18) The same year saw Harold Macmillan dismiss the hazards of cigarette smoking as "negligible compared with risk of crossing the street." The pipe-smoking prime minister was far more concerned by the prospect of losing tax revenue if Britons gave up smoking. He wrote in a memo: "Very serious issue. Revenue = 3/6d on income tax: not easy to see how to replace it."(19)

Most British newspapers did not view the smoking issue as one that deserved a great deal of coverage. Only *The Guardian* and *The Times* afforded it more than minimal attention, and only the former was inclined to view it as a suitable target for state intervention. *The Mirror* tended to take a light-hearted view of the whole business, and even when it reported compelling evidence about the lung cancer link it made sure the pill was sugared with stories about cigarettes being made safer and other promises of science saving the day. *The Express* was positively dismissive of the scientific evidence and only in the early 1970s did it begin to take the dangers of cigarettes seriously (20).

In 1962, the Royal College of Physicians (RCP) released the findings of its own commission on the subject and the British public was forced to accept that there was some truth in the 'smoking theory.' The RCP concluded that a 35 year old smoker had a 1 in 23 chance of dying before he was 45, and a 1 in 3 chance of dying before he was 65. Although the Commission added that "not all this difference in expectation of life is attributable to smoking,"(21) smokers were twice as likely to die before they reached retirement age than nonsmokers. Of tobacco's perceived benefits, the RCP found them to be "almost entirely psychological and social," although it accepted that smoking might help some people lose weight (22). With three-quarters of the adult male population still regularly smoking cigarettes, the RCP advised the government to limit tobacco advertising and force the tobacco industry to list tar and nicotine yields on cigarette packs.

A similar investigation into smoking and health was underway in the US. Soon after John F. Kennedy took office in 1961, representatives of the American Cancer Society, the American Heart Association, the National Tuberculosis Association and the American Public Health Association asked him to establish a commission to get to the bottom of the controversy. A committee was then set up under the aegis of the newly appointed Surgeon General, Dr Luther L. Terry. Its findings, published in the 1964 Surgeon General's Report, overwhelmingly found against the cigarette. Having studied 36 separate research documents on the association with lung cancer, Dr Terry estimated that smokers were nearly eleven times more likely to develop the disease than nonsmokers.*

The members of the Surgeon General's panel were forbidden to take up or quit the habit while it was in session, since they did not wish to give the media any indication of which way they were leaning. These meetings went on for over a year and as soon as they were over, Leonard Schumann - the heaviest smoker on the panel - immediately quit. He was not alone. One result of the 1964 Surgeon General's report was that cigarette sales fell by 2%.

The tobacco industry again protested its innocence and internal memos outlined what its response would be:

"Whatever qualifications we may assert to minimise the impact of the Report, we must face the fact that a responsible and qualified group of previously noncommitted scientists and medical authorities have spoken. One would suppose we would not repeat Dr Little's oft reiterated 'not proven'. One would hope the industry would act affirmatively and not merely react defensively.

We must, I think, recognize that in defense of the industry and in preservation of its present earnings position, we must either (a) disprove the theory of causal relationship or (b) discover the carcinogen or carcinogens, co-carcinogens, or whatever, and demonstrate our ability to remove or neutralize."(23)

Whatever doubts the industry tried to foster in the minds of its customers, the Surgeon General's report demanded "remedial action" and for the first time the American government took steps to inform the public about the perils of smoking. 'The Federal Cigarette Labelling and Advertising Act' was passed, placing limits on cigarette advertising to prevent it from appealing to minors or portraying cigarettes as sexy; a 'tar czar,' Robert Meyner, was appointed as the watchdog. The Act required explicit warnings, stating that smoking was a major factor

---

* The 1964 report has passed into legend as the first time a Surgeon General officially reported a link between cigarette smoking and lung cancer. The role of Terry's predecessor, LeRoy Edgar Burney, has been almost entirely overlooked. In November 1959, the *Journal of the American Medical Association* published Burney's 'Smoking and lung cancer: a statement of the Public Health Service' in which the then-Surgeon General provided a thorough, even-handed and astute summary of the evidence to date. He concluded that: "The weight of evidence at present implicates smoking as the principal etiological factor in the increased incidence of lung cancer."

in lung cancer, on cigarette packs and advertisements from 1965. Industry pressure resulted in this being scaled down in Congress. The deadline was put back to 1966, advertisements were excluded and the warning that was finally settled on did not mention cancer by name and merely warned: "Caution: Cigarette Smoking May Be Hazardous To Your Health."

The tobacco industry griped about excessive regulation but had no real cause for complaint. A further 17 liability suits had been lodged against the industry since the Surgeon General's report appeared and the industry desperately needed some kind of warning to be issued to the public as protection against future legal actions. Although tobacco executives would never admit to being relieved, the 1966 warning was sufficient to provide a measure of indemnity without sending a strong enough message to scare off too many customers.

As the world's biggest manufacturer of cigarettes, the United States had an unusually powerful tobacco lobby but government measures against the cigarette were no more lenient than in other countries. In Canada, the National Cancer Institute and the Canadian Medical Association had both confirmed that smoking caused lung cancer by 1961 but very little was done by the government to regulate the tobacco industry or its advertising, and consumption continued to rise, only peaking in 1966. In 1972, after years of inaction, the Canadian tobacco industry voluntarily put warnings on cigarette packs and stopped advertising on television and radio.

The British government banned tobacco advertising on television in 1965, something that was difficult for the American government to do thanks to the First Amendment's provision for freedom of speech. Generally, however, British governments preferred to negotiate with the tobacco industry rather than fight it. In 1970, the health secretary announced that the tobacco control policy would be made through voluntary agreement with the industry and health warnings appeared on packs for the first time. This voluntary measure was only legally enforced in 1990 and even then only because of EU law.

The USSR waited until 1971 before mandating warnings on cigarette packs and raising the legal age of purchase from 14 to 16.

France did next to nothing until 1976 when it restricted tobacco advertising and forced cigarette companies to display nicotine and tar yields on packs.

Anti-smoking measures in the countries of Asia were half-hearted at best. In Japan, four out of five adult males were smokers and the nation's *Hi-Lite* brand was one of the world's best selling cigarettes. The tobacco industry had been a government monopoly since 1905 and, with the state supporting pro-smoking adverts, the country's anti-smoking efforts inevitably lacked bite. Warning labels were introduced in 1972 with the less than compelling message that:

> "There are fears that smoking too much may be bad for your health, so be careful not to smoke too much."

But the Japanese were fanatical abolitionists compared with the Chinese. For years, Communist China was run by the chain-smoking Deng Xiaoping and there were no health warnings of any kind until 1979. For the Chinese, cigarettes represented modernity and good health. They were treasured because they provided an alternative to opium, a drug that symbolised the nation's paralysis and decline. Consequently China had, at one time, the world's most direct pro-smoking billboard ('Please Smoke a Cigarette') and anti-smokers were more likely to be lampooned than respected. When Deng Xiaoping finally died in 1997 one satirist wrote:

> "Deng is dead at the age of 92. Let us learn from this. Smoking kills."

In the mid-1960s, anti-smoking lobby groups had not yet resurfaced and in their absence, legislation focused on education, advertising and under-age smoking. There was little appetite for more draconian action. Smoking continued to be seen as an adult activity and while it probably carried a risk to health, it remained up to the individual whether they wished to take that risk. Australia's health minister captured the mood in government, saying, in the wake of the Surgeon General's report: "I do not believe a problem of this nature should be handled by arbitrary restrictions and prohibitions."(24) Instead, his administration launched a health campaign to make sure Australians were educated about the risks and could make an informed decision. As a result, the proportion of smokers in Australia fell from 43% to 37% between 1962 and 1967.

This decline was mirrored elsewhere. All around the world, information from government and the media about the hazards of smoking led to a sharp fall in smoking rates. In the US, smoking prevalence fell from 42.4% to 37.4% between 1965 and 1970 (25), largely as a result of education and reports in the press. The smoking rate had not dropped so greatly since the first lung cancer studies appeared in the early 1950s and no public health scheme since has been able to persuade so many smokers to quit in so short a period.

The return of the anti-smokers

The revival of anti-smoking as a mainstream movement began in a middle class living room in New York on Thanksgiving Day 1966. It was there, watching an American Football game with his parents (both of whom smoked), that a 25 year old part-time cruise-ship dancer named John F Banzhaf III suddenly became outraged by cigarette commercials appearing on television (26). Although he later claimed not to have had any previous interest in the smoking issue, he told *Readers Digest* that this was the moment he vowed to "do whatever I could to wipe out those evil commercials."(27)

Banzhaf had studied law at Columbia University and believed it might be possible to limit tobacco advertising without falling foul of the First Amendment. Under the Fairness Doctrine, television networks had an obligation to allow both sides of a debate to be heard. To Banzhaf, this meant broadcasting anti-smoking advertisements in reply to cigarette commercials. The Fairness Doctrine had never before been applied to advertising and had been created to ensure balanced coverage of political news. Banzhaf's interpretation had some obvious logical flaws (by the same rationale, the tobacco companies could demand free air-time every time a report about smoking and cancer was broadcast), but, seeing it as his best chance to stir things up, Banzhaf wrote to Henry Geller at the Federal Communications Commission (FCC) demanding the rule be applied to tobacco advertising and even requested that WCBS-TV give him air-time to personally broadcast anti-smoking messages to the nation.

Fortunately for Banzhaf, there were many within the FCC who also felt that cigarette advertisements were unethical but had been unable to find a legal way of putting a stop to them. Inspired by the young man's ruse, the FCC wrote to WCBS in June 1967 to demand free airtime for anti-smoking commercials. They had little time for Banzhaf himself, considering him to be brash, arrogant and egotistical and, as Geller said, "We never gave him a second thought - he was somebody we were using."[28]

In September 1967, the FCC ruled that one anti-smoking commercial must be shown for every four cigarette commercials. Banzhaf immediately appealed against the decision, complaining that the FCC had not gone far enough. Although it was a Saturday he flew to Washington and filed his appeal in the most liberal court he could find. He then requested $50,000 from the American Cancer Society to fight the case. They, too, were unimpressed by his manner and turned him down, informing him that they were "a medical and research institution" rather than a political action group. The tobacco industry, in turn, appealed against the original decision and against Banzhaf picking his own court. The television networks were also unhappy about having to give valuable air-time away for nothing and supported the industry's appeal, but in 1968 the court confirmed that the original ruling would stand.

In February 1968, flushed with success and having attained a welcome degree of fame, Banzhaf formed his own anti-smoking group, Action on Smoking and Health (ASH). With help from the Seventh Day Adventists, ASH monitored television stations to ensure that the FCC's ruling was being enforced. Finding that anti-smoking adverts were being given less than their allotted airtime and that a disproportionately large number of them were being run late at night, Banzhaf filed numerous complaints and at one point demanded WNBC lose its license.

The new federally mandated anti-smoking commercials had an immediate effect on the smoking behaviour of Americans. Per capita cigarette consumption had been falling rapidly since the Surgeon General's 1964 report but when the commercials began to be aired this decline accelerated. Encouraged by this, Banzhaf and the FCC felt that consumption would drop further if tobacco industry adverts were removed altogether. Supported by the American Cancer Society and the Consumers Union as well as anti-smoking Utah Senator Frank Moss and, briefly, Robert Kennedy, a total ban on cigarette advertising was proposed by the FCC and the Federal Trade Commission in 1968. This was not passed, although the same session led the government to force warnings on all cigarette advertisements, something the tobacco industry had avoided in 1965.

In 1970, the obstacle of the First Amendment was overcome when the Supreme Court ruled that the cigarette was a special case - a "unique danger" - because "it is harmful when taken as prescribed." Much to the dismay of the television networks, which stood to lose $200,000,000 in revenue, a blanket ban on broadcast cigarette advertising took effect on January 1 1971. The tobacco industry's marketing men launched a flurry of television ads in the last days of 1970. They had valued the exposure and respectability that broadcast advertising afforded them, but their disappointment was short lived.

With the cigarette commercials off the air, the Fairness Doctrine was no longer applicable and anti-smoking commercials disappeared with them. But the anti-smoking messages had been far more effective in deterring people from smoking than the cigarette advertisements had been in encouraging them to start. By one estimate, the televised health campaigns that ran between 1968-70 reduced annual cigarette consumption by 531 per person while cigarette advertising increased consumption by just 95 cigarettes a head. Anti-smokers rejoiced when the *Marlboro* man rode into the sunset at midnight on New Year's Eve 1970 but cigarette consumption, which had been falling for years, rose when the anti-smoking commercials disappeared and smoking prevalence remained at around 37% until the mid-1970s. The efforts of Banzhaf and the new generation of anti-smoking activists had backfired.

Of course, the tobacco industry increased its advertising and sponsorship in other areas but the loss of broadcast advertising - which had been taking up to 80% of their marketing budget - did not damage them financially. The industry had always argued that cigarette advertising was designed to persuade smokers to switch brands rather than to promote smoking *per se* and it was certainly true that the tobacco habit had spread to every corner of the globe centuries before the advertising industry was born. Anti-smokers argued that by allowing advertising, governments somehow legitimised or approved the product but removing cigarette advertising was no guarantee of reduced consumption. Britain's own ban on broadcast advertising was followed, in 1966, by 6 billion more units being sold than the year before (29). Although anti-smokers often assumed that cigarette advertising was the primary reason why people started smoking, Banzhaf had just snatched defeat from the jaws of victory by banning it.

Nonsmokers were largely unaffected by cigarette advertising and the broadcast ban had little or no effect on the number of people who took up smoking. For individual cigarette companies, however, advertising was paramount. There was essentially little real difference between brands of cigarettes. The only thing that could give a brand an edge was how it was perceived. For all the industry talk about taste and flavour, marketing men were primarily responsible for smokers switching brands.

Image and slogans have always been the making of tobacco companies. At one time or another *Fatima, Camel, Lucky Strike, Winston* and *Marlboro* have all been America's number one brand. American Tobacco controlled 92% of the world's tobacco business in 1911 but today both the company and its once mighty *Lucky Strikes* are also-rans.

For decades *Marlboro* was a woman's cigarette but from the mid-1950s Philip Morris radically changed the way in which its newly filter-tipped brand was marketed. The company employed a series of rugged, manly stereotypes in its advertising before deciding that a cowboy best represented the no-nonsense, all-American image it wished to convey. The brand seamlessly crossed the gender-divide and, in 1972, *Marlboro* became the world's best-selling cigarette. Advertising bans then swept the world and the anti-smokers' arch-enemy Philip Morris was fortunate enough to be top dog at a time when such laws effectively prevented its rivals from competing on anything other than price. Those brands that have made inroads into the market since the 1970s have either made a virtue of their low price, like *Lambert & Butler*, or their low yield, like *Silk Cut*.

As premium brands, *Marlboro* - and *Marlboro Lights*, which were launched in 1972 - have been untouchable market leaders for more than three decades, a feat never before achieved by a cigarette or a cigarette company. They owe their dominance, in large part, to advertising bans.

ASH

John Banzhaf's Action on Smoking and Health (ASH) did not have members as such, and relied on contributions from like-minded donors, of whom it had 5,000 in 1969, contributing a total of $90,227. When, the following year, Banzhaf succeeded in getting the "evil commercials" off the air for good, contributions fell to $58,381. With no television advertising to monitor, and with revenue dwindling, ASH's campaign looked to be running out of steam and in 1971 Banzhaf changed tack, declaring that ASH's aim was now to "defend the rights of nonsmokers."(30) This breathed new life into the group and Banzhaf, the self-styled "Ralph Nader of the cigarette industry," became the country's best-known anti-smoking activist. He was involved in the cigarette labelling act of 1970 which changed the warning on packs to a more decisive 'The Surgeon General has determined that cigarette smoking is dangerous to your health.' In the 1970s he campaigned for legally mandated no-smoking sections on public transport and he was an early proponent of the passive smoking theory. By 1979, ASH had 32,000 active donors contributing $358,509, of which Banzhaf drew $39,190 as its director.

ASH was not a traditional anti-tobacco group, nor was it purely a campaigning nonsmokers' rights group. Banzhaf's speciality was what he called 'legal activism'; challenging business and government in court to bring about social change. Banzhaf had a keen eye for the grey areas of the law and for legal technicalities ripe for exploitation. His lawsuits were by no means always successful but even the failures could be worthwhile when they generated publicity. ASH was professionalised at an early stage and was less reliant on volunteers than any previous anti-smoking group. By the late 1970s it was employing ten people, two of whom, significantly, were lawyers (31).

Unlike the Anti-Cigarette League, ASH did little campaigning at grass-roots level, finding it more effective to put its case directly to politicians, government agencies and judges. It did little in the way of health education, did not run stop-smoking clinics and its members did not tour schools or town halls. A study of articles in ASH's newsletters in the 1970s, found that only 1 in 10 were about health, while a full two-thirds concerned political or legal issues (32).

Lucy Page Gaston worked full-time for the Anti Cigarette League and lived in penury for most of her life. Banzhaf, by contrast, worked part-time for ASH, and drew a substantial salary for doing so, supplementing the income he received as a tutor at George Washington University Law School. He claims not to get "terribly worked up over his causes"(33) and yet he has pursued the smoking agenda for over forty years. On Banzhaf's office wall, alongside many clippings about himself, hangs the motto 'Sue the bastards!' and he has been called 'the man who tried to sue America.' The legal sale and advertising of a proven health hazard like cigarettes opened a Pandora's box of litigation and Banzhaf was one of the first to see its potential.

Business as usual

Keenly aware of the threat to their business, the tobacco companies continued to fight a rearguard action against the forces that were lining up against them. While the medical case against their product was looking increasingly water-tight, their vast profits provided ample consolation. Shortly after the Surgeon General's 1964 report, Cuyler Hammond revealed further results from the ACS study which showed that smokers were dying at twice the rate of nonsmokers and that they were around eleven times more likely to contract lung cancer. These results closely mirrored the conclusions in the Surgeon General's report. Even much of the tobacco industry's own private research strongly indicted their product. A 1963 TIRC report confirmed that smokers were more likely to die from heart disease and a subsequent report from the same institute indicated that women who smoked during pregnancy had babies that weighed less than those of nonsmokers.

The tobacco industry continued to keep the 'smoking controversy' alive and persisted with its policy of denial. No causal link had been established...many factors may be at work...the industry is looking into it... Business continued. Lawsuits were successfully defended. Philip Morris launched its long-running 'Come to *Marlboro* Country' campaign in 1964 and, in 1968, unveiled its *Virginia Slims* brand, aimed squarely at the female market. But by the end of the 1960s, both RJ Reynolds and Philip Morris had dropped the word 'tobacco' from their company names and had begun buying up less controversial companies like *7-Up* and *Miller* beer. Through all this, the industry's air of arrogant dispassion bordered on the blackly humorous. Questioned on television about the low birth weight issue in 1971, Philip Morris CEO Joseph F. Cullman III simply replied: "Some women would prefer having smaller babies."(34)

CHAPTER FIVE

'Smokers should be eliminated'

In 1972, Richard Nixon's new Surgeon General, Dr Jesse Steinfeld, published the latest report on smoking and health. It confirmed smoking as the major cause of lung cancer in the United States and implicated it as a contributor to coronary heart disease, low birth weights and premature birth. All of this had been suspected for some time. What set Steinfeld's report apart was the suggestion that 'secondhand smoke' was more than a mere nuisance and could be life-threatening to nonsmokers.

The report itself did not provide any solid evidence for this - there was none - but Steinfeld used the accompanying press conference to call for the creation of a nonsmokers' rights movement, saying:

> "Nonsmokers have as much right to clean air and wholesome air as smokers have to their so-called right to smoke, which I would redefine as a 'right to pollute.'
> It is high time to ban smoking from all confined public spaces such as restaurants, theatres, airplanes, trains and buses. It is time that we interpret the Bill of Rights for the nonsmokers as well as the smoker." (1)

With this statement, the Surgeon General went further than any of his predecessors had dared to go and the rabble-rousing may have been too much for the Republican administration. Steinfeld was not reappointed for Nixon's second term and no permanent replacement was made for another four years. Although it may have cost him his job, Steinfeld's rallying cry hit a nerve with disgruntled nonsmokers across America and the first significant wave of anti-smoking activity since the war began to take shape.

With cigarette advertising banned on television and with an unequivocal warning appearing on packets, the nascent anti-smoking movement focused its attention on public transport where unrestricted smoking was an annoyance to many.

Ralph Nader had made his name drawing attention to flaws in automobile safety and by campaigning against the pesticide DDT. In 1969, the young lawyer called on the Federal Aviation Administration (FAA) to ban smoking on all US flights. This was a bold request - even John Banzhaf was only suggesting separate sections for smokers and nonsmokers - and it fell on deaf ears. The FAA carried out a detailed risk assessment but neither they, nor the Civil Aeronautics Board, could find any evidence that the health of passengers was being compromised by smoke in the cabin. In fact, since the air in aeroplanes was ventilated every two minutes, it was found to be cleaner than in any other form of public transport.

The health of airline travellers was not, it seemed, being jeopardised and so the issue became one of consumer preference. A survey was carried out which found that 60% of respondents did not like to smell tobacco smoke on flights and, in 1973, the Civil Aeronautics Board segregated smokers and nonsmokers. It then banned cigars and pipes entirely, presumably because nonsmokers judged them to be particularly obnoxious and because pipe and cigar smokers were a smaller minority who would put up little in the way of resistance.

Nader pushed for a smoking ban on buses in 1970 but was defeated by the Federal Highway Commission. The following year, as a result of a further Nader petition, the Interstate Commerce Commission banished smokers to the rear 20% of buses (later extended to 30% due to smoking sections becoming overcrowded). In 1976, Nader succeeded in bringing about nonsmoking sections on trains but his momentum was finally halted a year later when the FAA drew the line at banning smoking in aeroplane cockpits.

The campaign for nonsmoking sections was relatively uncontroversial but it represented a significant shift in the fight against tobacco since it was not so much concerned with educating people as it was with segregating them. Today, this segregation would be put in terms of 'protecting' nonsmokers from being 'exposed' to secondhand smoke but such terminology barely figured in the early 1970s. Virtually no research had been published regarding passive smoking and the phrase itself was unknown. Public transport bans were brought about because nonsmokers were saying they did not like the smell of unrestricted smoking, not because they feared for their lives.

Smokers had little reason to protest, and few did. They were largely unaffected by the creation of nonsmoking sections. They were not yet forced to abstain for any period of time - and many of them were sympathetic to those who found smoke irritating and offensive. Some libertarians questioned the need for government action in an area that could just as easily be resolved by businesses listening to the needs of customers, but since public transport was usually run by the state, even that argument had little resonance.

The 'clean air' campaign goes global

The ongoing activities of public figures like Ralph Nader and John Banzhaf were complemented by concerned individuals taking action on their own doorstep. One of these was Betty Carnes, a respected ornithologist, who was in her sixties when she found herself seated next to a heavy smoker on an American Airlines flight. When the air filtration system broke down she became so nauseous that she was sick in a bag. A frequent flyer, Carnes requested that the airline designate the first three rows of seats nonsmoking and, in 1971, it agreed to do so.

Thereafter, Carnes became a vocal advocate of smoke-free places in her home state of Arizona. She set aside three floors of the hospital in which she worked for nonsmokers and campaigned for statewide smoking restrictions. In 1973, largely thanks to her lobbying, Arizona became the first US state to enact comprehensive 'nonsmokers' rights' legislation since the Second World War. Smoking was banned in elevators, libraries, theatres, museums and buses, just as the Surgeon General had recommended. Meanwhile, American Airlines increased its nonsmoking section to six, then twelve, rows of seats before banishing smokers to the back half of its planes.

In 1977, Betty Carnes gathered like-minded individuals around her to form Arizonans Concerned About Smoking (ACAS), a group that continued to escalate its demands after the death of its guiding light, ten years later, from stomach cancer. As part of her legacy she set up the Carnes Fund to give grants for female graduates through the auspices of the American Ornithologists' Union. Smokers were not eligible to apply.

A new wave of radical, direct action by militant anti-smokers was on the rise. In their book *The Legal Rights of Nonsmokers* (1977), the husband and wife team Alvan and Betty Brody called for smokers to be charged with assault and battery on the basis that exposing a person to smoke was intentional, harmful and offensive. In Connecticut, Dr Joseph J. Kristan put the theory to the test; he asked a smoker to put out his cigarette and, when the man refused, sprayed air freshener in his face. He was acquitted in court after claiming self-defence.

Another physician, Dr Alan Blum, was brought up by a passionately anti-smoking father - also a family doctor - who urged his son to tape record cigarette commercials in the 1960s, so confident was he that they would one day be regarded as curious period pieces. Dr Blum Snr was correct, and his son retained a lasting fascination for tobacco industry marketing practices. In 1977, he founded Doctors Ought to Care (DOC) with the express intention of parodying tobacco industry marketing practices. Turning *Marlboro* into *Fartboro* and rebranding *Virginia Slims* as *Emphysema Slims* hardly suggested that medicine's gain had been comedy's loss but Blum was one of the more thoughtful and pragmatic figures to emerge from the new wave of anti-smoking activity. While the American movement viewed a ban on tobacco advertising as a priority, Blum was one of the few to have learnt a lesson from Banzhaf's pyrrhic victory in putting an end to televised cigarette commercials; that counter-advertising is more productive than government restrictions. "The Devil," he said, "cannot stand to be mocked."(2)

A genuine grass-roots movement was spreading across the globe and it had the tobacco industry firmly in its sights. Australia saw the creation of the Non-Smokers Movement of Australia in 1977. The

Australian government had recently prohibited smoking on buses and trains and the group fought to extend these bans to airlines and indoor public places using the familiar tactics of letter writing, protests, publicity stunts and the publication of a newsletter: *The Clean Air Clarion*.

The Non-Smokers Movement of Australia's more youthful sibling was The Movement Opposed to Promotion of Unhealthy Products (MOP-UP), formed by Simon Chapman, an ebullient opponent of smoking still in his twenties (3). MOP-UP took on a host of unfashionable targets but it always viewed the tobacco industry as its greatest adversary and its members picketed the Australian Tennis Open for four years demanding that *Marlboro* be dropped as a sponsor. MOP-UP's campaigns were lively enough, but there was a yearning for still further radicalism and 1979 saw the formation of a militant splinter group whose unwieldy moniker - Billboard-Utilising Graffitists Against Unhealthy Promotions - made more sense when shortened to BUGA-UP.

Filled with quasi-anarchistic zeal, BUGA-UP members attacked advertising billboards for everything from beer and cigarettes to cars and air conditioning through the medium of vandalism, a favourite method being to spray-paint disparaging slogans across advertising hoardings. Cigarette billboards were the most inviting canvas since the product was heavily advertised, patently unhealthy and made by wealthy multi-national corporations. "The tobacco companies didn't know what to do," reminisced Chapman in 2004. "They were running round like headless chooks, and fulminating - 'This was vandalism! How immoral!' Well, that was pretty rich coming from them!" (4)

BUGA-UP was dominated by young, left-wing radicals but the appeal of defacing tobacco advertisements occasionally attracted more conventional characters. In 1982, for example, a Sydney surgeon was arrested for spray-painting a cigarette billboard. At times witty, at other times preachy and gratuitous, this subversive approach thrives in Australia to this day. The cigarette adverts have long-since been banned but visitors to the country's trendier areas will see billboards for everything from clothes to fizzy drinks attracting the paint of the nocturnal satirists.

GASP

The most influential anti-smoking group of the era was founded in the state of Maryland in 1971. Group Against Smoking Pollution (GASP) was the brainchild of Clara Gouin, a housewife and environmentalist, whose father had died of lung cancer and whose husband was acutely sensitive to tobacco smoke. Gouin set up the society with a handful of friends from her local church and immediately began publishing its newsletter *The Ventilator*, which was sent out to health charities and politicians up and down the country. With a $1 a year membership fee, GASP's early efforts were necessarily small-scale and local. Its members worked towards attaining nonsmoking sections in public places and, to that end, made badges, printed posters, petitioned politicians and, in time, published a pamphlet: *The Nonsmokers Liberation Guide*.

GASP's aims were, as Gouin later recalled, to "get nonsmokers to protect themselves" and "to make smoking so unpopular that smokers would quit."(5) It was an agenda that appealed to folk far beyond her immediate vicinity and new branches of GASP sprang up under like-minded individuals, first in Berkeley, then in Massachusetts. Within three years, GASP could boast more than fifty chapters, including two in Canada.

It was a loose coalition. All GASP branches were independent of its Maryland founder and Gouin had neither the ego nor the desire to become the face of a mass movement. But others did, not least Paul Loveday, president of GASP's Berkeley branch. Highly sensitive to tobacco smoke, a Mormon and a law graduate, Loveday was born to be an anti-smoking activist and he was at the centre of the West Coast's first major victory when Berkeley City council banned smoking in public places (ie. publicly *owned* buildings) and mandated nonsmoking sections in restaurants.

Buoyed by success and a measure of celebrity, Loveday demanded that his followers be given the power of citizen's arrest to apprehend those who flouted smoking restrictions. He was then joined by the zealous Stanton Glantz, a qualified aerospace engineer who had gained some notoriety protesting against the Vietnam war in his undergraduate days. Glantz made his mark as an outspoken anti-smoking activist in 1976 when he flew to Washington, DC to criticise Ted Kennedy's proposal to levy extra tax on high tar cigarettes. Glantz considered this to be a "dumb idea" and put forward the view that the best approach was to make smoking socially unacceptable - a policy that would later be known as 'denormalisation.'

GASP was constrained by limited funds and resistance from a tobacco industry that had not yet been fully discredited, but through hard-work, perseverance and an almost fanatical commitment to the cause, GASP was able to generate publicity that was disproportionate to its modest membership. Anti-smoking groups in this period received little or no government funding and the grass-roots movement attracted only a small number of followers. Advising fellow anti-smokers on how to form their own groups, Anne Morrow Donley of GASP said: "Don't expect crowds at your meetings. Expect maybe five to ten people at most."(6)

Like the Wizard of Oz, it was imperative that GASP appear larger and more powerful than its membership suggested. They made as much noise as they could and made friends in government, always recognising the importance of congratulating politicians after they had done something for them as well as haranguing them until they did. GASP's membership was predominantly young, white, suburban and middle-class but, through their press conferences and pamphlets, they claimed to represent nonsmokers - all of them, millions of them - and probably believed they were doing so. They wrote to the media and called up radio stations as the voice of the silent majority and this gave the impression that nonsmokers were far more passionate about being free from smoke than smokers were about having the right to smoke.

How much these "five to ten" local radicals represented average nonsmokers in the 1970s is a subject for conjecture. The lines had not yet been drawn between smokers and nonsmokers and it would take the belief that one group was directly harming the other for such a delineation to appear. This was still some years off but it was something that groups like GASP were already working on.

Although there was little to no proof that smokers were damaging the health of others, there was a tangible feeling that unrestricted smoking was often annoying and unnecessary. Irritation and intolerance of smoke was as old as smoking itself and the 'nuisance factor' began to play a part in anti-smoking legislation in this decade of renewed activism. In polls conducted in the early 1960s the percentage of US citizens who agreed with the statement that 'smoking is annoying' was around 45%. By the early 1970s this figure had risen to over 60% and by the late 1980s it stood at around 70%. Only when those who disliked smoking were in a clear majority were laws passed to restrict it; segregation on public transport being the earliest and most benign example.

As smoking rates fell and the number of smoking restrictions rose, surveys showed that nonsmokers were becoming increasingly intolerant of tobacco smoke in the air. It was something of a paradox that they were becoming more irritated by smoke the less they encountered it and this raised its own questions. Why did so many more people find smoking annoying in 1975 than they did in 1960 or 1945? Why, indeed, were there more complaints about tobacco smoke in 2005 than in 1975?

It may be that each generation is more delicate and irritable than the one before. The rise of asthma and allergies in the Western world over the last thirty years lends some support to this view. More prosaically, it may simply be because each generation produces fewer smokers than the last. In 1945, almost half of all Americans smoked. By the late 1970s this was down to a third. Millions had given up and ex-smokers were notoriously less tolerant of smoking than never-smokers.

On the other hand, it may be that, by the 1970s, it had become more socially acceptable to say that one found smoking annoying. Some sociologists have suggested that the reason for this lay, in part, with the rise of an anti-smoking movement which made hating tobacco smoke less a peculiar personal quirk and more of a reasonable preference. In effect, this meant that there had always been millions of 'closet' anti-smokers who only felt comfortable expressing their dislike of tobacco when others did the same in the 1970s. The number of people actively involved in anti-smoking groups during this period remained meagre but the snowball effect was becoming evident and public support was growing.

In January 1974, Lynn Smith organised a nonsmoking 'D-Day' in her home town of Monticello, Minnesota in which every resident was encouraged to abstain from smoking for twenty-four hours. It is not known how many smokers succeeded in this challenge, or how many even tried, but the idea garnered enough publicity for a similar event to be held across the whole state in November and a nationwide equivalent - 'The Great American Smokeout' - was launched by the government three years later.

Minnesota's growing reputation as a hotbed of anti-smoking activity was sealed in June 1975 when the state passed a law banning or restricting smoking in public places, shops, restaurants and hotels. The state of Utah passed similar legislation the following year, with employers facing up to three months in prison if they failed to create nonsmoking areas in their workplaces.

The nonsmokers' rights laws of Minnesota, Utah and Arizona were tame by today's standards. Businesses were obliged to listen to the views of their staff and implement a smoking policy that accommodated all employees. In Minnesota, smoking and nonsmoking areas had to be separated either by a four foot wide space or a four and a half foot tall barrier. Aside from these conditions, the legislation was relatively vague, with an emphasis on requiring "reasonable efforts" and "arrangements" in finding a satisfactory compromise between smokers and nonsmokers.

Most employers were able to comply with such legislation without spending a great deal of money and, as a result, there was little resistance from industry. Some took issue with the classification of privately owned restaurants and hotels as 'public places' and a few critics complained about what they saw as state-sponsored segregation, but the restriction on smokers' liberty was limited and only the tobacco industry put up much of a fight.

Over in California, GASP activists had the wind in their sails and a string of minor victories to their name when, inspired by events in Minnesota, they drew up a proposal for a statewide smoking ban that was officially known as The Clean Indoor Air Act but generally referred to as Proposition 5. This ordinance was more wide-reaching than the laws passed in Arizona, Minnesota and Utah but, with a vote due in 1978, GASP was wary enough of public opinion to make a number of tactical exemptions. This led to some strange anomalies. Smoking would be banned at jazz concerts, for example, but not at rock concerts even when performed in the same venue, presumably so as not to alienate younger voters. Banning smoking in bars was never mentioned.

Proposition 5 would require nonsmoking and smoking spaces to be partitioned, including in some outdoor spaces. Offences would result in criminal, not civil, prosecution and enforcement would be the responsibility of the police. GASP came up with the conveniently round number of $1 billion as being the total savings the state would make by passing the law, this supposedly coming from savings in health care and preventing lost earnings due to ill health. It was opposed by businesses worried about the costs, by the San Diego police, by the tobacco industry and ultimately by the public who voted 54% to 46% against it.

Two years later, GASP tried again with Proposition 10. Learning from their mistakes in the previous campaign, they proposed that the law be enforced by health inspectors rather than police officers and dropped the idea of partitioning spaces which had so alarmed small businesses. In this era of ASH, GASP and BUGA-UP, the tobacco industry, which had spent $6 million opposing Proposition 5, formed its own acronym-based lobby group - Californians Against Regulatory Excess (CARE) - and, again, the Californian electorate rejected the ordinance, with a barely unchanged 53% to 47% vote.

ASH (UK)

While the anti-smoking movement was gradually resurfacing in the US, grass-roots activity remained negligible in Britain. The National Society for Nonsmokers (NSNS) continued to be the only anti-tobacco association of any note and it had changed little since its inception fifty years earlier. As far back as 1948, its firebrand Lennox Johnston had called on the government to raise tobacco duty and found himself, not for the first time, widely ridiculed.

As much as he hated tobacco, Johnston was never unsympathetic to smokers themselves. After years of injecting himself with the drug, he knew only too well the power of nicotine addiction and he viewed nicotine lozenges, pills and, inevitably, injections as the solution. In 1957, the government set up the country's first smoking cessation clinic and Johnston himself set up a private clinic in Liverpool the following year. But that, for many years, was that.

Following the ground-breaking Royal College of Physicians report of 1962, several politicians proposed anti-smoking measures in vain. Most prominent amongst them was Enoch Powell, the Minister for Health, who fought for an increase in tobacco taxes with the express purpose of reducing consumption. The policy was never implemented because the Conservative government regarded any rise in cigarette prices as being unnecessarily punitive to the poor and the Labour government of the pipe-smoking Harold Wilson (1964-1970) took much the same stance.

Under Wilson, cigarette advertisements were pulled from television as part of a voluntary agreement with the tobacco industry but further action was considered illiberal and intrusive. It was not considered appropriate for politicians and doctors to tell the public how to live their lives and it was feared that to do so would not only threaten the £800 million that the government took each year in tobacco duty but would also encourage the anti-alcohol lobby to press for legislation against drinkers.

Calls for tax hikes, sweeping advertising bans and explicit warnings were contemplated by successive British governments in the 1960s but none of them came to fruition. Dictating where people could and could not smoke was almost unthinkable. In 1969, a request from the NSNS to ban smoking in public places was dismissed by an official at the Department of Health who wrote:

> "This society is particularly militant, even fanatical, and they write incessantly to various departments on the theme of abolishing smoking in practically every type of place imaginable."(7)

The NSNS had been a dogmatic irrelevance in British politics for decades and there were no effective anti-smoking groups of the type seen in America to push for fresh legislation. This lack of external activism was a source of frustration for those ministers who did wish to address the problem of smoking and so the Ministry of Health hatched a scheme to manufacture its own 'grass-roots' anti-smoking group. This novel idea had first been mooted as far back as 1962 when an employee of the Health Ministry wrote:

"There is at present very little in the way of an anti-smoking lobby... The most effective measure to limit smoking would be the promotion of a voluntary anti-smoking movement. It would be much easier for the Government and the local authorities to take regulatory measures against smoking if there is a body of opinion pressing them to do so." (8)

The concept floated around the corridors of power for nine years before George Godber, the Chief Medical Officer and chairman of the recently created Health Education Council, adopted it. Godber was the staunchest and most high profile anti-smoker in the land and had long viewed smoking as a vice that should be confined to consenting adults in private. He envisioned an activist group which would live on long after he left office and would lobby successive governments for ever tougher anti-smoking measures.

Several names were considered for this new organisation. These included the British Association on Smoking and Health and the Council for Action on Smoking and Health; but BASH and CASH were not sympathetic acronyms for an organisation which would receive charitable status. In the end he decided to borrow a name that had worked elsewhere and in January 1971 the British version of Action on Smoking and Health was launched.

ASH (UK) was a unique creation in British politics. It would masquerade as, in Godber's words, a "voluntary group" but was staffed by full-time government employees. It would accept donations but would never be reliant upon them since it was funded by the taxpayer. It was created by elected politicians but it would be staffed by people who would never have to stand for election. The public would be allowed to become members but it had no need for volunteers since it would speak directly to the media and lawmakers (its membership never exceeded more than a few hundred people in any case). ASH did not exist to set up stop-smoking clinics or to provide help for smokers who wished to quit. Instead it was designed from the very outset to be a professional pressure group and by the end of its first decade it had become set on an agenda of eliminating smoking throughout the United Kingdom (9).

A milder smoke

In the United States, the threat from the growing anti-smoking movement was sufficient for the tobacco industry to assume the mantle of custodians of American principles of liberty and freedom. The Tobacco Institute made the case that smoking bans were essentially unAmerican and warned of a new era of Prohibition. With its new slogan 'Freedom of choice is the best choice,' the Tobacco Institute set about accusing its enemies in the anti-smoking lobby of being killjoys and puritans. On National Public Radio in 1979, its formidable spokesman William F. Dwyer launched a scathing attack:

"The anti-smokers are a small but vocal corps - I have to say it - of neo-Prohibitionists; they are reformers; they are those people, essentially a joyless tribe...who want to manage everyone else's life, perhaps because they have been incapable of managing their own." (10)

The industry spent the 1970s casting doubt on the notion that cigarettes were harmful without explicitly denying it. A Tobacco Institute memorandum of the time (which came to light twenty years later) described the strategy of prevarication and confusion as "brilliantly conceived and executed over the years" for its use of "variations on the theme that 'the case is not proved.'"(11)

Over the course of the decade, the proportion of American adults who smoked fell from 37.4% to 33.2%. Sharp though this drop was, tobacco executives might have reflected that since they were selling a product that had been officially branded deadly, business could have been a good deal worse. Besides, per capita consumption only dropped from 10.97 to 10.57 a day (12) over the same period, the international market remained lucrative and the number of young people smoking remained unchanged.

One key question for the tobacco companies was whether it was worth pursuing the low-yield market more vigorously. In the 1930s and 1940s, they had begun to reduce the amount of tar and nicotine in their cigarettes in an attempt to allay the public's health fears. The trend towards lower yields accelerated during the 'tar derby' of the early 1950s, in which tobacco companies competed to produce the 'lightest' cigarette available, but came to an abrupt end in 1954 when the Federal Trade Commission (FTC) prevented the tobacco industry from advertising tar and nicotine yields. Thereafter, yields drifted upwards, partly because there was no financial incentive to reduce them and partly because the increasingly popular filtered brands required higher yields to offer the same nicotine 'kick.' After years of reducing yields, the 1960s saw the triumph of 'full flavour' (ie. strong) brands such as *Winston* and *Marlboro**.

The American 'tar czar' Robert Meyner maintained that showing yields would send a message to the public that one cigarette was 'safer' than another but, in 1967, and with the blessing of the Surgeon General, the FTC reversed its decision and allowed cigarette companies to once again list the amount of tar and nicotine that was found in their products. The FTC did not, however, *require* them to do so and America's tobacco industry was thereby given a choice not available to its counterparts abroad. (In Europe, the favoured approach was for government to force the industry to display tar and nicotine levels.)

Not all cigarettes were advertised with their yields after 1967 and, unsurprisingly, it was the low tar brands that did so first. 'Light' and

---

*A 1938 *Consumer Reports* study of cigarettes found nicotine yields of between 1.4mg (in *Lucky Strikes*) and 2.3mg (in *Marlboro* and *Chesterfield*). The tar yield invariably came out at about 10 times the nicotine yield and, despite industry efforts, it was very difficult to reduce tar without reducing nicotine. Levels of both rose after the FTC's 1954 ruling. In the 1950s, the average nicotine level in US cigarettes was 3 mg nicotine (and 43 mg tar) and remained at this level for much of the 1960s. By way of comparison, a modern full strength *Marlboro* in the UK contains just 0.9 mg nicotine and 8 mg tar.

'ultra-light' cigarettes scaled new heights of popularity during this period. These included Lorillard's long-running *Kent* as well as their more recent addition, *True*. Philip Morris introduced *Merit* (9 mg of tar) and, in 1972, *Marlboro Light*. By 1980, average tar and nicotine levels in cigarettes were a third of those found in their 1950s cousins.

For a time, lowering yields became a legitimate public health issue. Thomas Whiteside of *The New Yorker* asked the Food and Drug Administration to coerce the tobacco industry into reducing tar and nicotine levels and John Lindsey, the mayor of New York, proposed a "disincentive tax" of 4 cents per pack for all cigarettes containing over 15 mg tar. Low yields were considered so important that, in 1976, the Senate held hearings to discuss taxing cigarettes according to their tar and nicotine contents. These hearings - which GASP's Stanton Glantz gate-crashed - saw Senator Frank Moss recommend a legal limit of 21 mg tar but the committee could not reach agreement and the idea had to be shelved.

There was a strong scientific case to be made for lower yields. The results of Cuyler Hammond's twelve year study showed that people who smoked low tar cigarettes (then defined as those with under 17.7 mg tar) were 26% less likely to contract lung cancer than those smoking full strength brands. He also found a 14% lower risk of heart disease and an overall lowering of premature death of 16%. Cigarettes were still dangerous, to be sure, but this research suggested that 'lighter' cigarettes made a real difference to the risk undertaken by those who continued to smoke. Hammond's research suggested that a wholesale shift to low tar brands would save the lives of 1 in 6 smokers.

On the other hand, Robert Meyner spoke for many when he warned that listing low tar yields was akin to advertising health benefits and could encourage people to keep smoking. Faced with a choice between withholding information that might help smokers minimise the risk to their health and the possibility of slowing the quit-rate, the medical establishment was split on the issue. The hard-liners who aimed for the total elimination of smoking saw it as a question of sending out the right message: no form of smoking could be condoned and no cigarette should be seen as safer than another. But the pragmatists, including Ernst Wynder and the American Cancer Society's medical director Arthur Holleb, recognised that mass abstinence was unlikely to be achieved in their lifetime and felt that the tobacco industry had an obligation to reduce the dangers as far as possible.

Ultimately, the pragmatists were defeated and Hammond's research has now been largely forgotten since it does not fit the orthodox view that all cigarettes are equally evil. Still, evidence continues to show that light cigarettes are indeed less harmful. In 1981, the US Surgeon General accepted that lower tar yields reduced incidence of lung cancer and legislation around the world has reflected that view. The British government, for example, banned tobacco advertising in 1986 but only for cigarettes with tar levels over 18 mg and current European Union laws limit tar yields to 14 mg.

In 1995, two studies in the *British Medical Journal* concluded that lower yield cigarettes were significantly less harmful, with one reporting that: "About a quarter of deaths from lung cancer, coronary heart disease, and possibly other smoking related diseases would have been avoided by lowering tar yield from 30 mg per cigarette to 15 mg."(13)(14)

The dominant view in anti-smoking circles, then as now, had no time for such talk. Public health bodies, which would soon be providing free syringes to heroin addicts to minimise the risks of their dangerous (and illegal) habit, held to the quit-or-die approach when it came to cigarettes (15). Dr John Slade, an influential anti-smoker from New Jersey, wrote in 1990 that he wished the US government had stopped cigarette innovation in 1950 because then "the only cigarettes on the market would be unfiltered 70 mm smokes, and far fewer people would be smoking."(16) A higher proportion of smokers would have died in the process, but for those who expected every smoker to quit, that was perhaps beside the point.

The 'safer' cigarette

The search for the 'safer' cigarette led America's National Cancer Institute (NCI) to set up 'The Less Hazardous Cigarette Working Group' in 1968 to research the possibility of minimising the health risks associated with smoking. Knowing that the tobacco industry had spent millions of dollars attempting to do the same, the NCI invited industry scientists to contribute to the sessions. The industry accepted, with one proviso. Ever wary of making an admission that their products were hazardous, it had the organisation's name changed to the more benign 'Tobacco Working Group.'

The research team was led by Dr Gio. B. Gori, the deputy director of the NCI's Smoking and Health program, who announced, almost from day one, that the creation of a significantly safer cigarette was not just possible but imminent. Gori's ambitions were not, however, matched by his rather pedestrian methods even if these methods did have a certain simple logic. Gori's plan was to remove as much tar as possible from cigarettes without making them unsatisfying to the smoker. It was much the same strategy as the tobacco industry had been pursuing for decades.

Anti-smokers have since portrayed Gori as 'pro-smoking' by giving smokers the hope of a 'safe' cigarette. In truth, he never pretended that it was possible to eliminate all risk from smoking and he made it clear that he was targeting only those "who wish to overcome the smoking habit but are unable to do so 'cold turkey.'"[17] This was a view shared by Surgeon General William Stewart and his successor Jesse Steinfeld. The former never expected a 'safe' cigarette but he anticipated reducing the risks "to a level which the average knowledgeable smoker might be willing to tolerate."[18] The latter prefaced his 1972 report with a call for smoking cessation but added: "We must also, however, work towards reducing the dangers of smoking for those who have not quit by developing less hazardous cigarettes." [19]

There was, then, nothing controversial about the government's attempt to make cigarettes safer, nor was it considered unseemly for the tobacco industry to collaborate in these efforts. It was always made clear that the $6,000,000 spent by the NCI in this endeavour would be accompanied by a campaign to promote total abstinence, lest their work be viewed as a green light to carry on smoking.

Gori worked on the assumption that two cigarettes a day represented a "tolerable risk," that is to say it made dying of a smoking related disease very much less likely than smoking twenty a day. This was borne out by the evidence and no one disputed that there was a dose-response relationship between smoking and disease. Gori based his estimates on pre-1960 (unfiltered) cigarettes which had, on average, 43 mg of tar in them. Cigarette yields had fallen significantly since then but since he was making his estimates of risk based on the 1964 Surgeon General's report it seemed reasonable to use pre-1960 cigarettes as the gold standard.

Gori worked out that the 1970s equivalent of two of these cigarettes was 9 *Benson and Hedges Lights* or 27 *Carlton* menthol cigarettes and he endeavoured to reduce tar levels further, thus creating an 'ultra light' cigarette. The National Cancer Institute's biostatistician said that this would still represent a doubling in risk for lung cancer but this was still a huge improvement on the eleven-fold increase reported by the Surgeon General.

Meanwhile, Liggett & Myers were using rather more creative methods to develop a cigarette that appeared to drastically reduce lung cancer risk. By scattering the rare metallic element palladium into tobacco they produced a cigarette which appeared not to cause lung cancer at all. Liggett scientists working for the project - code-named 'Operation Tame' - painted cigarette tar on mice, just as Ernst Wynder had done in his damning tests of the 1950s, and found a reduction in tumours of 95-100% compared with regular cigarettes. If the same results appeared in humans it would be a sensational breakthrough and Liggett began stockpiling huge quantities of palladium in preparation for the launch of its new brand of cigarette. It was to be called *Epic*.

Why *Epic* never appeared is one of the great mysteries in the history of the tobacco industry. For years, Liggett had been selling a product that could be lethal and would sooner or later result in massive liability suits. The problem it faced was that *Epic*, or any other 'safer' cigarette, would not alter the past. Even if it was completely harmless, the company might still be liable for the damage done by its conventional brands. If, on the other hand, *Epic* proved dangerous - and it had only been tested on animals - the company would be in an even more desperate situation.

In the worst case scenario, the use of palladium could make the cigarettes even more hazardous - as had happened when Lorillard experimented with the asbestos filter - and, if so, Liggett would be stranded. It would not benefit from the honour-amongst-thieves agreement with the other tobacco companies; its competitors were more likely to turn on it for releasing a 'safer' alternative and thereby implicitly condemning the other brands as lethal.

Nor was there any guarantee that *Epic* would sell. Even if it was genuinely safer, it might still flop. In 1975, Brown & Williamson had released *Fact*, with several compounds - such as cyanide - removed but it had failed in the marketplace and had to be withdrawn. The same thing happened when British tobacco companies launched cigarettes containing tobacco substitutes in 1977.

Then there was the problem of how to market it. The law prohibited the tobacco industry from advertising supposed health benefits and, even if the law was changed, they could not risk implicating their other brands as unsafe. Hoisted by their own petard, Liggett proposed advertising *Epic* with the provocative tag-line:

"We don't believe that mice-painting tests can be extrapolated to humans. But *you* may believe. And we think you deserve a choice" (emphasis in the original) (21).

All these problems worked against innovations in cigarette design, although Liggett cannot have believed them to be insurmountable otherwise they would never have begun research in the first place. What really put an end to *Epic*, and all the other attempts to launch significantly safer cigarettes, was internal pressure from the rest of the industry and external pressure from the tobacco control movement (22).

An article about the *Epic* breakthrough was sent to the journal *Cancer Research* but was rejected because the editor felt that it would encourage smoking. The American Cancer Society, public health officials and most of the medical community were against *Epic* for the same reason, to say nothing of the nonsmokers' rights groups which were uniformly hostile since it would do nothing to reduce 'stinking' smoke in the atmosphere, whether dangerous or not. After lobbying from health groups, the Food and Drug Administration declared that new cigarettes would need to prove safety and efficacy, an impossibility for any tobacco product, and *Epic* was dead in the water.

Gio Gori faced hostility from the same quarters in 1978 when he published the fruits of his work in the *Journal of the American Medical Association* in a paper entitled 'Towards less hazardous cigarettes: current advances.' Ernst Wynder urged him not to publish, predicting it would "bring down a firestorm."(23) He was correct. The anti-smoking lobby went berserk when they heard that a scientist was proposing that people smoke safer cigarettes rather than giving up.

President Carter had recently appointed Joseph Califano as Secretary of Health, Education and Welfare. A former 60-a-day man, Califano had recently quit at the request of his son and had come to view cigarettes as 'public health enemy number one.' Appealing for a "second health revolution," Califano recommended a tax hike on cigarettes and smoking bans on all aeroplanes. Only a few months earlier he had launched the biggest federal anti-smoking campaign to date. Gori's paper could not have been published at a worse time.

Siding with the anti-smoking lobby, Califano diverted the National Cancer Institute away from risk-reduction projects like the Tobacco Working Group and demanded that Gori be fired. Sacked at the moment when he expected to be most appreciated, a dejected Gori later commented: "The new policy was: Smokers shouldn't be helped - smokers should be eliminated."(24)

CHAPTER SIX

'Nonsmokers arise'

By the late 1970s, the race was on to find credible evidence that secondhand smoke posed a health risk to nonsmokers. When the Surgeon General first brought the passive smoking theory to the public's attention in 1972, it was almost entirely hypothetical. It did, however, seem to many people, as Richard Kluger remarked, only "common sense" that if tobacco smoke caused disease in smokers then it was possible, even probable, that it could do the same to those who breathed it involuntarily. On the other hand, it was also not unreasonable to assume that, although tobacco contained carcinogens, they only provoked disease in a minority of smokers after decades of heavy, continuous and direct use*. Even the most potent toxins could be safely encountered at low enough levels. Why not tobacco?

Several of the biggest names in smoking research believed the threat from Environmental Tobacco Smoke (ETS), as it was known, to be illusory from the outset. Cuyler Hammond pointed out that even as GASP and ASH were promoting the passive smoking theory in the mid-1970s, there was "no shred of evidence"[1] to support it. Ernst Wynder, who had spent twenty-five years researching smoking and health, told a cancer conference in 1975 that "passive smoking can

---

* Nonsmokers also breathed the smoky air through their noses, providing added protection. One of the main reasons why scientists found it so difficult to induce cancer in animals was the animals' reluctance to breathe through their mouths. In 1958, the researcher R.D. Passey reported: "Our failure during the past five years to induce lung tumours in mice, rats and hamsters by exposure to strong concentrations of cigarette smoke is a striking negative result." Wynder finally managed it by performing tracheotomies on dogs.

provoke tears or can be otherwise disagreeable, but it has no influence on health [because] the doses are so small."(2) Even some anti-smoking groups were sceptical. In 1973, ASH (UK) set up a committee to look at the evidence and concluded that "there is virtually no risk to the healthy nonsmoker apart from exceptional exposure to tobacco smoke in an unventilated room or a close car."(3)

Plausible or not, it was a theory with obvious and immediate appeal to the anti-smoking lobby and they were quick to spread it. John Banzhaf wrote in 1972: "I have little understanding for those men and women whose nasty nervous habit forces me to breathe carbon monoxide. Quite frankly - as well as literally - they make me sick."(4) In the same year, *Readers Digest* printed an article by one Max Wiener entitled 'Nonsmokers, arise!' in which he opined that "smoking should be confined to consenting adults in private" because of the threat to nonsmokers' health (5).

All laws restricting smoking had so far been based on the preference of some nonsmokers to have smoke-free spaces but mere preference was insufficient to justify more far-sweeping legislation. Nonsmoking sections had been created in the spirit of compromise, with the rights of nonsmokers never given any greater weight than those of smokers. The passive smoking theory presented the anti-smokers with a golden opportunity to depict tobacco smoke as a serious health threat to all, rather than a mere nuisance to a minority. Most importantly, it would help bypass the awkward issues of civil liberties and property rights that had so far stymied the anti-cigarette bandwagon.

Neither the tobacco industry nor the emerging anti-smoking movement were under any illusion about the political value of the passive smoking theory. The Surgeon General, in his 1972 report, combined the announcement of the ETS hazard with a call for an anti-smoking movement; one must follow the other. The cigarette companies, meanwhile, considered the passive smoking theory to be the "most dangerous development to the viability of the tobacco industry that has yet occurred."(6)

To risk one's own health may be reckless but it was a matter for the individual. If he endangered the health of others, however, the state might be obliged to intervene. In this new paradigm, smokers became killers and nonsmokers victims. For the anti-smoking movement to be able to put the debate in these terms was priceless and, with this in mind, Sir George Godber announced at the 1975 World Conference on Smoking and Health: "We must foster an atmosphere where it is perceived that active smokers would injure those around them."[7]

The anti-smoking groups took such pronouncements as a rallying cry. They did not wait for proof that passive smoking was dangerous. For propaganda purposes, it was enough that the Surgeon General had identified it as such and they assumed it would only be a matter of time before solid evidence appeared. As one activist later remarked: "We were just waiting for science to tell us what we already knew."[8]

By the late 1970s, this science was still nowhere to be found.

Scientific experiments

The Surgeon General specifically identified carbon monoxide, tar and nicotine as the most likely hazards in secondhand smoke, with acrolein, hydrogen cyanide, nitric oxide, nitrogen dioxide and phenol named as 'probable' hazards. The first laboratory experiments into ETS focused on carbon monoxide, and Banzhaf's comments about being forced to inhale the gas reflected the prevailing belief amongst anti-smokers that it was the most dangerous part of secondhand smoke.

But the awkward truth was that even the smokiest rooms had lower carbon monoxide levels than many outdoor locations. The limit set by the US Environmental Protection Agency (EPA) for outdoor carbon monoxide concentration was 9 parts per million (ppm), but this was regularly exceeded in everyday life without anyone being unduly concerned. Readings from sidewalks showed carbon monoxide concentrations of 61 ppm during heavy traffic, 20 ppm during moderate traffic and 6 ppm in light traffic [9]. Even the people *inside* the cars on a typical street were subjected to a level of 12 ppm, rising to 23 ppm when the windows were opened. In underground car parks readings could reach as high as 700 ppm.

Smoky bars and offices were relatively free of carbon monoxide by comparison. When the Surgeon General reviewed the evidence in 1979 he found low concentrations of 3.4 ppm in a theatre, 2.7 ppm in an office and 7 ppm on a train. In the context of the 1970s, when smoking aboard aircraft was one of the key battlegrounds, it is interesting to note that carbon monoxide readings inside passenger planes were usually below 2 ppm (10).

A quiet city street, therefore, had twice the carbon monoxide of a smoky room, and when scientists measured blood carboxyhaemoglobin (COHb) levels - which show how much carbon monoxide is absorbed into the blood stream - they found the same story.

The Channel Island of Sark provided scientists with the perfect control group since there was virtually nothing on the island to contaminate the air with carbon monoxide. Society ran much as it had for centuries; only the Dame of the island owned a car and the only other possible sources of carbon monoxide were lawnmowers. Concentrations in the air were below 1 ppm and COHb levels amongst nonsmokers averaged 0.68%. By contrast, nonsmokers in Washington and Chicago had COHb readings of 1.4% and 2.0% respectively (Stewart et al. 1974) (11). Someone would have to be exposed to 105 cigarettes for two hours in a tiny unventilated room for their COHb reading to match these levels (Harke, 1970), and in neither scenario was there a realistic threat to health.

In 1982, the scientist Roy Shephard wrote a book titled *The Risks of Passive Smoking* to sum up the evidence for the passive smoking theory to date. A carbon monoxide expert and a passionate anti-smoker (as he made abundantly clear in the book's preface), Shephard evaluated the evidence against carbon monoxide as a hazard in secondhand smoke but was highly ambivalent about the risks posed. By the time he wrote his monumental text-book Carbon Monoxide: The Silent Killer the following year, he had accepted that it did not pose any threat to nonsmokers (12). Again, it appeared that walking down a city street exposed an individual to more carbon monoxide than sitting in a smoky office. The worst Shephard could say was that if the office worker arrived to a smoky office, his COHb level would drop slightly slower than if he arrived to a smoke-free one.

This left the second of the compounds that the Surgeon General had identified as most likely to cause disease: nicotine. A strange choice, this, as nicotine had never been linked to any disease since Louis-Nicolas Vauquelin identified and isolated it in 1828. It is, so to speak, the active ingredient in cigarettes and it is the only part of tobacco that is unique to that plant. Like every other substance in the universe, it is deadly at high enough doses - one 19th century scientist discovered that a single drop of pure nicotine was enough to kill a cat - but it is very doubtful whether the amounts of nicotine found in tobacco smoke are dangerous to heavy smokers, let alone those around them.

The EPA's 'safe level' threshold for nicotine is 0.5mg/m3 and it is a level that has never been reached in even the smokiest rooms. In the 'worst-case' real life situation (a submarine) nicotine readings only reach 0.032mg/m3, or 8% of the EPA's 'safe' level. There was no evidence whatsoever that nicotine (or, for that matter, acrolein) in secondhand smoke posed any kind of health threat to nonsmokers and few suggested otherwise until the 1990s when the US Centers for Disease Control published a pamphlet titled *Facts about Second Hand Smoke* which stated: "At high exposure levels, nicotine is a potent and potentially lethal poison. Second hand smoke is the only source of nicotine in the air."[13] The agency failed to add that while secondhand smoke may be the only source of nicotine in the air, it is never present at anything approaching "high exposure levels" to make it "potentially lethal."

Unhappily for anti-smoking campaigners, clinical experiments were proving unhelpful in showing secondhand smoke to be a health hazard. Unable to show the long-term effects on the health of passive smokers, scientists tried to demonstrate short-term symptoms like shortness of breath, coughing and wheezing. Known effects of smoking included diminished blood flow to the skin, a small rise in blood pressure and an increased liability to abnormalities of heart rhythm. If any of these symptoms could be shown in involuntary smokers it would suggest that they were absorbing enough from the smoke to be of some concern.

However, as Roy Shephard noted with an almost audible sigh, "the evidence that similar changes occur during passive smoking is not particularly strong."[14] Indeed. Forty 10 year olds were placed in a smoke filled room by Dr Luquette in 1970 while their heart rate was monitored. There was an insignificant rise in their heart rates and what increase there was in blood pressure was put down to the excitement of having been shown anti-smoking films prior to the experiment.

In 1978, Dr Pimm and his team seemed to be getting closer to finding some sort of effect from secondhand smoke when his sample group of women registered a 5 to 10 beat per minute increase after being exposed to smoke (and without even being shown anti-smoking films!) but the male sample failed to get as excited as their female counterparts and did not replicate the increase.

That the subjects were displaying a psychological response to being part of an experiment rather than a pharmacological one was evident. In one of the more unusual experiments described by Shephard, 23 nonsmokers were placed in chambers filled with cigarette smoke and then called upon to perform vigorous physical exercise. After two hours, only one reported any wheezing or tightness in the chest. Evidence that passive smoking had any significant effect on the respiratory system of nonsmokers was, as Shephard glumly concluded, "meagre and somewhat inconsistent." (15)

The dose makes the poison

With laboratory experiments being of little assistance to the anti-smoking cause, a young physicist in Maryland used mathematics to prove that passive smoking was a killer. James L. Repace's involvement in the battle against tobacco was perhaps inevitable. He was an asthmatic, as were two of his children, and was unusually sensitive to tobacco smoke and other airborne particles. His father had died of lung cancer, aged 59, and Repace campaigned for nonsmoking sections in the restaurants of his hometown. He felt intuitively that secondhand smoke was a killer and, when he found no evidence in the literature to back up his gut instinct, he went out to find it himself. In 1978, Repace put his faith in a machine called the piezobalance which purported to show air impurity - 'respirable particulate matter' - per cubic foot. The device was crude: it didn't measure or identify specific impurities and, crucially, it was left to the user to make his own mind up as to whether the pollutants it measured were dangerous or not.

Repace took his contraption to local restaurants, bowling alleys and other smoky public places and compared the data from these locations with his samples from nonsmoking venues. Working as an amateur and with limited resources, he was forced to make some broad assumptions and simplifications as he carried out his work over a ten week period. When he analysed his data, Repace found that the places which allowed smoking had between 10 and 100 times more respirable particulate matter than those that did not. Based on the assumption that secondhand smoke was carcinogenic, he extrapolated that these locations posed a lung cancer risk of 250 to 1,000 times greater than would be legal if the Environmental Protection Agency's outdoor air regulations applied to indoor areas (which they did not).

Repace wrote up his findings with the assistance of the theoretical chemist Alfred H. Lowrey and GASP founder Clara Gouin, in a paper that concluded: "Clearly indoor air pollution from tobacco smoke presents a serious risk to the health of nonsmokers" (16). This was an audacious claim considering the shortcomings of the raw data. Even if it was reasonable to assume that the differences in respirable particulate levels between, say, a bowling alley and a library were due to tobacco smoke, it was a huge leap to claim that this heavily diluted tobacco smoke could cause lung cancer. The data collected with the piezobalance equipment essentially said no more than that smoky places were smokier than smoke-free places. The rest of the conclusions were based on Repace's own *a priori* hypothesis that secondhand smoke was a public health menace. The paper therefore suffered from its circular and self-serving assumptions while ignoring the basic scientific principle that "the dose makes the poison."

Repace, who had a degree in physics but no medical qualifications, was working in the electronics division of Washington's Naval Research Laboratory when he carried out this research but, while he was writing up the paper, he was offered a job at the Environmental Protection Agency. His new employment gave him some much needed credibility when he submitted his work to *Science* magazine in 1979. Its editors, after some hesitation, agreed to publish it in May 1980 and, finally, eight years after Steinfeld's Surgeon General report had warned of the threat of secondhand smoke, the first piece of supporting evidence was published. It naturally generated excitement in the public health community but was elsewhere condemned for its sweeping assumptions and lack of conventional scientific practice and rigour. Repace became the darling of the anti-smoking movement overnight and the 1980 study launched his career as a professional anti-smoker, testifying in court cases and appearing at anti-smoking conferences around the world.

For all the drawbacks of Repace's *Science* article, it had the virtue of at least containing some original field research. The same could not be said of his second study, published in *Environmental International* in 1985, which merely extrapolated from existing statistics. The paper - 'A Quantitative Estimate of Nonsmokers' Lung Cancer Risk from Passive Smoking' - was again layered with his own idiosyncratic preconceptions; for example, that the average smoker consumed 32 cigarettes a day. Having set himself the task of estimating the number of deaths due to passive smoking, Repace used a 1980 study of the strictly nonsmoking Seventh Day Adventists as the control group. The rate of lung cancer deaths amongst Adventist women was 7.4 per 100,000, lower than the 12.7 per 100,000 rate found amongst nonsmoking women in the general population.

The authors of the original 1980 study had never suggested that passive smoking was a factor in this difference in lung cancer mortality but Repace surmised that it was the only factor, something that the Office of Technology Assessment, reviewing the research to date in 1986, considered "inappropriate." That the Adventists might not be a wholly representative sample group - they did not drink alcohol and most were vegetarians - seemed not to have occurred to Repace. His aim was to estimate how many lung cancer deaths were attributable to passive smoking and, by extrapolating his data onto the whole population of the USA, he came up with a figure of 5,000.

Repace conducted his research in his spare time, and it was in no way connected with the EPA. In line with the agency's regulations, a disclaimer was published alongside the study to made it clear that

Repace's views were not necessarily shared by his employer. Nevertheless, there was room for confusion which was not helped by Repace publishing the EPA's address as the point of contact for reprint requests. Sure enough, when the study was reported in the press, it was announced with headlines such as 'EPA Study Links Deaths of Nonsmokers to Cigarette' (*New York Times*).

It was an article of faith for Repace that any amount of smoke, no matter how small, could cause cancer. Perhaps because of his own extreme physical reaction to tobacco smoke, he assumed that there were sufficient people vulnerable to contracting cancer in the general population that even a microscopic amount of secondhand smoke could kill thousands. Essentially, Repace believed that it was not the dose that made the poison but that tobacco was always a poison, and while a very low dose would not kill as many people as active smoking, it would still kill.

In science, this theory is known as 'linear risk extrapolation.' It dictates that there is no threshold to risk and that even one molecule or particle can be enough to kill if it comes in contact with vulnerable human tissue (17). It is a contentious theory amongst scientists and its relevance to the issue of secondhand smoke is, in any case, doubtful. It is rather like assuming that if drinking 40 shots of vodka kills 80 people out of 100, then drinking one shot of vodka must kill 2 people. Or, as Joe Dawson put it: "This is like saying that if a million people cross a body of water 10 feet deep and 100,000 of them drown then 1,000 would drown if the water were an inch deep." (18)

No biological evidence has ever surfaced to back up Repace's view that such a low dosage is enough to cause cancer (19). Research to date, notably Gio Gori's work in the 1970s, had suggested quite the opposite. Nevertheless, Repace felt that his reading of the Seventh Day Adventist study showed that he was correct. The 5,000 deaths he had extrapolated from that study was at the top end of - but still just inside - his own previous estimate of 500 to 5,000 deaths based on "five deaths per 100,000 per milligram of tar absorbed per day per smoker."(20)

Epidemiology

If one took Repace's figures seriously, the deaths attributable to passive smoking were still so small in number that they would not be observable to doctors, coroners or anyone else. They could only be shown using the largest nationwide studies. With clinical experiments failing to turn up the goods, passive smoking researchers turned to epidemiology.

Epidemiological studies were sometimes accused - not always unfairly - of being glorified surveys, but the work of Doll and Hill had demonstrated the potential of the science in the 1950s and it would later be used to decipher the mystery of why people were dying of a disease then known only as GRID (Gay Related Immune Deficiency) but today known as AIDS.

There had been a real and observable rise in the number of gay men dying before their time in the 1980s, just as there had been a sharp rise in lung cancer cases amongst smokers in the 1940s. But no one had noticed an epidemic of lung cancer amongst nonsmokers and this was the critical difference between traditional epidemiology and passive smoking epidemiology. Doll and Hill had been employed to explain an epidemic. The secondhand smoke researchers had their theory but needed to find the bodies. Epidemiology - literally, 'the study of epidemics' - was being used for the first time to identify, rather than explain, an epidemic.

If deaths from passive smoking had ever been observable to the naked eye, the best period in which to witness them would have been when smoking was widespread amongst men but taboo amongst women. If secondhand smoke was life threatening, one would expect lung cancer rates amongst nonsmoking women married to smokers to increase sharply. Such an increase was never identified in America or Europe and those days were now gone, but science was given another chance in Japan. Throughout the 1960s and 1970s, smoking continued to be socially unacceptable amongst women whilst smoking rates for men remained sky high. In 1981, the epidemiologist Takeshi Hirayama of Tokyo's National Cancer Center published the results of his study of nonsmoking wives married to smokers. It caused a sensation.

Hirayama began his study of 91,540 nonsmoking wives of smoking husbands in 1965, monitoring cases of lung cancer, emphysema, asthma, cervical cancer and stomach cancer until 1979. He asked their husbands how much they smoked and divided them into three categories: those smoking less than 14 cigarettes a day, those smoking 14-20 a day and those smoking over 20 a day. By the end of the study, 346 of the women had contracted lung cancer, including 174 who had not smoked but had been married to smokers.

When the results were written up and published in the *British Medical Journal* in January 1981, Hirayama showed increased risks of 1.4, 1.61 and 2.08 for the wives of light, average and heavy smokers respectively. That is to say, these women had a 40%, 61% and 108% greater risk of developing the disease than those not regularly exposed to tobacco smoke. These were not the strongest of findings but they were statistically significant. Epidemiologists generally treated anything less than a doubling of risk with scepticism. Ernst Wynder regarded anything less than a relative risk of 3.0 as a weak association (21) and the editor of the *New England Journal of Medicine* said (in 1995) that, in epidemiological studies, "we are looking for a relative risk of 3 or more."(22) Nevertheless, an association was apparent, there was a dose-response relationship and the 2.08 figure for those women most exposed was certainly suggestive.

But such was the rarity of lung cancer amongst nonsmokers that even if Hirayama was correct, the absolute risk remained very small, with the annual lung cancer mortality risk rising from 0.012% to 0.025% for the most heavily exposed women (23). Whilst these kind of odds may have been too small to concern the individual, they were of interest to those working in public health and Hirayama's paper provided a strong enough indication of harm to warrant further research. If subsequent studies showed a stronger association, or at least replicated the best of Hirayama's findings, the anti-smoking movement would indeed have a powerful new weapon.

Hirayama's paper was greeted with delight by anti-smoking groups and derision by the Tobacco Institute. Criticism of his work was not confined to those in the pay of a worried tobacco industry, and even the head of Hirayama's own research institute remarked that Japanese men did not spend enough time at home to subject their wives to much cigarette smoke. Certainly, the paper threw up some odd results. Nonsmoking women married to farmers who smoked, for example, had a higher lung cancer rate than the women who actually smoked, a finding that Hirayama admitted was "puzzling."

Could the difference in lung cancer risk be the result of factors other than secondhand smoke? It was hard to say. Diet was one well-established risk factor in lung cancer: high fruit and vegetable intake had been shown to reduce lung cancer risk by around 50% (24). It was no secret that smokers tended to have a poorer diet than nonsmokers and it was reasonable to assume that the women in the Japanese study ate much the same food as their husbands, and yet Hirayama asked no questions about their diet. Nor did he enquire about whether the wives used traditional Asian coal-fired cooking methods which, in themselves, were known to at least double the lung cancer risk (25).

There was also concern that some of the wives presented themselves as nonsmokers when they were not. Smoker misclassification was almost inevitable in surveys of this kind (26). Smokers felt the urge to identify themselves as nonsmokers in even the most innocuous of studies. The scientists who took carboxyhaemoglobin readings from the aforementioned residents of the island of Sark found an average reading of just 0.68%. In some people, however, it was as high as 2.6% and this was almost certainly because they were undeclared smokers. This, bear in mind, was in a study that had nothing to do with smoking and in which there was no obvious reason for them to lie. Such problems were magnified in the case of Japan. The very fact that smoking amongst women was taboo made it particularly likely that they would conceal their habit from researchers, employers and even from their own husbands. If even a relatively small number of subjects did this, the results of Hirayama's study would be skewed beyond all recognition.

Doubts about Hirayama's methodology grew when it was revealed that he had put women who admitted to being occasional smokers into the nonsmoker category. This was a staggering oversight, all the more so since the whole premise of the passive smoking theory was that low dosages of tobacco could be carcinogenic.

Hot on the heels of the Hirayama study came some research from Greece that appeared to corroborate his findings. Dimitros Trichopoulos' paper, also published in 1981, was a modest and tentative investigation designed to inspire more rigorous research. While Hirayama had conducted a 'cohort' study (ie. he had followed a group of healthy subjects over a period of years paying particular attention to those who became ill), Trichopoulos conducted a 'case-control' study in which he asked existing lung cancer patients to recall their exposure to secondhand smoke in the past. This was a less reliable approach since it expected elderly, critically ill people to remember their exposure to tobacco smoke decades ago. There was also the problem of 'recall bias'. With the association between tobacco and lung cancer now well-known, there was a real danger that ill nonsmokers would exaggerate their past exposure to tobacco as they sought to find a reason for suffering from what was widely viewed as a smokers' disease.

Trichopoulos's sample group was much smaller than Hirayama's, consisting of just 40 nonsmoking lung cancer cases but he found nonsmokers married to smokers had a relative risk of 2.4 - ie. they were 140% more likely to contract lung cancer than those who were married to never-smokers (27). The results were inconclusive due to the small sample group and Trichopoulos freely admitted that the study had "obvious limitations." Nonetheless, his findings were not so far away from those recently provided by Hirayama and it was at least enough to suggest that secondhand smoke was a public health hazard. Researchers around the world began to design their own studies to confirm the threat.

The era of public health begins

With secondhand smoke taking centre stage, and the smoking rate failing to drop as quickly as many had hoped, the medical establishment underwent a profound change in the 1970s as a distinct public health movement took shape. Mainstream health organisations began to feel the influence of strident grass-roots groups like GASP and ASH, not least because so many of these young radicals were beginning to find work within their institutions. Just ten years earlier, the American Cancer Society had told John Banzhaf that it was strictly a research institution, but now it became more proactive on the smoking issue. In 1977, it formed the National Commission on Smoking and Public Policy which publicly rebuked the US medical community for not doing more to lobby the government:

"The American Lung Association has used some of its volunteers to campaign for state legislation restricting smoking in specified public areas; however, neither the American Heart Association nor the American Cancer Society have participated in this activity to any substantial degree. State legislators have testified before this Commission that they rarely hear from either organisation when legislation is introduced or when hearings on bills are held."(28)

This kind of criticism spurred public health authorities and charities to take a more political role, endorsing laws against smoking and smokers for the good of public health. This brought them closer to the single issue anti-smoking pressure groups and further from their roots as neutral scientific bodies. In 1980, the AHA, ALA and ACS joined forces to create the Coalition on Smoking or Health to push for bigger warning labels on cigarette packs, an increase in tobacco taxes and an end to the tobacco price support program.

The campaign was further bolstered by the belated involvement of the American Medical Association which finally accepted that smoking caused lung cancer in 1978, some 25 years after the American Lung Association had come to the same conclusion. The AMA had been strangely quiet on the subject since 1964, when it had accepted millions of dollars from the tobacco industry to carry out a prolonged investigation into smoking and health, something this august body would today prefer to forget. When this fourteen year process finally ended with a report of unoriginal and bland conclusions, they began to make up for lost time.

In Britain, a long-standing belief in the sovereignty of the individual had hampered efforts to force people to stop smoking but this was beginning to show signs of waning. The policy of successive British governments had been based on providing information about smoking and helping those who wanted to give up to do so with the help of the NHS and, after 1987, the Quit organisation (the latter being an offshoot of the National Society of Non-Smokers). By the early 1980s, ASH (UK) had become wed to an absolutist agenda of eradicating tobacco (29) and began to explicitly challenge the *laissez-faire* approach of the Thatcher government.

ASH lobbied for tougher government action to coerce smokers into giving up and, in 1981, after two tax rises pushed the price of a pack of twenty beyond the £1 mark, cigarette consumption fell by 10 billion units (30). ASH then appealed to the British Medical Association to take a harder stance on the smoking issue. As a direct result of this pressure, the BMA announced its new position in 1984, dismissing the argument for freedom of choice by portraying smokers as helpless victims of the voracious tobacco industry's advertising campaigns.

The era of public health was at hand. Increasingly, doctors emphasised prevention over cure. Gio Gori's safer cigarette project represented the final attempt to find a technological solution to the smoking problem. Thereafter, modification of behaviour - the 'quit-or-die' approach - was viewed as the only answer. From the 1970s, changing people's habits became the overriding aim of a resurgent public health movement which did not limit itself to the issue of smoking - where abstinence was clearly the best advice - but to controlling salt, sugar, fatty foods, alcohol, poverty and environmental pollutants; all of which were regarded as medically suspect.

This was a momentous shift in emphasis for a medical community which had until recently believed in treating the sick and leaving the well alone, but it was one which, in large part, was forced upon them as the number of genuine medical breakthroughs dwindled. The birth of the first test-tube baby in 1978 was arguably the last in a series of dramatic advances which had begun with the discovery of penicillin in 1941 (31). The post-war era had been a golden age for medical science, with the development of vaccines practically wiping out infectious diseases in the Western world, but the days of miracles and wonder were coming to an end. With the battle against contagious diseases all but won, Europeans and Americans survived long enough to die of old age - most often through heart disease or cancer.

Vaccines, antibiotics and X-rays were insufficient to tackle the complex and ill-understood diseases of ageing which were now the leading causes of death. Open-heart surgery and chemotherapy were available but the former was an expensive and risky last resort and the latter was a miserable and usually futile experience for both patient and doctor. Lacking the ability to cure cancer and heart disease, the medical community turned to prevention. It was, on the face of things, an impossible job to track down the biological causes for the myriad cancers that afflicted humanity but the discovery of the smoking-lung cancer link encouraged them in their belief that similar carcinogens were out there and could be eliminated. The battle against tobacco thereby became the template for a new war on cancer and the public health movement once again turned to epidemiologists to fill the knowledge vacuum.

The ambitious campaign to rid society of the diseases of ageing rested on three key assumptions: that external or environmental factors were at work, that epidemiologists could identify them, and that, once identified, the public could be persuaded to avoid them. It hinged on the belief that cancer and heart disease were fundamentally unnatural and that their causes must, therefore, be man-made. This is was what James Le Fanu called the 'social theory' of disease and it assumed that the modern world was in some way responsible for the upsurge in cancer and heart disease.

Again, the smoking-lung cancer association appeared to validate this presumption. The invention of the cigarette - that great symbol of modernity - allowed tobacco smoke to be absorbed into the lungs without any thought of what the consequences might be for the health of the smoker. Thalidomide and industrial asbestos had also been tragically brought to market before they had been adequately tested for safety. Was it not conceivable that other technological innovations (such as food additives and pharmaceuticals) were to blame for the rise in cancer and heart disease seen in the 20th century? Was it not also possible that products which were proven carcinogens at high doses (such as tobacco smoke or dioxins) were also deadly in trace quantities? It was, as we shall see, a theory with serious limitations but, for public health groups, the social theory reinforced their belief that changing people's behaviour was the most effective way of saving lives.

Central to this school of thought was the belief that Westerners were victims of their own wealth. Cancer and heart disease were redefined as 'diseases of affluence.' Rich foods, red meat, sugary snacks and TV dinners were assumed to be responsible for higher cholesterol levels and various forms of cancer. This theory was given credibility when, in 1981, Richard Doll and Richard Peto co-authored a book - *The Causes of Cancer* - which claimed that, apart from those caused by smoking, 70% of cancers were caused by diet.

Paradoxically, in light of the supposed role of affluence in the cancer epidemic, poverty also became a public health issue. This, as Dr Michael Fitzpatrick explains, was not so much a response to the health of the working class as it was a means of bringing in left-wing policies by the back door:

"The new public health movement was a product of the wider decline of the left. After a period of significant influence in Western societies from the late 1960s to the mid-1970s, the left subsequently experienced a series of defeats, culminating in its collapse following the disintegration of the Soviet bloc in 1989-90.
One consequence of the disillusionment which had set in much earlier was the tendency for activists to retreat from public activity to attempt to pursue political objectives through their professional work, usually in some public service occupation, often in education or health."(32)

Fitzpatrick is one of a number of writers to have pinpointed the World Health Organisation's Alma-Ata conference, held in the USSR in 1978, as the start of the socialisation of medicine. It was here that the definition of health - previously considered to be the absence of illness - underwent a radical revision. The WHO now defined health as "a state of complete physical, mental and social well-being" and called it "a fundamental human right."(33)

The Alma-Ata Declaration committed the worldwide medical

profession to achieving 'Health for All by the year 2000,' a noble aim, but one that could only be brought about, wrote Fitzpatrick, "through a comprehensive programme amounting to the reconstruction of the world according to socialist principles of redistribution and equality." This was followed, three years later, by a British report entitled *Inequalities of Health* which recommended introducing a maximum wage, increasing state benefits and forcing a "greater redistribution of wealth."(34)

Inequalities of Health had been commissioned by a Labour government that had since been voted out of office and it received a cool reception from Margaret Thatcher (who pointedly released it on a bank holiday). Those who advocated the redistribution of wealth on the pretext of creating 'health equality' were given short shrift on both sides of the Atlantic in the 1980s and, lacking the power to implement their policies at the highest level, many of them drifted towards the public sector where they found an opportunity to influence attitudes at a gentler, but sustained, level.

When the long winter of the left finally ended in the mid-1990s, these activists, campaigners and social reformers would re-emerge with a far-reaching public health agenda. For the time being, however, both the British and American government were uneasy about intruding too heavily into the private habits of their citizens, and that included smoking. In the US, Joe Califano's 'second health revolution' came to an abrupt end when president Carter asked him to quit in the run up to the 1980 election, so unpopular had he become with smokers and tobacco farmers.

When Ronald Reagan took office in January 1981, the feeling that anti-smoking legislation would be sacrificed in the name of deregulation seemed to be confirmed when the new president announced that his staff would be "far too busy with substantive matters to waste their time proselytising against the dangers of cigarette smoking."(35) Writing in the early 1980s, the sociologists Troyer and Markle predicted that, in this political climate, "voluntary action groups such as ASH will be hard-pressed to hold the ground they have previously gained, let alone press for the further stigmatisation of smoking."(36)

This forecast proved to be spectacularly inaccurate.

The galvanisation of the movement

"Voluntary action groups," as Troyer and Markle called them, may still have been several hundred thousand people short of a mass movement but they continued to grow in number and were becoming increasingly belligerent. At the dawn of the Reagan era, GASP claimed to have 10,000 members and its Californian branches were gearing up for another campaign to ban smoking in public places. 1978 saw the creation of the American Council on Science and Health (ACSH). Its president, Elizabeth Whelan, was a Republican with degrees in medicine from both Yale School of Medicine and Harvard School of Public Health. The ACSH was formed as a consumer advocacy organisation that aimed to hold the tobacco industry accountable to the same regulation expected of other corporations. Smoking was its primary target and Whelan wrote two forthright books denouncing the tobacco industry. The appearance of ACSH provided a political balance to a movement that had previously been dominated by the left-wing.

Various other anti-smoking groups emerged in the late 1970s, the names of which seemed to be largely dictated by how they would appear as acronyms. They included Smoking Makes Oxygen Go (SMOG), Fresh Air for Non-Smokers (FANS) and, most tenuously, the Society for Mortification And Smoker Humiliation (SMASH). Such wordplay was not solely the preserve of the anti-smoking fraternity; their opponents formed People United to Fight Fanatics (PUFF) and Growing Resentment Over Anti-smoking Noises (GROAN).

Fuelled by fears about passive smoking and emboldened by numerous local victories, a new militancy entered the American anti-smoking movement. Nowhere was this more evident than in California, where GASP activist Stanton Glantz was rising to prominence. Having spent ten years studying mechanical engineering, Glantz abandoned the subject in 1973 and embarked on a two year course in cardiology. In 1977, he was installed as an assistant professor of medicine at the University of California, San Francisco (37).

With his bushy hair, spectacles and array of brightly coloured tee-shirts, Glantz looked every inch the nonconforming West Coast academic. Having been twice defeated at the ballot-box, the Californian branch of GASP became Californians for Nonsmokers Rights in 1981, with Glantz as president. Glantz was well aware of the passive smoking theory's potential to stiffen the resolve of those who did not enjoy the smell of cigarette smoke and to mobilise those who had previously shown no interest in the issue. As he told the delegates at an anti-smoking conference:

"The main thing the science has done on the issue of ETS, in addition to help people like me pay mortgages, is it has legitimised the concern that people have that they don't like cigarette smoke."

He added, presumably referring to the tobacco industry (or was it smokers?):

"The bastards are on the run and we are on a roll."(38)

This kind of emotive language became increasingly common in the first years of the 1980s. James Repace did his utmost to present himself as an impartial researcher but the mask slipped when a new anti-smoking bill was rejected in Washington, saying:

"You're going to start seeing nonsmokers becoming more violent. You're going to see fights breaking out all over."(39)

CHAPTER SEVEN

'A smoke-free America by 2000'

In July 1983, a thousand delegates from over 70 countries descended upon the Canadian city of Winnipeg to attend the Fifth World Conference on Smoking and Health. More than 100 meetings were held over six days and everyone who was anyone in the anti-tobacco movement took to the stage to rally their supporters. Like the Olympics, these conferences were held every four years and, since their inception in 1967, had been characterised by reviews of scientific literature and debate over how to inform the public about the hazards of smoking. In Winnipeg, however, there was a tangible sense of renewed purpose and an unprecedented thirst for action.

Donna Shimp appeared twice to tell her story of being the first person in the US to be legally compensated for having to work in a smoky office. Representatives from the UK's Health Education Agency talked about their aim of reducing smoking prevalence to 20% by 1993 (it stood at 36% at the time). John Banzhaf III gave a speech in which he described smoking as a "stupid, smelly and socially unacceptable practice that should be restricted to consenting adults in private." He claimed that smoking cost America $50 billion a year, urged the victims of fires caused by cigarettes to sue the tobacco industry and demanded that smokers ("no matter how poor") pay more than nonsmokers if they needed to visit a doctor [1].

Barely two years had passed since the first epidemiological study fingered passive smoking as a hazard to nonsmokers but the concept had taken firm root with those on the platform. Takeshi Hirayama once again presented his study of nonsmoking Japanese wives and Stanton Glantz told his audience that "the effects of involuntary smoking on nonsmokers probably holds the key to controlling and reducing primary smoking."(2)

Some speakers were more circumspect. Richard Doll's colleague, Richard Peto, said that Hirayama's findings were "difficult to believe"(3); James Repace admitted that the evidence for the passive smoking theory was "conflicting" and Dr Roy Shephard conceded that "for the moment, the most readily justified complaints of the nonsmoker are annoyance and irritation."(4) In contrast with Banzhaf's claim that smokers were a drain on the economy, Robert Leu, of the Swiss Institute for Social Sciences, explained how smoking did not place a financial burden on society since smokers were less likely to draw pensions or require expensive treatment for geriatric diseases.

Amongst the delegates at Winnipeg were a handful of tobacco industry representatives who were trying desperately hard to blend in. The industry was explicitly referred to as "the enemy" throughout proceedings and the undercover observers were shocked by both the new militancy and the whole 'clean-life' ethos which pervaded the conference. In a sardonic report to his employers at Philip Morris, one 'industry monitor,' Hans Verkerk, described what the "missionaries" - as he called them - got up to:

"What normally are coffee and tea breaks at every other conference were in Winnipeg called 'exercise and nutrition breaks.' A young girl in gym attire would appear in front of the audience, the music was switched on, and led by the gymnast, the audience started jumping up and down. The industry monitors, who were under strict orders to remain inconspicuous, could be seen jumping around like maniacs.
This would then be followed by the consumption of health foods and soft drinks."(5)

The policies agreed upon in Winnipeg set the template for the international anti-smoking movement for the next twenty years. They included a total worldwide ban on all forms of tobacco advertising, progressively higher taxes on cigarettes, limits on where and when tobacco could be legally sold, a ban on the sale of high-tar cigarettes and the initiation of a global No Smoking Day (which began in 1984). Above all, the primary policy objective - as stated in the 819 page book which documented the event - was "to establish NON-SMOKING AND THE RIGHT TO A SMOKE-FREE ATMOSPHERE AS THE NORM" (capital letters in the original)(6).

In his closing address, Dr Delarue told the delegates:

> "Mobilisation of resources is just beginning. An enormous resource of personnel is required, as well as a major increase in available funding." (7)

Another speaker let slip the prohibitionist intent of the whole enterprise when he said:

> "It is time to call a spade a spade, and announce our final goal:
> the eradication of the problem...
> Cigarettes started to invade the industrialised countries at the beginning of this century.
> It should be possible to get them out before we have gone too far into the next." (8)

The industry monitors were lucky to get out alive.

Proposition P

By this time, two more states - Nebraska and Montana - had passed laws mandating nonsmoking areas in public buildings and some privately owned places. In California, after two failed attempts, Californians for Nonsmokers Rights (CNR) decided to concentrate not on the whole state but on San Francisco, with an ordinance that would only affect office workplaces. This was a canny move. If passed, the door was opened to extending the definition of a workplace to other indoor settings, perhaps even to bars and restaurants. The proposal - the San Francisco Smoking Pollution Control Ordinance (1983), better known as Prop P - stated that tobacco ("or any other weed or plant") was dangerous to health and was a "cause of material annoyance."(9)

Like the state-wide law passed in Minnesota, Prop P offered to "accommodate" smokers but with the crucial difference that if a satisfactory compromise could not be reached - in other words, if even one nonsmoker complained - smoking would be banned throughout.

CNR promised employers they would be under no obligation to spend money creating nonsmoking sections but this was somewhat disingenuous since the creation of nonsmoking and smoking areas would very likely require expenditure. In reality, as CNR knew all too well, employers could only get away with spending nothing if they banned smoking completely.

By limiting its scope to offices and by targeting a city where opposition to smoking was strong, the San Francisco ordinance gained more support than Prop 5 and Prop 10. Spurred on by CNR president Stanton Glantz, the campaign took an openly anti-tobacco industry stance, with one ad saying: 'Tell the cigarette companies to butt out of San Francisco.' Throughout his career Stanton Glantz tended to see his crusade as more of a David and Goliath battle between the American public and the tobacco industry than as a struggle between smokers and anti-smokers. A sympathetic journalist once asked him what his ultimate goal was, and was surprised by his response:

> "...he didn't say, 'to have fewer people get sick and die from smoking.' The first words out of his mouth were, 'To destroy the tobacco industry.'" (10)

The 1983 campaign was the first of what Glantz saw as pitched battles with the "merchants of death" and CNR capitalised on growing resentment of industry profits and power. The ordinance was passed, albeit by just 1,259 votes. Not for the last time, politicians exempted themselves from the ordinance by excluding "any property owned or leased by state or federal government entities." Spurred on by this triumph, Glantz, like Lucy Page Gaston before him, indicated his expansionist plans by renaming his organisation and Americans for Nonsmokers' Rights was born.

On the trail of secondhand smoke

Some readers may want to skip the next few paragraphs and simply accept that the evidence against Environmental Tobacco Smoke (ETS) in the 1980s was, as Richard Kluger delicately put it, "hazy at best." However, the brief explanation of epidemiological practice below may be useful in understanding what is to come. A more extensive discussion can be found in the Appendix.

Epidemiology is based on statistics. When studying disease, epidemiologists use one of two approaches. In a cohort (or prospective) study, they find a group of people who are suspected to be at risk by virtue of, for example, their diet. The epidemiologist then finds a control group which is similar to the first in every way except that they do not eat the same food. Having been thoroughly interviewed, both sets of subjects are left to get on with their lives until such time when the researcher reappears and observes how many of them have been stricken with disease. If there are more cases of disease amongst the first (case) group than in the second (control) group, then his hypothesis may be correct.

The second method is the case-control (or retrospective) study. Here the epidemiologist finds people who are already ill and asks them about their past habits, work, exposure to pollutants or whatever else he believes might be a risk factor. He then finds a group of otherwise similar people who are not afflicted with the disease and interviews them. If the subjects who are ill recall markedly different behaviour, exposure or habits to the control group then, again, his hypothesis is supported.

Put in simple terms, this is how epidemiology works. But random sample groups naturally produce random associations which are due only to chance and may not be indicative of a general pattern in the population as a whole. How to distinguish causation from fluke? To minimise the risk of misinterpreting chance results, epidemiologists use upper and lower limits of probability - the confidence interval - which act as a margin of error. The control group's risk factor is always 1.0. Results for the other group is shown with the estimated risk first, followed by the upper and lower confidence limits in brackets.

For example, if a study of red meat eaters shows a relative risk of bowel cancer of 2.5 (1.4-4.0), we are being told that if all other things are equal, they have between a 40% and 300% greater chance of developing the disease over someone who never eats red meat. In this instance, the best guess (the first figure) is that, on average, the red meat eater is two and a half times more likely to fall victim to the disease and the hypothesis that red meat causes bowel cancer is supported because, even at the low end of the confidence interval, there is an increase in risk. It does not prove the hypothesis but it is a *statistically significant* finding - it is probably not the result of chance.

Anything below 1.0 represents a reduction in risk. And so, if the meat-eater's relative risk is 1.2 (0.8-1.4), then the finding says nothing and can be disregarded. Although the headline figure shows an increased risk of 20%, the confidence interval indicates that it could as easily be a reduction of risk of 20% (or an increased risk of 40%). Since the risk straddles 1.0, it is of no statistical significance. It does not disprove the hypothesis - the hypothesis can never be disproved - but nor does it support it. It is a null finding and the epidemiologist goes back to the drawing board. Statistical significance is, therefore, the method used to distinguish the random from the real.

In the five years following the groundbreaking studies of Hirayama and Trichopoulos, a further eleven epidemiological papers were published on the subject of secondhand smoke. They, too, surveyed nonsmokers married to smokers but they provided scant evidence that passive smoking posed a health hazard to nonsmokers. In Hong Kong, Chan and Fung's study of 84 female lung cancer victims found that only 34 had been married to smokers, and the resulting relative risk of 0.75 (0.43-1.30) gave the unlikely suggestion that those exposed to secondhand smoke were 25% *less* likely to develop lung cancer than those who were not (11). The finding was nonsignificant, as were two American studies of 1984 which also found negative associations, one of 0.79 (Kabat), the other 0.80 (Buffler et al).

But another US study, conducted by Pelayo Correa and published in *The Lancet* in 1983, suggested that secondhand smoke doubled the risk of lung cancer in nonsmoking wives. However, the numbers of cases involved were so small that the study could draw no firm conclusion (12); of the 302 female lung cancer patients involved, only 14 were nonsmokers married to smokers. The results were even less compelling when men were studied. Of 1,036 male lung cancer patients, only one was a nonsmoker married to a heavy smoker.

In contrast with Correa's limited sample group, Lawrence Garfinkel was given access to the vast database of the American Cancer Society's long-running nationwide survey - initiated in 1959 - which held information about 375,000 female nonsmokers. Having studied the data, Garfinkel found "very little, if any, increased risk of lung cancer" for those exposed to passive smoke and not even "a slight increase" in lung cancer risk for nonsmokers who lived with smokers (13). Four years later, Garfinkel used a database from four hospitals and questioned 134 nonsmoking lung cancer patients. He found a slightly stronger link between ETS and lung cancer, with an average risk of about 1.31 (0.94-1.83) but the association remained weak and, again, it was of no statistical significance. It later transpired that 8.5% of the women who had initially claimed to be nonsmokers were in fact smokers, something that undermined what little evidence Garfinkel had gathered together and served as a reminder of the confounding factors that often blighted studies of this kind (14).

Of the remaining papers, neither Wu (1985) nor Akiba (1986) found any statistically significant increase in risk from passive smoke and the only British study of the period found a risk of 1.03 - effectively zero - and concluded that the risk to nonsmokers was "at most small, and may not exist at all."(15)

For those who actually read the medical journals, the passive smoking theory was already running out of steam. When the National Research Council assessed the data in 1986 at the behest of the Office on Smoking and Health, it pointed to the paucity of evidence and, in a comment that showed its panel was well aware of the motives of those who would overstate it, concluded that more research was required if "policies are to be based on possible adverse health effects and not solely on the discomfort that passive smoking causes among the two-thirds of Americans who do not smoke."(16) But the new Surgeon General was not listening.

C. Everett Koop

In 1986, Surgeon General C. Everett Koop issued his report on smoking and health. Since taking office under Ronald Reagan, Koop had become a passionate and articulate opponent of smoking and the tobacco industry, and was already well on his way to becoming the world's most famous advocate of the passive smoking theory. In 1984 he announced his aim of 'A smoke-free America by the year 2000,' a slogan that unwittingly echoed Lucy Page Gaston's unrealized dream of 'A smokeless America by 1925.' The 1986 report was an opportunity to reach out to the American public directly and was guaranteed to generate publicity. "It is certain," he told the press, "that a substantial proportion of the lung cancers that occur in nonsmokers are due to ETS exposure." He spoke of the "relative abundance" and "cohesiveness" of the data which was, to say the least, an idiosyncratic interpretation of evidence that the Office of Technology Assessment had recently called "equivocal."(17)

Koop, like many anti-smokers, believed that it did no harm to overstate the evidence against secondhand smoke as part of the wider effort to ban smoking in public places and abolish smoking by the end of the century. It could be argued that even if white lies were told, they were nothing compared to the stream of deception and misinformation the tobacco industry had been spewing for decades and, for Koop, the noble end of reducing cigarette consumption justified the means. It was in this spirit that he summed up the patchy and contradictory evidence that had so far come to light in the passive smoking debate. His comments to the press were not borne out by the report itself and the devil was, as ever, in the detail. Those few who read it in full found that, far from being "certain," the relationship between secondhand smoke and lung cancer was described as merely "plausible" and the conclusions of Hirayama were deemed suspect because "misclassification of exposure to ETS is inherent."(18)

There is little doubt that Koop was aware of these shortcomings, although he would later comment that "we felt we had enough to go on."(19) The 1986 report was as much a political document as a scientific one, written by a Surgeon General who urged nonsmokers to "get involved...push for local and state laws that restrict or ban smoking in public places." Koop even described his mission as an anti-smoking "crusade," a word that even anti-smoking crusaders were reluctant to use.

There was a desire to make the 1986 report a watershed moment equal to that of 1964; a report that would resound across the world and launch the next wave of legislation against smokers. The bans and restrictions Koop called for would not be possible unless the majority believed that passive smoking was a threat to their health and that smokers, therefore, were a menace. Charles Whitley, a politician from North Carolina, called the report "a very deliberate attempt to turn nonsmokers into anti-smokers"(20) and if that was the intention, the report was an unqualified success. The following year a poll conducted by the Centers for Disease Control recorded that three-quarters of Americans believed secondhand smoke presented a physical danger to nonsmokers.

Koop may have believed that he was pre-empting, rather than deliberately distorting, the evidence. He may have felt he was only following in the footsteps of Dr Jesse Steinfeld, who had used his position as Surgeon General to kick off the passive smoking controversy in 1972. Nonetheless, it was an extraordinary report. Even strong opponents of tobacco like the historian Richard Kluger have expressed surprise at Koop's reading of the evidence. Calling the evidence against ETS "murky," Kluger wrote:

"Without a doubt Koop was on the side of the angels, but without much doubt, either, he was in this instance using dubious means - shaky science - to justify the worthy end of achieving a healthier society." (21)

Ultimately the report was more effective as a substitute for the evidence than as a summary of it. When questions were asked about the credibility of the passive smoking theory, anti-smoking groups around the world were able to assert that none other than the Surgeon General of the United States had explicitly identified it as a clear and present danger. Few people were inclined to delve further.

The changing face of the anti-smoking movement

Anti-smoking activists were naturally swift to endorse the views of the Surgeon General and the transformation that had begun in Winnipeg was reflected in an article published by Stanton Glantz in 1987. Titled *Achieving a Smokefree Society*, its author recommended that anti-smoking campaigners adopt a new persona. They should see themselves, he said, as "not 'anti-smoker' but rather environmentalists."

"The issue should be framed in the rhetoric of the environment, toxic chemicals, and public health." (22)

Anti-smoking groups sprung up all over America in the 1980s. Joe Tye set up Stop Teenage Addiction to Tobacco (STAT) after his five-year old daughter spotted a *Marlboro* billboard and squealed "Look daddy, horses!" Citizens Against Tobacco Smoke (CATS) was formed by the inimitable Ahron Leichtman, an ex-smoker who suffered from acute sensitivity to tobacco smoke and claimed that even the briefest exposure brought on headaches. Leichtman had been a member of ASH since the 1970s and campaigned for Prop 5 and Prop 10 in California. In 1980, he relocated to Cincinnati where he became further radicalised and founded that state's own branch of GASP, launching a vigorous campaign for smoking bans and gaining some local notoriety after an angry confrontation with a smoker at a fish counter. He formed CATS in 1985 as a vehicle for his militant agenda of bringing down the tobacco industry.

A large number of lawyers continued to be drawn to the cause, following in the footsteps of Nader and Banzhaf. One of them, Edward L. Sweda Jr., had joined GASP in Massachusetts where he was known to protest in a grim reaper suit declaring, with no little hyperbole, that "if you work near smokers, your lungs suffer the same harm as if you smoked up to 10 cigarettes a day."(23) The president of his GASP branch, fellow law graduate Richard A. Daynard, was inspired by the collapse of the asbestos company Johns-Manville and resolved to bankrupt the tobacco industry in court. To that end he formed the Tobacco Products Liability Project and by 1990 Daynard had filed 150 suits on behalf of smokers who had become ill with 'smoking-related' diseases. A similar organisation, Ciglit, was formed by lawyers in Texas.

Meanwhile, the man who had started it all, John Banzhaf III, continued to teach at George Washington University where he encouraged his students to engage in 'legal activism.' Amongst other achievements, Banzhaf's students pounced on a gentleman's club and forced it to accept women members. The following year, three students from his class found dry-cleaners charging more to wash women's 'oxford-style' shirts than they did for the men's variety. There was a reasonable explanation: women's shirts were too small to be put on mechanical presses and had to be washed by hand, but that was not good enough for Banzhaf's prodigies. They formed a group called the Coalition Against Discriminatory Drycleaning and submitted a complaint to the Human Rights office before filing lawsuits against two of the offenders.

Soon, it became a news story and journalists flocked to find out more. The owners of one shop were Korean immigrants with little grasp of English and were shocked and bewildered at having their lives turned upside down by a group of law students working on an assignment. With no money to fight the case, their lawyer explained that they had agreed to charge the same prices from now on and told the press that "they just want the media attention to go away and end the disruption to their lives." One of the students who brought the case was starry-eyed from his first experience in legal pedantry: "This is my first legal action," he said, "and the fact that it's had so many real-life implications is really satisfying."(24)

Banzhaf gave all the students A grades and the following year supported his new class in prosecuting hairdressers for charging men and women different prices.

No smoking in the sky

In the late 1980s, anti-smoking groups saw a total ban on smoking in aeroplanes as matter of priority. And yet all the available evidence, as assessed by the aviation authorities, showed that aeroplanes were less smoky than almost any other indoor environment, thanks to almost continuous air changes. Besides which, smokers and nonsmokers were already segregated and had been for years. The fervour displayed by anti-smokers towards aeroplanes when so many other places allowed unrestricted smoking perhaps owed more to psychology than reason: aeroplanes were confined spaces and the appearance of under-ventilation made them an obvious test-case for total smoking bans.

Individual airlines had resisted banning smoking without a 'level playing field,' that is to say, without a law forbidding other airlines from allowing smoking. Some took this as evidence that airlines were pro-tobacco. Nothing could have been further from the truth. They stood to gain from savings in cleaning costs, not having to empty ashtrays and, above all, less frequent and therefore cheaper ventilation. They would also be free of the administrative headaches involved in delegating seats to smokers and nonsmokers while making sure all flights were fully booked. Their reluctance to impose a ban voluntarily was born only of a fear that smokers would exercise their right to choose a rival carrier. If smoking was banned by law, however, they knew that very few smokers would opt to stop flying altogether and when a bill arrived to ban smoking on all flights they put up very little fight.

Senator Richard J. Durbin (Dem) had lost his father to lung cancer when he was 14 and led the campaign, amending an appropriations bill with a clause to ban smoking on domestic flights of two hours or under. This mirrored the law that had been passed in Canada the previous year but in the US it had already been defeated twice before it reached the House. By this time Americans for Nonsmokers' Rights had got their 15,000 members to make their voices heard and had enlisted the support of many flight attendants.

The bill was narrowly passed in April 1988 - by 198 votes to 193 - but was immediately criticised by some anti-smokers, not least Citizens

Against Tobacco Smoke, for its limited scope. They were missing the point. Total bans were politically unpopular and could only be carried by increments. Calling for a ban on short flights was a master stroke because it made the bill politically palatable - it did not seem unreasonable to ask smokers to go without a cigarette for two hours - while making a total ban virtually inevitable.

Having overcome the first hurdle, it was a simple matter to argue that, since the first law had been passed with the health of cabin staff in mind, it was nonsensical to limit the ban to short flights. Never mind that many of those who had gone along with the law originally had done so because it seemed churlish not to, rather than because they believed that secondhand smoke was a killer. Once the precedent had been set, the anti-smoking groups pointed to what they now described as a "loophole" in the law and achieved inch-by-inch what they could not have hoped to achieve in one stroke. Sure enough, smoking sections were abolished on all US flights in 1990. The tactic of drawing up limited but politically acceptable anti-smoking legislation with inherent loopholes that could be dealt with later became a distinctive feature of the anti-smoking movement around the world.

One curious and unintended consequence of the aeroplane ban was that airlines began to save money by changing the air in the cabin less frequently. Traditionally, this was done every two minutes and old air was never recirculated, but with no tobacco smoke to draw attention to the quality of air, the carriers reduced air changes to once every twenty minutes. This led to a musty aroma on board and, according to a report in *The Lancet*, contributed to the appearance of Deep Vein Thrombosis, a disease unknown in airline passengers until the 1990s (25).

With this battle won, Ahron Leichtman's aspirations rose considerably and he signposted his intention of eliminating tobacco from the country, and perhaps the world, by changing his organisation's name from Citizens Against Tobacco Smoke to Citizens for a Tobacco-Free Society. Inspired by Banzhaf's novel use of the Fairness Doctrine, Leichtman now demanded that newspapers and magazines give anti-smoking groups free ad space equal to that paid for by cigarette companies. He insisted that smoking cost America $100 billion a year, talked about the "forces of darkness" lined up against him (26) and, in 1991, sued radio host Andy Furman for assault after having cigar smoke blown in his face.

In 1994, Leichtman wrote a pamphlet titled *The Top Ten Ways to Attack the Tobacco Industry and Win the War against Smoking.* He was, one might conclude, something of a hard-liner. Comparing smokers to people who spray poison, slap or spit, he asked readers of *USA Today*:

> "Would you calmly suggest these folks be placed in a separate section where they couldn't harm you? No, you'd probably want them arrested and put in jail. That's where people who commit assault and battery are sent." (27)

After the total ban on airlines, the message from the anti-smoking movement was that nonsmokers did not merely have the right to smoke-free air but that they had the right to it at all times and in all circumstances. That smoky environments might be avoidable to a reasonable person was not enough. The idea of nonsmokers' rights, combined with the notion that nonsmokers were being actively assaulted and murdered by smokers, nourished their belief that they were having their rights violated if people smoked anywhere they might conceivably wish to go. Striking a balance between the rights of smokers and those of nonsmokers was, in the eyes of groups like ASH, no longer necessary nor desirable.

As the 1980s came to an end, those on the cutting edge of the movement put their weight behind the policy of 'denormalisation,' which portrayed smoking as deviant and unacceptable behaviour. One of its chief proponents was Stanton Glantz, who explained the policy as "implicitly defining smoking as an anti-social act." (28) By regarding smokers as abnormal, social pressure could be brought to bear which, combined with the smoking bans which made them literally outsiders, would 'encourage' them to quit. The line between 'denormalisation' and stigmatisation was a thin one, as was the line between 'encouraging' and 'forcing.' It would become thinner as the years went on.

Surgeon General C. Everett Koop called smoking a 'disorder' and the Centers for Disease Control added tobacco use to its list of diseases.

This uniquely classified a mode of behaviour as a sickness. It was official confirmation of something that had been first mooted by Lennox Johnston in the 1940s: that smoking was itself an epidemic which had to be fought until it was wiped out.

A mode of behaviour had never before been officially defined as a disease and for good reason. Like over-eating, drinking and gambling, smoking is a behaviour, not an ailment. It does not have the symptoms of a disease, nor is it contagious, but for those who liked to believe that they were fighting a war on smoking rather than smokers, it was a convenient redefinition.

If smoking was an epidemic then what was lung cancer? A symptom? Well, yes, according to Dr John Slade in a 1985 issue of the *New York State Journal of Medicine*:

> "The cancer or myocardial infarction or emphysema are only signs
> of an underlying disease: chronic cigarette use."(29)

One might question the wisdom of a medical philosophy which considered heart attacks and cancers to be little more than side-effects but, for the anti-smokers, it was expedient to do so.

One of the most unfortunate consequences of the quit-or-die approach was the appalling underfunding of lung cancer research. Seeing it as more of a behavioural problem than a medical one, the US federal government, by 2005, was funding lung cancer research to the tune of just $1,830 for every case, in contrast to the $14,370 spent on each case of prostate cancer and $23,475 spent on each case of breast cancer (30).

With lung cancer research seemingly going nowhere, it was easier to practise preventative medicine by lobbying for legislation to control behaviour. By reclassifying smoking as an epidemic, smokers became both victims and carriers. It made it possible to view perfectly healthy people as diseased by virtue of their lifestyle and it was they, rather than the genuinely sick, who would henceforth be 'treated' by public health policies.

Windfall

The tobacco industry was still able to outspend its opponents, even if the media were less inclined to publish industry statements without extensive rebuttal. In 1988, Americans for Nonsmokers' Rights and GASP fought a campaign to increase tobacco taxes in the form of a new ordinance known as Prop 99. Few denied that a rise was overdue. Only six states had a lower rate than California and the tax had last been increased in 1967, since when it had naturally fallen behind the rate of inflation. Passed with 58% of the vote, the real achievement of Prop 99 was not to bump up the tax on a pack of cigarettes from 10 to 25 cents but to secure a commitment from the state's politicians to funnel 20% of the money raised towards anti-smoking projects.

It had taken fifteen years but the Californian activists finally had the financial power to match their passion. In its first year, $175 million was given to anti-smoking causes and this soon rose to over $500 million, including $44 million spent on tobacco research at Stanton Glantz's University of California. $30 million was set aside for anti-smoking commercials and since the newly enriched anti-smoking groups were keen advocates of denormalisation, this meant that California became the first state in America to force smokers to, as Jacob Sullum put it, "pay for their own vilification."(31)

Prop 99 created an almost bottomless pit of money for anti-smoking organisations and long-serving activists were well placed to take up full-time jobs in tobacco control and receive lucrative commissions for tobacco research. Notice that the bank was open for business was given in newspaper ads asking:

> "Are you involved in a nonprofit program looking for money?
> If your work can incorporate tobacco prevention, there may be funding available."(32)

With tobacco control 'project directors' able to earn $265 an hour, there was no shortage of veteran anti-smokers rushing to get in on the action and the President of the California Medical Association was candid enough to admit that health groups were "fighting for this money like jackals over a carcass."(33)

Prop 99 explicitly prohibited funds from being used to encourage "the passage of any law, including public ordinance and regulations," but lobbying for legislation was the *raison d'être* of the Californian anti-smoking groups. Americans for Nonsmokers' Rights could hardly pretend not to be a lobby group but by forming the Americans for Nonsmokers' Rights Foundation, it became eligible for grants. The foundation was awarded $1,200,000, much of which was spent compiling a hit-list of perceived "enemies."(34)

In any case, activists did not have to carry placards to sway the public to vote for tougher anti-smoking measures. Prop 99 money paid for research into passive smoking that was often conducted by people who were, to put it mildly, emotionally involved in the debate. One such researcher was Stanton Glantz who, by 2005, had produced more than 150 papers on every conceivable aspect of tobacco control and who said that he asked himself one question when conducting his research:

"If this comes out the way I think, will it make a difference? And if the answer is "yes," then we do it, and if the answer is "I don't know" then we don't bother. Okay? And that's the criteria."(35)

The case crumbles

Despite the input of such conspicuously partisan researchers as Stanton Glantz and James Repace, the case against passive smoking was far from closed. Epidemiological studies into secondhand smoke continued to act better as demonstrations of chaos theory than of any kind of cause-and-effect between secondhand smoke and lung cancer.

Quite how fine the line between proving and disproving the passive smoking theory was can be illustrated by two papers published in the 1980s. In 1984, the obscure *European Journal of Respiratory Disease* published David Hole and Charles Gillis's epidemiological study of 16,171 residents of the west of Scotland (36). The study involved middle-aged people who were classified as either 'exposed' or 'not exposed' to secondhand smoke. It ran for ten years and in that time just 8 female lung cancer cases were identified. Unfortunately for the passive smoking theorists, the women who were exposed to secondhand smoke were found to be no more likely to contract the disease than those who were not.

Gillis and Hole announced, rather grandiosely, that their study showed that the female lung cancer rate was 4 per 10,000 and they concluded their paper with a thinly veiled plea for more funding, which must have been granted since they continued to monitor the Scottish residents for a further five years. In that time, just one more woman died of lung cancer. This sad but unexceptional death had a dramatic effect on Gillis and Hole's study since the unfortunate woman happened to be listed in the 'exposed' category (as were most of the women). A statistical correlation between passive smoke exposure and lung cancer could now be shown. Consequently, the whole paper was rewritten and, in August 1989, brought to the world's attention, not - this time - in a little-known specialist publication but in the *British Medical Journal* (37). The age standardised lung cancer mortality rate for 'unexposed' women remained at 4 per 10,000 while the rate for 'exposed' women had now risen to 5 per 10,000. Or, to put it another way, being exposed to secondhand smoke raised lung cancer risk for female nonsmokers by, after adjustments, 37%. And all because of the death of a one woman in the west of Scotland.

It was becoming clear to neutral observers that if there was any risk from secondhand smoke it was too slight to be identified in small studies. Although Surgeon General Koop presented secondhand smoke as a proven health hazard in his comments to the press, the text of his 1986 report called for new research to be carried out on larger sample groups and, by the early 1990s, seven such studies had been carried out. Taken together, they appeared to show that passive smoke was wholly benign. The largest of them - Fontham (1991) and Wu-Williams (1987) - directly contradicted each other, with the former showing a 29% increase and the latter a 30% decrease in risk for women married to smokers. These were the only studies that found statistically significant associations. Of the rest, Wu (1985) and Stockwell (1992) found nonsignificant elevations in risk, Gao (1988) and Janerich (1990) found nonsignificant reductions in risk and Brownson (1990) found a relative risk of exactly 1.0.

With three results higher than 1.0, three lower than 1.0 and one exactly 1.0, one could hardly ask for a more even spread and the obvious conclusion was that the true risk must be 1.0 (zero). This, of course, was not what the anti-smoking groups or the medical community wanted to hear and they allied themselves with the only one of the seven studies to have shown a significant increase in risk. It received the lion's share of media coverage.

Published in late 1991, Elizabeth Fontham's study was unquestionably a newsworthy piece since it was the first (and, as it turned out, last) time a study from the United States found a statistically significant association between secondhand and lung cancer, albeit by a whisker and albeit only in certain scenarios (childhood exposure, for example, showed a consistent negative trend). It was a sizeable study of over 600 proven lung cancer cases, and the issue of smoker misclassification was addressed by measuring cotinine (a biomarker for nicotine) from patients at random. Although cotinine does not remain in the body for long and it was highly probable that many of the smokers in the group would have quit once they were diagnosed with lung cancer, this process still managed to weed out one or two secret smokers. Recall bias was addressed by using colon cancer patients as the control group, the idea being that they would be as likely to exaggerate or downplay their past exposure to tobacco smoke as the lung cancer victims.

There was no statistically significant link between exposure to secondhand smoke and lung carcinoma but there was a small association with adenocarcinoma - a particular type of lung cancer most often associated with nonsmokers - and Fontham focused her attention on this area. The figure that came to be quoted was a 29% increase in risk for lung cancer (38) but since Elizabeth Fontham has never made the raw data used in the study available it is impossible to analyse her methodology further.

Ross Brownson's 1992 study also used a sample group of over 600 proven lung cancer cases and found that those exposed to their parents' smoke in childhood had a statistically significant *reduction* in lung cancer risk of 0.7 (0.5-0.9). Those who lived with a spouse who smoked one or two packs a day were also 30% less likely to contract the disease than those who did not. When workplace exposure was studied there was, again, no evidence of harm and the overall risk ratio for passive smokers was found to be exactly 1.0 (0.8-1.2), the most compelling evidence yet that the passive smoking theory was erroneous.

In the same year, Heather Stockwell and her team published the findings of their study of 210 female lung cancer victims. Like Brownson, she found no increase in risk from workplace exposure but found statistically insignificant increases in risk for nonsmoking wives of 1.6 (0.8-3.0) and for children of smoking fathers of 1.2 (0.6-2.3)(39).

The way in which these null findings were presented to the public was perhaps even more revealing than the findings themselves. Funded by the National Cancer Institute, Stockwell did not attempt to explain why those exposed to secondhand smoke at home were dying of lung cancer while those exposed at work were not. Not only did she not ask the question, she did not tabulate any of the figures for workplace exposure and the finding was brushed off in a single sentence, leaving her free to spend the remaining five pages of the report discussing the positive associations in detail.

Brownson, funded by the same organisation but without even the scantest positive associations to report, simply ignored his own evidence and wrote up his paper as if his research somehow supported the passive smoking theory. Incredibly, he reported that there was "a small but consistent increase in lung cancer risk from passive smoking," a statement utterly at odds with the tables of evidence he presented, before concluding that "comprehensive action to limit smoking in public places and worksites are well-advised."*(40)

The story of Dwight Janerich's paper is the most illuminating of all. Janerich had gathered his data of 439 lung cancer patients in the early 1980s, thanks to another NCI grant. They showed no association

---

* In his comments to the press, however, Ross Brownson accepted that the study did not support the passive smoking theory: "I wish our findings had gone in the exact pattern the public health community would like. But one of the criticisms of medical research is that the only thing findings ever show is some kind of health risk. I feel it's important to publish findings, no matter what they show." ('Risk studies differ on passive smoking,' *Washington Post*, 20.11.93)

between secondhand smoke and lung cancer and, perhaps because of this, he was given no further money to pursue it. Only when a PhD student approached Janerich for permission to use the data was it written up (as a doctoral thesis) but it was never published and, once completed, was forgotten about. It took a Philip Morris employee, who was suspicious that secondhand smoke studies were being buried if they did not support the anti-smoking cause, to discover the thesis preserved for posterity on a University microfiche (41).

Once he brought its null findings to the attention of the media, the NCI suddenly renewed its interest in the research and provided Janerich with a grant to rewrite the study. Published in the *New England Journal of Medicine* in 1990, he found two statistically significant results. One indicated that exposure to very large amounts of secondhand smoke during childhood slightly raised the risk of developing lung cancer in later life and the other indicated that exposure to smoke in social settings helped *protect* against lung cancer. Neither association was particularly strong and the one clearly ran contrary to the other. (42)

Janerich emphasised the one positive association (with children) and did all he could to brush over the rest. Like Brownson, he brazened it out, simply asserting that "the evidence we report lends further support to the observation that passive smoking may increase the risk of subsequent lung cancer."(43) And also like Brownson (and Stockwell) this misleading conclusion appeared in the summary of the report - the only part any quizzical journalist might bother to look at. With only a tiny minority of people inclined to read these studies in full, it was exactly the kind of sound-bite that kept the passive smoking theory alive in the public's mind even as the science crumbled.

The Environmental Protection Agency on passive smoking

In 1989, The Environmental Protection Agency (EPA) took on the unenviable task of drawing together the epidemiological evidence on passive smoking to build a case that would support Koop's controversial and premature assertion that it killed nonsmokers. There was never any doubt what its verdict would be. Almost as soon as the task was set for them, members of the EPA panel told the press that secondhand smoke was "cancer causing," with one confidently announcing: "Whether or not there are health effects associated with ETS is no longer in question."(44) It would be three years before the EPA published its report and yet by May 1990 the New York Times was able to report that the agency had "tentatively concluded that it [secondhand smoke] causes 3,000 or more lung-cancer deaths annually."(45)

John Banzhaf appeared on television to proclaim that secondhand smoke was more dangerous than asbestos, radon "or any other air pollutant"(46) and fellow lawyer Richard Daynard predicted a spate of lawsuits in which employees would sue their bosses for allowing them to be exposed to passive smoke. All these pronouncements served a purpose. The EPA only regulated outdoor air quality and was powerless to bring in indoor smoking restrictions whatever its final conclusions may be. It therefore relied on employers worrying about future lawsuits should their employees became ill; if that happened the EPA's report could be cited in court. Not a single case had ever been brought against anyone on the grounds that secondhand smoke had harmed them, but this gambit was effective in scaring companies into bringing in smoking restrictions voluntarily.

The important thing was that secondhand smoke be condemned by an official government agency. It did not have to be the EPA. In 1964 the Surgeon General and his team had carried out a painstaking and thorough investigation into smoking and it was conceivable that a similar expert panel could be assembled again. The Surgeon General chose not to do so, perhaps because he understood what would be required to bring a case against secondhand smoke and did not want his department tainted by it.

Besides, the EPA had a long track record of overstating environmental dangers and a high public profile. Above all, it had professional anti-smoker James Repace, who was now charging $800 a day as an 'expert witness' on secondhand smoke, and who had his feet under the desk at the EPA's Indoor Air Division. According to Repace, it was he and his staff who "were able to convince EPA top management to initiate a request for research office staff to produce the now-famous

1992 EPA risk assessment on passive smoking, to put the Agency as a whole on the record."(47)

The most effective method of making the feeble evidence against secondhand smoke appear threatening was to cherry-pick the most favourable studies and multiply the weak associations they reported by America's vast population. Statistically insignificant findings might be scientifically meaningless to epidemiologists but extrapolating them across nations of millions could make it appear that hundreds, even thousands, of lives were being lost each year. By so doing, complex and conflicting epidemiological data could be simplified for the public who would be unaware if such figures were hypothetical estimates or real figures based on death certificates and coroners' reports.

A null study is a null study and gathering ten or twenty of them together does not change that fact but this is precisely what the EPA did, using the process of meta-analysis which, to quote 'junk science' expert Steve Milloy, takes "individual studies that don't stand up on their own from a statistical point of view and combines their statistics to construct a new statistically stronger and newsworthy study."(48)

With 31 disparate studies and so many flaws to deal with, the EPA gave more weight to some studies than others; a reasonable idea in principle but one which the agency employed haphazardly. For example, Gillis and Hole's 1989 study of just nine lung cancer cases had found an insignificant relative risk of 1.37 (0.29-6.61) and, considering the miniscule sample group, had arguably been a pointless, and certainly inconclusive, exercise and yet it was put in the top tier. Wu-Williams' large study of 417 cases, on the other hand, found a significant reduction in risk of 0.7 and was put in the bottom tier even though the agency described it as "large and basically well-executed."(49)

The fact remained that only 6 of the 31 studies assessed by the EPA showed a statistically significant relationship: Hirayama's Japanese study, two Greek studies co-authored by Trichopoulos, an obscure paper from China and two studies from Hong Kong, one of which was an unpublished University thesis.

And so the EPA took the 11 studies that best suited their hypothesis, combined their findings and discarded the rest. Even then, the results remained statistically insignificant using the 95% confidence interval that the agency had always used in the past, and so it was lowered to 90%, thereby giving statistical significance to null studies and very weak associations. This naturally raised eyebrows but the EPA was at least candid in explaining why it had to be done:

> '..the justification for this usage is based on the a priori hypothesis...that a positive association exists between exposure to ETS and lung cancer.'(50)

This admission comes from the fruits of the EPA's extensive investigation, a report of over 700 pages entitled *Respiratory Health Effects of Passive Smoking* (1992). In it, secondhand smoke was labelled a group A carcinogen, the term bestowed on any pollutant which kills 1 in 100,000. The EPA found passive smoking to present an increased risk of just 1.19, a relative risk that epidemiologists would normally dismiss as a very feeble association, if they considered it at all.

Even if true, nonsmokers who lived with smokers only had a 0.015% chance of contracting lung cancer compared to the 0.012% chance taken by those married to nonsmokers. Meaningless to individuals, this risk was extrapolated over the population of America to arrive at - as the *New York Times* had predicted - 3,000 lung cancer deaths a year. And so it was that the EPA concluded that passive smoke was a "serious and substantial public health risk."

The report was immediately criticised from all quarters for its shoddy methodology and shameless bias. To quote Richard Kluger:

> "The government agencies seemed nearly as capable in this instance of blowing smoke at the public to cloud the scarcity of cold, clinical public-health risk as the cigarette companies had habitually been in denying and distorting the overwhelming scientific case against the direct use of their product."(51)

The tobacco industry took legal action against the EPA and the revelations that came to light in the ensuing court case revealed a culture of arrogance, deception and cover-up within the agency that few could have guessed at. Of the EPA's moving of the goalposts to realise its objectives, the judge remarked:

> "Results did not confirm the EPA's controversial a priori hypothesis.
> In order to confirm its hypothesis, EPA maintained its standard significant
> level but lowered the confidence interval to 90%.
> This allowed EPA to confirm its hypothesis
> by finding a relative risk of 1.19, albeit a very weak association."(52)

And of its conduct during the course of its hearings between 1989 and 1992:

> "EPA publicly committed to a conclusion before research had begun;
> excluded industry by violating the Act's procedural requirements;
> adjusted established procedure and scientific norms to validate
> the Agency's public conclusion...
> disregarded information and made findings on selective information;
> did not disseminate significant epidemiologic information;
> deviated from its Risk Assessment Guidelines;
> failed to disclose important findings and reasoning;
> and left significant questions without answers.
> EPA's conduct left substantial holes in the administrative record.
> While so doing, produced limited evidence, then claimed the weight of the
> Agency's research evidence demonstrated ETS causes cancer." (53)

This damning verdict came in 1998, too late to prevent the cavalcade of smoking bans based on the EPA's suspect conclusions and it did little to change public perceptions, largely because it was barely reported. The New York Times had previously put secondhand smoke stories on its front page but when the judge tore apart the EPA's case in court, it was reported on the bottom of page 23. Anti-smoking campaigners continued to quote from the EPA report as if the judge had never spoken and the public were largely unaware of - or indifferent to - the fact that the Environmental Protection Agency had just been exposed, in court, of deceiving the American public on a grand scale.

It was a turning point not just in the history of tobacco but in that of science. John Brignell described it in *The Epidemiologists* as "the greatest statistical fraud ever" and its influence would endure well into the next century:

> "There is no doubt about it - every study of passive smoking, if evaluated on the basis
> of statistical probity, shows that it is harmless; but probity had been jettisoned.
> It was a deeply symbolic and decisive moment in time.
> Once you could get the world to accept a relative risk of 1.19 at a
> significance level of 10%, you could prove that anything caused anything.
> The scientific era that had started with Bacon four centuries earlier had come to an end
> and the world was ready to return to the rule of mumbo-jumbo." (54)

CHAPTER EIGHT

'This is a crusade, not a lawsuit!'

John Banzhaf once compared the anti-smoking movement to a three-legged stool. One leg consisted of telling smokers that they were harming themselves. The second leg was the belief that secondhand smoke was harmful to nonsmokers. The third leg was the idea that smokers placed an unfair financial burden on the general population by obliging them to pay for the treatment of their diseases through higher taxes and medical insurance costs. This economic argument, which, at the Winnipeg conference, Banzhaf called the "new weapon," came to the fore after Bill Clinton became US President in 1993 (1).

Without really trying, Ronald Reagan had already done more than any of his presidential predecessors to reduce cigarette consumption. In 1982, he doubled the federal tax on cigarettes to 18 cents a pack. This was not intended as an anti-smoking measure. The federal cigarette tax had not risen for thirty years and Reagan, like his ideological counterpart Margaret Thatcher, needed to raise money to make up for lowering other taxes. The British had seen this policy at work in 1947 when post-war privations dictated a 43% jump in tobacco duty. That tax had resulted in a 14% drop in consumption and Reagan's efforts also provoked a significant drop (of 6.7%) as the combination of the tax hike, tobacco industry price gouging and inflation resulted in the price of a pack of cigarettes jumping from 62 cents to 96 cents in the space of two years.

This seemed to confirm that raising prices was the single most effective way of bringing down the smoking rate. Keenly aware of the potential of taxation as a weapon, the anti-smoking lobby pleaded with Reagan to raise tax on cigarettes again but he refused to do so. Federal tax on a pack of cigarettes remained at 18 cents until 1991 when, with the budget unbalanced once more, George Bush Sr. increased it by 4 cents. This time, however, a fall in consumption failed to occur; the smoking rate actually rose for the first time in years.

Bill Clinton promised to be tougher on tobacco. Hillary Clinton described the interests of the tobacco companies as being "in transparent conflict with those of the Clinton administration" and she sent out a message by banning smoking in the White House as soon as she and her husband moved in (2). This met with a mixed reception from the dignitaries and ambassadors from countries where smoking had yet to been denormalised. King Hussein of Jordan congratulated Mrs Clinton on banning smoking with the ambiguous compliment that it would "guarantee short meetings."(3)

Clinton raised the federal tax on cigarettes by a further 4 cents in 1993 but much greater sums of money would be needed if he was to fund his ambitious health care reforms and he made it known that he was considering going much further. A touch hopefully, the American Medical Association joined former Surgeon General Koop in demanding a two dollar rise. In a survey, 74% of the public agreed with a one dollar hike. By a remarkable coincidence, this was exactly the same percentage of Americans who were nonsmokers.

The Coalition on Smoking or Health, Citizens for a Tobacco-Free Society and various other anti-smoking groups claimed that smoking cost the country $100 billion a year. If true, a $3.90 per pack tax rate would be required if smokers were to pay their way. Closer examination of the mathematics showed that the cost of smoking was not $100 billion or anywhere close to it. According to those who came up with the figure, $47 billion - nearly half the total - was put down to 'lost productivity' and a further $40 billion was made up of 'foregone earnings of those dying prematurely,' 'lost income tax' and, rather tenuously, 'lost housekeeping services.'

Happy enough to include lost income tax and foregone earnings on the debit side, the anti-smokers were less eager to balance the account with the tobacco industry's $50 billion contribution to the economy (4) or the savings in medical care, pensions and benefits from smokers dying younger. When one also took into account the $28 billion that smokers were already shelling out on private health care and tobacco duty, it was more accurate to say that smokers were subsidising the health care of nonsmokers. This was not a proposition that anti-smokers liked to dwell on. Jeffrey Harris testified before Congress to say that smoking cost society $88 billion a year but when it was put to him that smokers might actually save the taxpayer money by dying prematurely, he retorted: "This is not the kind of calculation in which civilised society engages. This is not a matter of cold economic calculation, but a matter of health."(5) Fair comment perhaps, but it was anti-smoking advocates like Harris who had brought up the economic argument in the first place. Having insisted that government policy on smoking be based on the amount of money that could be saved, they could hardly complain when it was pointed out that, as a "matter of cold economic calculation," it would be best if everybody dropped dead at their retirement party.

The average lung cancer patient is diagnosed at the age of 70 and most die within a year of diagnosis. The idea that smokers deprive society of their productivity and income tax when most perish beyond retirement age is immediately suspect. The fact that they die, on average, several years before nonsmokers - but still in old age - indicates that they are departing this world at a time at which they are becoming most costly. A "cold" fact, for sure - and certainly not a reason to encourage smoking - but nor is it a sound basis to discourage it, at least from an economist's point of view.

How much, then, were nonsmokers costing smokers? In a thorough study published in the *Journal of the American Medical Association*, William Manning took account of savings made from smokers' premature, and relatively quick, deaths and calculated that the total cost to society amounted to 15 cents a pack - 23 cents less than the average state and federal tax on cigarettes. The Congressional Research Service endorsed Manning's findings and all independent research confirmed that smokers paid more in tax than they received in health care and had done so for many years. *Preventive Medicine*, in 1990, reported that nonsmokers required more medical treatment than smokers and the Congressional Research Service found that "reduced smoking probably would cause an increase in net budgetary costs."(6)

In the UK, the facts were even clearer. Raising the price of tobacco had long been the cornerstone of British attempts to cut the smoking rate. Margaret Thatcher had no particular axe to grind with tobacco and her own husband was a prolific smoker (until his death at the age of 88) but she found cigarettes, along with petrol, to be the least contentious commodity to tax. As her Chancellor, Nigel Lawson, remarked: "Such is the success of the anti-smoking lobby that the tobacco duty is the one tax where an increase commands more friends than enemies."(7) So enthusiastically did the treasury raise tobacco taxes, that by the mid-1980s, cigarette duty was paying for a third of the National Health Service. By the late 1990s, excise tax on a pack of cigarettes made up over 80% of the retail price and was providing the government with over £11 billion a year. On the debit side, even ASH (UK) could not pretend that smoking-related diseases were costing the country any more than £1.5 billion a year.

Despite all the evidence to the contrary, the myth of smokers being a drain on the economy persisted in Britain and elsewhere for years. The reason is not hard to fathom, for it extended the idea of passive harm beyond the wafts of smoke and declared that smokers harmed the wealth of nonsmokers, as well as their health.

Back in America, Clinton announced that he would raise the tax by 18 cents; a 75% increase but far less than the anti-smoking groups had hoped for. In 1994, after a long and bitter fight, the Clinton health reforms collapsed and with them went the proposed tax rise. Still no friend of cigarettes, the President legislated for a 10 cent and 5 cent rise to be introduced in 2000 and 2002 respectively. With characteristic political savvy, this left him free to complete his term in office - which ended in 2000 - without risking any backlash from smokers.

Smuggling

The anti-smoking movement has been cursed through the ages with the problem that, no matter how many man-made laws they created, the natural laws of supply and demand, and the law of unintended consequences, always got in the way. Never was this more true than with the issue of smuggling.

After the passage of Prop 99, other states began taxing smokers to pay for anti-smoking campaigns. The traditionally anti-tobacco states of Massachusetts and Arizona passed laws that were based on the Californian ordinance in 1993 and 1994 respectively. Michigan tripled tobacco duty in 1994 and Washington State increased its already hefty cigarette tax two years later. None of them saw a fall in the smoking rate like that seen on the West coast. They did, however, witness a drop in cigarette *sales* while their neighbours across the state-line noticed a sudden surge in demand. It was not difficult to see what was going on. Smokers were going across state to buy their cigarettes and for the first time in years, cigarette smuggling was becoming a serious problem in the USA.

The unintended consequences of raising taxes were first witnessed in California, where the Prop 99 price hike resulted in a suspicious 24% increase in cigarette exports to Mexico, from where smugglers brought them straight back into the state for illicit sale. Legislators in Michigan cheered when their own tax increase resulted in a 19% fall in over-the-counter cigarette sales but it was matched by a significant rise in consumption in neighbouring Wisconsin, Indiana and Iowa plus a 14% boom in low-tax North Carolina. All told, cross-border cigarette sales in the US are estimated to have risen fivefold between 1980 and 1994 (8).

Escalating tobacco taxes in Britain resulted in 1 in 5 cigarettes being smuggled into the country by the late 1990s. The arrival of the European Union and the opening of the Channel Tunnel gave smokers a ray of hope, since EU trade laws allowed them to buy unlimited quantities of cigarettes at the tax level of the country from which they were purchased. The UK government agreed with the concept in principle but the reality of millions of Britons travelling to France and Belgium to buy cigarettes and alcohol at much reduced prices mortified the Treasury and a new law was quickly brought in to curtail this particular piece of European harmonisation.

The British government restricted its citizens to buying only enough cigarettes on the continent to satisfy 'personal use' but it was left to customs officials to decide what constituted 'personal use' and, shorn of clear guidelines, they regulated the system in the most arbitrary and haphazard fashion. By 2002 they had reputedly impounded 20,000 cars and there were stories of little old ladies being arrested with a handful of cigarettes in their handbags. It took several national newspapers to campaign against the system before the government finally buckled and allowed 3,200 cigarettes or a kilo of rolling tobacco per person, enough to keep a 20-a-day smoker going for three months.

It was in Canada that the problem of cigarette smoking really came to a head. Canada's anti-smoking activities had lagged behind those of its neighbour to the south until 1974 when its own Nonsmokers' Rights Association was born. Over the next ten years Canada built a reputation as one of the world's least tobacco-friendly countries.

Although fast becoming a model for the tobacco control movement, Canada was inescapably positioned next door to the world's largest exporter of cigarettes. As part of its war on smoking, the Canadian government raised tax on cartons of 200 cigarettes by $2 in 1985 and by a further $4 in 1989. With prices already at an all time high, the government added another $6 to a carton in 1991 and it was at this point that Canada's normally law-abiding citizens snapped. The smuggling began in earnest. Canadian brands were being exported to America's northern cities in massive quantities before being brought straight back into Canada by smugglers in upstate New York via the Akwesasne Indian Reserve on the Quebec border. In 1989, Canada exported 1.26 billion cigarettes and just 1.8% of all the cigarettes in the country were believed to be contraband. By 1993, it was exporting 18.6 billion units and a quarter of all cigarettes were being smuggled in.

The response of the Canadian government was to stem the flow of cigarettes going out of the country by levying an export tax of $8 per carton. This led to a significant drop in exports but only served to anger the Canadian tobacco industry and did nothing to appease smokers. Thousands of tobacco farmers, workers and retailers protested on Parliament Hill and the Canadian tobacco industry threatened to move out of the country and take its jobs with it. The government backed down and suspended the export tax but kept the sales tax in place. The smuggling continued. Cigarettes were now being sold on the black market for $20 a carton, less than half their official retail price. More people were smoking, children found it easier to get hold of cigarettes, tobacconists were losing money to black marketeers and the law was being systematically undermined.

The situation was reaching the level of a national crisis and tobacco tax became a major issue in the run up to the 1993 election. In Quebec, where most of the contraband was arriving, The Movement to Abolish Tax on Tobacco was formed, and by January 1994, retailers across the province were openly selling contraband in protest at the government's refusal to bring down tobacco duty.

In Canada, this amounted to little short of anarchy. Two-thirds of all cigarettes smoked in Quebec were now thought to be contraband. Choosing between an unworkable public health initiative and overt civil disobedience, the Prime Minister Jean Chretien finally relented, lowering the federal tax by $5 a carton and agreeing to meet any further reduction made by local politicians. With Quebec lowering its local tax by $3, this meant tax in the province fell by $11 a carton. Order was restored.

As all this went on, the Canadian Cancer Society, rather than blaming the smugglers (or their own policy) for the problem, condemned the tobacco industry for having the temerity to export cigarettes to the US. When the climb-down finally came, the Canadian Council on Smoking and Health and the National Strategy to Reduce Tobacco Use were livid. In the midst of the crisis they had funded advertisements in 30 publications to declare that the Prime Minister would be personally responsible for 250,000 deaths if he dropped the tax. As it transpired, per capita consumption actually fell once the rollback came into effect, but to placate the health lobbyists, the government banned packs of ten - what the anti-smokers called 'kiddie packs' - and increased tax on tobacco company profits to pay for a national health drive. To this day, there are many in Canada's anti-smoking movement who feel that the original tax hike was the right move and would have succeeded had it not been for the pesky tobacco industry getting up to its old trick of legally exporting cigarettes to buyers in the United States.

The safer cigarette (slight return)

The behaviour of the tobacco industry worldwide followed a depressingly familiar pattern. Interviewed for a British television programme, a Philip Morris spokesman maintained that he did not believe that cigarettes caused cancer and, when challenged, stretched the rhetoric of doubt to surreal new lengths:

PM spokesman: Anything can be considered harmful. Apple sauce is harmful if you get too much of it.

Interviewer: I do not think too many people are dying from apple sauce.

PM spokesman: They are not eating that much.

Interviewer: People are smoking a lot of cigarettes.

PM spokesman: Well, let me put it this way. The people who eat apple sauce are dying. The people who eat sugar die. The people who smoke die. Does the fact that the people who smoke cigarettes die demonstrate that smoking is the cause? (9)

With cigarette advertisements taken off the television, the industry took to negotiating deals for product placement on the big screen and paid to have their brands smoked in dozens of Hollywood films including *The Living Daylights*, *Apocalypse Now* and *Beverley Hills Cop*. Sylvester Stallone accepted $500,000 to smoke Brown & Williamson cigarettes in five films but the most notorious example was the 1979 payment by Philip Morris of $42,500 to the producers of *Superman II*, in which the super-hero's girlfriend, Lois Lane, suddenly becomes a smoker of *Marlboro* cigarettes (the *Marlboro* logo appears no fewer than 22 times in the film). However, by the end of the 1980s, movie executives had decided - without any government intervention - that such deals provided poor value for money and product placement arrangements died out.

The search for a safer cigarette, however, continued. Cigarette companies spent hundreds of millions of dollars looking for this holy grail and unearthed some promising areas for research, but success in the market place continued to elude them. Selling a known carcinogen remained a more viable business proposition than trying to remove the cancer-causing agents.

Reynolds piloted its near-smokeless *Premier* brand in a few US states in 1988. It was a complex facsimile of a cigarette which released very little smoke and heated the tobacco with an aluminium rod that ran down the middle. This, it was claimed, reduced tar levels by 90% and reduced or eliminated the carcinogenic effects of tobacco smoke. As a near smokeless device, *Premier* was tailor-made to lead the counter attack against an anti-smoking lobby that was successfully touting the supposed perils of passive smoke. But *Premier* had so little in common with conventional cigarettes that it required its own instruction manual to use and those who tried it out in the test-cities of St Louis and Phoenix found it as unsatisfying as it was unusual. Having spent the best part of a billion dollars on the product, RJ Reynolds abandoned *Premier* before it had a chance to be rejected by the rest of the nation.

Philip Morris made similar efforts with brands called *Next* and *Accord* and Reynolds would try again in 1996 with *Eclipse*. In the case of *Eclipse*, even the doggedly anti-tobacco Senator Henry Waxman accepted that it was "safer" but all the major US health organisations - bar the Institute of Medicine - rejected it without trial, in the case of the American Cancer Society because of the tobacco industry's "long history of deception."(10)

The Food and Drug Administration (FDA) did not, much to its chagrin, have the authority to regulate cigarettes but it was able to regulate any new 'nicotine delivery device'. Increasingly staffed by tobacco control advocates and former activists, the FDA had become wedded to the precautionary principle which led it to wage a war against saccharine after experiments demonstrated that large doses led to bladder cancer in rodents (it was years before the FDA finally accepted that it was not carcinogenic for humans).

Thwarted in its attempts to get the Supreme Court to give it authority to regulate conventional cigarettes, the FDA was never likely to approve variations of a product that was a proven killer, unless its safety was proven through decades of research. This posed an ethical dilemma. Demanding safety and efficacy from new products was a reasonable requirement but it made less sense in the case of cigarettes. Here was an exceptional instance of a known health hazard already on the market and the only criterion for new innovations should have been that they were not *more* dangerous. If it was no safer, it would be just another hazardous cigarette brand out of hundreds. If, however, it proved less carcinogenic, it could be a major boon to the health of smokers.

But reducing the hazards of smoking was no longer the priority for anti-tobacconists, including those within the FDA. They wanted smokers to give up altogether and the safer cigarette was at odds with the 'quit or die' policy that had prevailed since the abolition of the Less Hazardous Cigarette Working Group in the late 1970s. As far as anti-smoking groups were concerned, a safer cigarette would not remove the nuisance of secondhand smoke, would not lead to the destruction of the tobacco industry and might work against their efforts to persuade smokers to quit. They persisted with the rhetoric that all cigarettes were equally dangerous and even criticised one innovation for "only" reducing cancer risk, a shortcoming that many smokers would have gladly overlooked (11).

The non-appearance of the safer cigarette allowed the anti-smokers to have their cake and eat it. While they mocked the idea that cigarettes could be made less dangerous, they could not resist the opportunity to paint the industry as indifferent to the health of its customers by not releasing safer alternatives. ASH (UK) asserted that "the hunt for a so-called safer cigarette is farcical...inhaling smoke is so dangerous that the particular blend of toxic constituents will not make much difference."(12) This was at odds with one of its other widely reported press releases in which it ASH (UK) announced: "the tobacco industry has investigated and patented technologies that would reduce the substances in cigarette smoke that cause cancer, heart disease and emphysema...even a small improvement could save thousands of lives."(13)

Between 1975 and 2000, at least 150 patents for safer cigarettes were lodged by tobacco companies (14) but every new development was hampered by opposition from government and public health groups. In the belief that worldwide abstinence could be achieved within a generation, the anti-smoking movement was not prepared to dilute its message by conceding that safer smoking alternatives might be available. This left the industry with few options beyond reducing nicotine and tar yields whilst promising research, such as the palladium project and Philip Morris' work in eliminating cadmium, was aborted. Assuming such work had any merit and that safer alternatives existed, there was clearly a balance to be struck between reducing harm to the individual and the ideal of mass abstinence. Such subtleties sat awkwardly with the black-and-white world-view of anti-smoking pressure groups, particularly when they involved cooperating with their foes in the tobacco industry, and the safer cigarette remains one of the great what-ifs in tobacco's story.

Back in the dock

Herbert Osmon was the man charged with monitoring the anti-smoking movement for the tobacco giant RJ Reynolds. A feisty character, Osmon had nothing but contempt for the "zealots" who sought to destroy the industry he loved. In 1991, he gave a speech to RJ Reynolds employees to warn them that the 1990s would be the industry's toughest decade:

> "Bear in mind that the goal of the anti-smoking zealots is
> 'a Smoke-Free Society by the Year 2000.'
> That is nine years from now.
> We will see a frenzy of activity over the next few years
> as we get close to the new century."

But Osmon remained hopeful:

> "I believe with determination we can prevent the anti-smoking movement from
> achieving its goal and ensure that the tobacco business will still be
> here in strength in the year 2000. And then what?
> How much emotional energy will the zealots have expended,
> only to have failed to meet their goal?
> Can they really get fired up by a new slogan which says
> 'a Smoke-Free Society by the Year 2010'? I don't think so." (15)

One reason for Osmon's optimism was that, although it was under siege, the industry remained undefeated in the court room. Bolstered by armies of lawyers, its decades old policy of solidarity through denial continued to protect it in an increasingly hostile environment. The industry took some bloody noses in the 1980s but came away from several tightly fought liability suits financially unscathed.

The most memorable of these began in 1983 when Marc Z. Edell filed a law suit against Liggett & Myers on behalf of Rose Cipollone. Edell had seen his colleagues in the legal profession make millions from the collapse of the asbestos industry and was tipped off that Cipollone would make an ideal plaintiff for a liability suit against the tobacco industry.

Cipollone had begun smoking *Chesterfields* in 1942 at the age of 17 and in 1955 switched to another Liggett brand, *L & M*. As the evidence about the health hazards began to mount she continued to smoke cigarettes, changing to Philip Morris's *Virginia Slims* and *Parliament* brands in 1968. In 1974, aged 49, she switched again, this time to Lorillard's *True*. Seven years later she lost a lobe in her right lung to cancer and in 1982 had to have the lung removed completely. Still she kept smoking and did not manage to quit until Edell's lawsuit was filed. At that point, her changes in brand allegiance became an important legal issue since, if found responsible for her cancer, three different manufacturers would have to share liability.

She died in 1984, aged 58, and her case finally went before a jury in 1988. Edell told the court that the tobacco industry had knowingly misled Mrs Cipollone into believing that cigarettes were safe in the years before the Cigarette Labelling Act and forced it to reveal internal documents which hinted at the scale of the industry cover-up. Part of the case against Liggett was based on the company's failure to release the *Palladium* brand in the 1970s, after it had been shown to virtually eliminate tumours in mice. Still denying that cigarettes were dangerous to health - and that tests on mice had no bearing on human biology - Liggett's CEO was forced into tacitly, and absurdly, accepting that his company had spent millions of dollars looking into ways of protecting rodents from getting cancer (16).

After a long and gruelling court case, the jury ordered Liggett to pay Rose Cipollone's widower $400,000 in damages. For the first time, a cigarette company had lost a liability case but it fell short of being an unequivocal endorsement of the prosecution's argument that the industry had been responsible for Cipollone's death. The jury, like those before them, believed that smokers should bear most, if not all, of the responsibility for the consequences of their actions. This was reflected in the relatively small amount awarded and the fact that the damages were given in Rose's husband's name rather than as posthumous compensation to her. This distinction soon became academic when the Cipollone verdict was reversed on appeal and the tobacco industry's 100% record continued.

The near-miss of the Cipollone case gave lawyers hope of a major victory. "You can use whatever analogy you want," said John Banzhaf, who knew a thing or two about lawsuits, "flies to honey, vampires to blood - but we've got a glut of lawyers out there just looking for someone to sue."(17) New lawsuits were filed all over America and, in 1990, a jury came to another ambiguous conclusion in the case of the late Nathan Horton, a heavy smoker who had died of lung cancer, against American Tobacco. The Mississippi court found the cigarette company and Horton equally culpable for his death but awarded no damages.

It was not until 1994 that the wheels really began to fall off the industry bandwagon. In February, the age-old campaign to have the Food and Drug Administration regulate cigarettes as 'nicotine delivery devices' found an advocate in FDA Commissioner, David Kessler. Kessler announced his intention to bring tobacco under his jurisdiction and proposed that nicotine levels be reduced to such a degree that they would have little to no pleasurable effect on the user, rather like removing alcohol from beer.

In March, the industry faced its largest class action yet, in the form of Castano versus American Tobacco. Involving 60 attorneys, the case was ambitious beyond words, purporting as it did to act on behalf of every "nicotine-dependent" person in the US, past and present, plus "the estates...the spouses, children, relatives, and 'significant others' of those nicotine-dependent cigarette smokers and their heirs and survivors," a list that seemed to include virtually every American to have drawn breath in the 20th century (18). They chose Diane Castano - whose husband Peter had died of lung cancer aged 47 - as the lead plaintiff and openly sought to bring down the tobacco industry for their own financial gain. With the prospect of billions of dollars in damages, the legal vultures began to circle and the case attracted lawyers who saw it as a meal ticket. One cheerfully admitted: "I am a pirate...I have been described as an ambulance chaser, and I don't disagree."(19)

Success promised untold riches but proving cause and effect in a single case was notoriously tricky and suing on behalf of millions was doomed to failure. Demonstrating in court that cigarettes caused disease required detailed medical information about every one of the plaintiffs and was an impossibility in a class action of this scale. The Castano lawyers' approach was therefore not to sue on the basis of disease but for "economic loss and emotional distress." In an important departure from previous cases, they emphasised addiction rather than health. The cigarette companies had long denied that cigarettes were addictive and no one had been able to prove that they knew otherwise. In this, the Castano lawyers were about to be given a helping hand.

Mr Butts

In April 1994, Henry Waxman, now chairman of the House Subcommittee on Health and Environment, subpoenaed the CEOs of the country's largest cigarette companies and asked them - under oath - if they thought that tobacco was addictive. In a clip endlessly replayed on television, each in turn stood, raised their right hand and said they did not.

In May, Stanton Glantz received a parcel containing 4,000 pages of secret tobacco industry documents from an anonymous source calling himself 'Mr Butts'. Unbeknownst to Glantz, these had been stolen from the offices of Wyatt, Tarrant & Combs, a law firm which represented Brown & Williamson, the makers of the popular mentholated *Kools* brand. The man who stole them, Merrell Williams, had worked for the company in a minor capacity since 1988. The law firm prosecuted

Williams - whose father had smoked *Lucky Strikes* and died of a heart attack - for the theft but neither they nor Brown & Williamson were able to prevent the documents being leaked.

The box of papers sent by Mr Butts contained internal memos, letters and details about research and marketing tactics which showed the tobacco industry had deliberately misled the public for decades. Most relevant to the Castano case was the evidence that at least one senior tobacco industry executive had been acutely aware that cigarettes were addictive as far back as 1963. The documents were also mailed to the *New York Times*' journalist Philip J. Hilts, who published a front-page story which let its readers know, in general terms, what lay in their pages. By the following year, the documents had become so widely distributed that the Supreme Court ruled they could not be suppressed because they were already in the public domain. They appeared on the internet the very next day.

1994 was turning into a miserable year for the cigarette companies and it was not yet summer. On May 23, the state of Mississippi sued the tobacco industry to reclaim hundreds of millions of dollars spent treating patients with smoking related diseases. Two weeks later, the state of West Virginia filed a similar lawsuit and in August, Minnesota went the same way, holding 'Big Tobacco' accountable for failing to admit that nicotine was addictive.

David Kessler then wrote to the Coalition on Smoking or Health to tell them that there was "mounting evidence" that nicotine was addictive. The FDA immediately made this three-page letter public and it kick-started a storm-in-a-teacup controversy. On the face of it, the sudden emphasis on addiction was puzzling. Of all the statements made by the industry to keep itself afloat in the previous forty years, its insistence that cigarettes were not addictive was the least credible.

That tobacco was addictive had been appreciated by Christopher Columbus before the weed had even made it to European shores. Anyone who smoked or knew a smoker could see that it was often a difficult habit to give up. Lennox Johnston had demonstrated tobacco's addictive nature in 1942 and various studies of humans and animals had confirmed his conclusions. The FDA itself had recently approved the nicotine patch, a product which owed its very existence to the addictive power of tobacco, and yet here was the FDA's director writing to the Coalition on Smoking or Health to tell them that there was only "mounting" evidence that nicotine was addictive.

Whether Kessler was naive or feigning naivety is hard to tell. To this day, Kessler maintains that the tobacco industry knew that its products were addictive "long before the FDA" found out. Even if he had only recently noticed that cigarettes had something of a hold over their users, did he really believe that the chairman of the Coalition on Smoking or Health was unaware of this fact? What is certain, however, is that the upcoming class actions had less chance of success if juries believed that the addictive nature of nicotine was a matter of long-standing common knowledge.

Had the tobacco industry been making cigarettes more addictive than natural tobacco? This certainly seemed to be the implication. In March 1995, ABC's *Day One* news programme misrepresented reports about the tobacco industry manipulating nicotine levels by claiming that cigarettes were being 'spiked' to keep smokers hooked. This showed a woeful ignorance about how cigarettes were manufactured. Nicotine was certainly 'manipulated' by the tobacco industry but only insofar as they reduced it. Nicotine levels were lower in cigarettes than in raw tobacco and it was no secret that cigarettes had less tar and nicotine than ever before. The most basic research would have confirmed this. Nicotine yields had been printed on cigarette packs for years and the industry had been lowering tar and nicotine yields since the 1960s.

Philip Morris immediately sued ABC for $10 billion (the age of silly money being demanded by both sides had truly begun) and the network settled out of court for a reported $16 million. The company even gave FDA officials a tour of one of its plants to educate the agency on the cigarette-making process. ABC apologised but the original 'spiking' report garnered far more publicity than the retraction and the belief that tobacco companies added nicotine to tobacco stayed around in the public consciousness for years.

Whether the lawyers bankrupted the tobacco industry or the FDA made its products illegal, the focus on addiction offered anti-smoking activists a new justification for their crusade against smokers. It shook the conventional argument that people had the choice whether or not to smoke and the potential for those who wanted to take the anti-smoking crusade to the next level was enormous. Coercion and force could officially be substituted for persuasion and education. As Iain Gately put it: "Helpless addiction was the best chance the anti-tobacco movement had against the citadel of freedom of choice."[20]

And yet, while nicotine dependence was self-evidently a very significant factor in explaining why many people smoked, it was a stretch to give it as the *sole* explanation for smoking's popularity. Why, if this was the case, did smokers find nicotine gum and nicotine patches so unsatisfying?

Viewing smoking purely as an addiction bolstered the anti-smokers' belief that people only smoked because of peer pressure when teenagers and only continued because they were hooked. Anti-smokers like Kessler began to call smoking a "pediatric disease" which, as Jacob Sullum noted, justified treating smokers like children [21].

The tobacco industry on the ropes

If 1994 was the tobacco industry's *annus horibilis*, 1995 brought no respite. Having received Mr Butts' stolen tobacco documents, Stanton Glantz went into a frenzy of photocopying and teamed up with Dr John Slade, a soft-spoken former GASP president who was the proud owner of a personalised car number plate which read 'NO CIGS.' The pair spent much of 1995 submitting articles to the *Journal of the American Medical Association* (JAMA) which used excerpts from the documents to expose the duplicity of the tobacco industry through its own words. Slade then led the campaign to have nicotine regulated by the government and, in 1995, the FDA finally succeeded in bringing cigarettes under its jurisdiction*. Abolitionism was suddenly in the air.

Hard-liners had never disguised their intention of destroying the tobacco industry but were more cagey when it came to publicly supporting prohibition. And yet, even if prohibition remained a dirty word, why break the tobacco industry of today if another would be allowed to take its place tomorrow? The former president of the American Cancer Society, Dr Benjamin Byrd, had already gone on the record to say he would like to see Congress make cigarettes completely illegal. When smoking was at its height of popularity such a declaration would been tantamount to treason and, for years, even zealots in the ANR had been fearful of being viewed as cranks by demanding the criminalisation of tobacco. Now, with the industry besieged on all sides, prohibition seemed nothing more than the logical conclusion to twenty years of activism.

The Brown & Williamson documents had mobilised popular support. The man in the street could tolerate an industry selling a lethal product but he would not tolerate a liar. Hatred of the tobacco industry rose to a level never before seen. It was not a time for understatement.

---

*This judgement was given by Judge William Osteen who has since been accused of being a tobacco industry sympathiser by anti-smoking groups after he savaged the EPA's secondhand smoke report. The evidence for this rests entirely on his brief employment by a tobacco company in 1974 when he was a private attorney (he was based in North Carolina). His presiding role in the anti-industry FDA decision appears to have been forgotten.

The attorney general of Texas said that "history will record the modern-day tobacco industry alongside the worst of civilisation's evil empires." Stanton Glantz compared the industry to Timothy McVeigh and the *New York Times*' Philip J. Hilts equated industry executives with Nazi concentration camp guards (22). In 1995, *JAMA* dedicated a whole issue to the 'cigarette papers' and concluded that "we should force the removal of this scourge from our nation."(23)

It was in this bilious atmosphere that Philip Morris prepared to defend another huge class action brought by the soon-to-be-crowned king of anti-tobacco lawsuits, Stanley Rosenblatt. Begun in 1991, Rosenblatt was suing the industry on behalf of a woman called Norma Broin and several thousand fellow flight attendants who, he claimed, had suffered as a result of secondhand smoke. Since no court had yet found the tobacco industry culpable for the death of a single smoker, it was ambitious to be suing on the basis of secondhand smoke but Rosenblatt was banking on a jury being more sympathetic to nonsmokers than they had traditionally been to smokers.

Although he stood to earn hundreds of millions of dollars from a guilty verdict, Rosenblatt displayed all the conviction of a dedicated anti-smoking activist when he declared that his ultimate ambition was to "destroy the industry and thereby save millions of lives."(24) Set on bringing the cigarette companies to their knees, he told the press: "This is a crusade, not a lawsuit!"(25)

The tobacco industry was hovering inches from destruction but if it went, what would follow it? Stanton Glantz envisioned a state-owned tobacco industry manufacturing what he called "plain cigarettes" with reduced nicotine content and bland packaging (26). He, at least, seemed to take into account the obvious problems of smuggling, organised crime, lawlessness and contempt for the law that his own grandfather would have remembered from Prohibition days.

But Glantz's dream of nationalising the industry - and even then, he said, only for the last generation of die-hard smokers - was never a realistic proposition in the US. State ownership of the tobacco industry would make the government liable to criticism from an anti-smoking movement which would never disperse and, more importantly, it would leave itself open to the massive class actions that the Clinton administration had itself encouraged. The government had no desire to get into bed with the world's most hated industry and it is doubtful whether politicians ever seriously entertained the idea.

Prohibition was even less workable. Even if the American government could outlaw tobacco production, the rest of the world would only buy its tobacco elsewhere and it would take a Herculean effort of law enforcement to prevent cigarettes being brought in from Canada or Central America by newly enriched organised criminals. The government would not let prohibition happen.

Endgame

The huge, unwieldy Castano case collapsed in 1995, a victim of its own monumental ambition, but there was no respite for the tobacco industry. With the Brown & Williamson documents in the public domain, the company's former research director, Jeff Wigand, came in from the cold to testify that his former employers had known cigarettes to be addictive. Sacked for "poor communication skills," Wigand proved himself an able communicator when he appeared on CBS's *60 Minutes* television show to tell the American public that Brown & Williamson executives were liars (a story later played out to millions more in the Hollywood movie *The Insider*).

Once its private memos appeared on the internet for all to see, it was only a matter of time before Brown & Williamson lost a personal injury suit. The moment came in Jacksonville, Florida, where a jury found the company liable for the lung cancer of Grady Carter, a man who had smoked for 44 years. The jury found for the plaintiff on the basis that American Tobacco (which was now owned by Brown & Williamson) had not told him that *Lucky Strikes* were addictive. Disgusted by the tobacco industry's duplicitous and Machiavellian behaviour, the jury admitted that the leaked memos had been an influence on a case which otherwise had no more chance of winning than previous liability suits. "We wanted to send a message to the tobacco companies," said one juror: "We ain't gonna take it no more."(27) The court awarded $750,000 to Grady Carter and his wife but, once again, the decision to compensate the plaintiff was reversed on appeal. The killer blow had yet to be delivered.

Nonetheless, the tobacco industry was surviving by the skin of its teeth and it knew its hour was at hand. Massachusetts became the tenth state to launch a massive legal action against it for conspiracy to "mislead, deceive and confuse" its residents. Florida's governor Lawton Chiles made doubly sure of a successful outcome for his own state's class action by stripping the tobacco industry of its defence with the Medicaid Third-Party Responsibility Act. This new law held manufacturers responsible for *any* harm their products caused, regardless of the known risks, and did not hold the individual at fault even if he admitted to being primarily responsible for the damage done. Furthermore, prosecutors would no longer have to show harm to individuals; aggregated statistics would suffice.

The Medicaid Third-Party Responsibility Act was passed with the sole purpose of bringing down the tobacco industry but the implications of such a law naturally worried the business community since it left them liable to lawsuits for any idiotic misuse of almost any product. To calm their fears, Chiles issued a statement assuring them that the law would only be used against cigarette companies; a remarkable admission to come from a legislator and a clear affront to the rule of law. The Act was patently unjust and Florida's Supreme Court said it was "completely arbitrary" and "violate[d] due process" when it overruled it a year later (28). Undeterred, Chiles used his powers as governor to force the Act through and, as a result, won the state of Florida $11 billion in compensation from the tobacco industry.

With the writing on the wall, Liggett & Myers was the first to crack. In March 1996, the company conceded that cigarette smoking caused lung cancer, heart disease and emphysema. Over the next twelve months it settled with 27 states and paid billions in reparations. By the time it had paid out, it was common knowledge that RJ Reynolds and Philip Morris were discussing terms with Attorneys General about coming to a similar settlement.

Hard-liners in the anti-smoking movement were vehemently

opposed to any deal. They believed that, given time, the class actions would overwhelm the industry and that cigarette companies should not be given any protection from future actions. But the US government wanted the industry's money, not its destruction. In any case, even if the private lawsuits succeeded - and they had all failed so far - future court cases would benefit individuals rather than the state.

By June 1997, all the tobacco companies had agreed to a deal known as the Master Settlement Agreement (MSA), and the Senate held hearings on how much the industry should pay the state by way of compensation. The government bandied around a figure of $368.5 billion but even this colossal sum fell short of what anti-smoking groups demanded. ASH testified to say that, on the basis of smoking's supposed $100 billion a year cost to the country, the industry owed $20 trillion ($20,000,000,000,000,000)(29).

Ultimately, the settlement amounted to $246 billion to be paid over 25 years, including the $40 billion that had already been secured by four states which had already sued. In exchange, the industry would be protected from liability suits, including those made by state and federal governments, and the FDA was prevented from tampering with nicotine levels in cigarettes until 2009. The industry was obliged to cease billboard advertising, close down the Tobacco Institute and release 45 million pages of previously unseen documents. Additionally they had to admit publicly that cigarettes caused lung cancer and several other diseases and place warnings on packs saying, for the first time, 'Smoking is Addictive.'

The Master Settlement Agreement set the industry the target of reducing underage smoking by 30% within five years, 50% within seven years and 60% within ten years and further financial penalties would follow if these targets were not reached. For the legions of anti-smoking groups who would soon be enjoying the spoils of the settlement, this was money in the bank. Forty years of campaigning had done little to reduce teenage smoking and there was no expectation that the tobacco industry - without any legal authority or powers at its disposal - would be able to halve it in the space of a decade.

The MSA turned the financial affairs of the anti-smoking movement upside down. $1.45 billion went to the newly formed

American Legacy Foundation which, with a $250 million grant in its first year, became the wealthiest anti-smoking organisation in history, and a further $500 million a year was put aside for anti-smoking and stop-smoking campaigns. While cigarette companies continued to make hefty profits, they were now the David to the anti-smoking industry's Goliath. For every pack of cigarettes sold at $3.50 the government received $1.61 in tax; the cigarette companies made 28 cents (30).

The Master Settlement Agreement was, by a wide margin, the largest compensation pay-out of all time. The tobacco giants had to own up to being systematic liars while simultaneously handing over billions of dollars to anti-smoking groups who would spend every cent trying to grind them into the dust.

It was not enough for Stanton Glantz who wrote an article for the *Los Angeles Times* with the self-explanatory title 'What deal? We got suckered,' nor did it satisfy the equally zealous Ahron Leichtman of Citizens for a Tobacco Free Society who began a campaign called 'No immunity to kill with impunity.' The lawyers involved were criticised for making so much money out of the deal by, of all people, ASH's John Banzhaf, and the Advisory Committee on Tobacco Policy and Public Health said that the target of reducing underage smoking by 60% was a let down and should have been raised to 100%. Banzhaf agreed, claiming that the tobacco companies could reduce underage smoking to "any level they want" by "raising taxes," a facile and naive comment which suggested the tobacco industry could do something that successive governments, and organisations like ASH, had conspicuously failed to.

If anti-smoking groups were not happy with the Master Settlement Agreement - and many of them clearly were not - they should have been, for while it left the tobacco industry still breathing, it was battered, bruised and too cowed to adequately fight the battle over passive smoking that was coming to a head. The settlement never threatened to bankrupt the cigarette companies. Decades of ever-rising taxation on cigarettes had shown the ability of consumers to absorb price rises, and the costs of the settlement were swiftly passed on to smokers. Financially intact, the industry was nonetheless humiliated and disgraced and was still licking its wounds when laws were passed around the world that reflected the new zero-tolerance policy towards smokers.

CHAPTER NINE

'I have a comic book mentality'

For the ground troops of the anti-tobacco war, the next achievable objective was to get rid of smoking areas from restaurants. There was even talk of extending smoking bans to that last refuge of the smoker: public bars. This upped the ante considerably, taking the battle out of the workplace and into recreational settings. Previous anti-smoking laws had never defined bars and clubs as public places for the very good reason that they were privately owned. Smokers had accepted smoking restrictions in their offices, believing there to be an unspoken agreement that their social life would be unaffected. Now, said the anti-smokers, bars were both public places and workplaces and those within them should be protected from secondhand smoke.

There was, if anything, even less evidence of passive smoking being harmful to nonsmokers in the workplace than there was of it being a health hazard in the home. While the EPA was constructing its 1992 report, two large US studies - both funded by the National Cancer Institute - found that exposure to passive smoke in the workplace was no threat to nonsmokers (1). In fact, no epidemiological study had ever found any statistical link between lung cancer and secondhand smoke in social settings (or the workplace). Statistically non-significant associations abounded but with very mixed results. Five had shown an increase in risk but six showed a reduction.

The evidence could not have been more flimsy but a new ordinance was proposed in California all the same. Named - none too poetically - AB13, it would criminalise smoking throughout all bars, restaurants and offices. The passive smoking theory could tenuously be used to justify much of this law on the basis of workers' health and safety, albeit only if one first accepted that people had no choice over where they worked. Where AB13 broke new ground was in demanding that smoking rooms also be consigned to the dustbin of history. Since nonsmokers had no reason to be in smoking rooms and every opportunity to avoid them, a new rationale was required and Americans for Nonsmokers' Rights began to shake off its origins as a nonsmokers' rights group and talked more openly about forcing smokers to do what they thought was best for them.

The 'denormalisation' programme was entering its next phase. Stanton Glantz talked about destroying the "social support network" that normalised smoking, a network he described as something "the tobacco industry had spent decades and billions of dollars building."(2) This was palpable nonsense. In so far as such a network existed at all, it was one that predated the tobacco industry by centuries. People had been smoking freely in social surroundings since tobacco was discovered. Permission to smoke had always been granted or withheld by the host and, by demanding that the government override the rights of proprietors to set their own rules, the anti-smokers were not returning to a mythical age that predated Philip Morris but were removing a right that had been implicit in society since time immemorial.

Glantz's sworn enemies in the tobacco industry knew they stood to lose money if AB13 was enacted and they responded by bringing Proposition 188 before the Californian electorate. In other countries, or in other times, Prop 188 would have been considered a draconian anti-smoking measure but in California in the mid-1990s it was nothing more than a damage limitation exercise. Prop 188 mandated nonsmoking areas in all buildings but also made the provision of smoking areas a legal right that could not be removed by local ordinances.

To promote Prop 188, Philip Morris formed Californians for Statewide Smoking Restrictions and funded it to the tune of $9 million. This sum was dwarfed by the Prop 99 funds available to California's anti-smoking organisations who created another group - Bar and Restaurant Employees Against Tobacco Hazards (BREATH) - to fight the industry's spoiler law. The tables were turned on the tobacco industry. It had been reduced to campaigning for a far-reaching smoking ban - admittedly the lesser of two evils - and was financially outgunned by people who had adopted its old tactic of forming front groups. As if that were not bad enough, they were using the industry's own money to do it. In a private memo, RJ Reynolds executive Tim Hyde accepted that the industry was bailing water out of a sinking ship: "Even if we should win," he wrote, "it doesn't solve the problem. The real problem is the hundreds of millions that the other side have in Prop 99 money to fight us."(3)

The battle over Prop 188 was fought in terms that appealed to Glantz and Americans for Nonsmokers' Rights - a pitched battle between themselves and the tobacco industry. After the Brown & Williamson documents came to light, disgust at the industry became the movement's trump card and the Coalition for a Healthy California adopted the pithy 'Stop Philip Morris' as its campaign slogan. Supporters of AB13 urged voters to "tell the tobacco industry to butt out of California" and their television commercials put the tobacco industry centre-stage.

The anti-industry sentiment was in keeping with a wider anti-smoking advertising campaign that had been launched with $200 million from the Prop 99 treasure-chest. Describing these commercials, in which he and the ANR had a hand, Glantz said: "Far from running a traditional 'smoking will kill you' campaign, the Californian effort viewed tobacco as a social and political problem and went after the tobacco industry directly and aggressively."(4) This was true enough. One proposed advert parodied the Marlboro Man by showing a cowboy lassoing a frightened child, dragging him across the ground and branding him - lest the point be missed - with the words 'Tobacco Industry'(5). Another showed footage from the Waxman hearings in which the CEOs of the big six tobacco companies testified that they did not believe nicotine to be addictive. The words 'under oath' were repeated again and again by a voice which, at the end, added: "Now the tobacco industry is trying to tell us that secondhand smoke isn't dangerous. Do they think we're stupid?"(6)

Such advertisements were emphatically not part of a "traditional 'smoking will kill you' campaign," in fact they provided no health information of any kind. Denigrating the enemy rather than addressing the issue, the 'Under Oath' commercial was the very definition of an *ad hominem* attack and it resulted in RJ Reynolds swiftly threatening legal action. The commercial was withdrawn before the end of its scheduled run, as was the cowboy ad.

When, in other commercials, medical or scientific data was presented, it was usually wildly exaggerated. One radio ad, entitled 'Save a Waitress', began: "Hi, I've been a bartender for a long time. When I worked in a smoky bar, it was like smoking a pack of cigarettes a day..."(7)

Using taxpayers' money to vent spleen against the tobacco industry was no doubt satisfying for many within the anti-smoking movement but it was not necessarily the best way to persuade smokers to give up cigarettes. Of all the reasons people gave for why they smoked, admiration for cigarette companies tended to feature low in the list. Commercials which showed cackling tobacco executives in darkened rooms plotting to hook children on cigarettes (another ad from the same period) were more valuable as tools for appealing to nonsmokers than to smokers. The cigarette firms naturally disputed the passive smoking theory and, from a scientific point of view, were often speaking from a position of strength. But by reminding the public that they had lied in the past, the new wave of television adverts sought to persuade them that secondhand smoke must be deadly simply because 'Big Tobacco' said it was not. This was no accident. *Ad hominem* attacks on the industry were explicitly part of the anti-smokers' strategy, as Michael Siegel, a senior figure in Americans for Nonsmokers' Rights, told fellow activists:

> "Do not get into arguments with the industry about the scientific evidence. This is exactly what the industry wants... Instead, the best approach is to expose the tobacco industry ties of the so-called scientists making the arguments."(8)

Consequently, anti-smoking activists never sought a debate about the sketchy evidence for the passive smoking theory, and while insults and insinuation helped to shield them from answering awkward questions, it was a facile and intellectually stifling response. It was, however, highly effective. The industry-sponsored Prop 188 was defeated by 71% to 29% in November 1994 and AB13 was allowed to prevail. Of those who voted against Prop 188, 22% said that their main reason for doing so was "because it was sponsored by the tobacco industry." Only 38% put it down to a desire to "protect smoke-free public places."(9) All workplaces in California were made smoke-free in 1995 and smoking rooms were banned. On January 1 1998, smoking in bars and clubs also became a criminal offence.

Good versus evil

After the controversial television advertisements, California's governor Pete Wilson began to divert Prop 99 money away from denormalisation and anti-industry projects, and instead spent $5.7 million on smoking cessation programmes. A third of Prop 99 money was spent on research, medical care and stop-smoking campaigns. For Glantz and the ANR, such efforts were secondary to the main task of vilifying, ridiculing and attacking Big Tobacco and Wilson now assumed the role of villain. Almost from the day it was passed, Prop 99 had been a source of in-fighting between what Glantz called the "health groups" (the anti-smoking activists) and the "medical groups" (the doctors), with the latter preferring to treat the sick rather than tend to the healthy. Americans for Nonsmokers' Rights considered the mainstream health organisations too timid to adequately tackle the smoking issue and were openly resentful towards the Californian Medical Association when it requested Prop 99 funds be used on medical treatment (10).

This enmity first came to the surface in 1989 when $20 million (of the $600 million available from Prop 99) was spent on the Child Health and Disability Prevention Program, an unarguably worthwhile project which screened young children for diseases. Glantz, who had a lifelong tendency to assume that anyone who disagreed with him was linked to the tobacco industry, once again sensed the invisible hand of Big Tobacco. In his book *Tobacco War*, he wrote of "the tobacco industry and its allies among the medical service providers"(11) in reference to the Californian Medical Association. In 1996, the ANR accused Governor Wilson and Steve Thompson of the Californian Medical Association of being "tobacco industry heroes" and ran newspaper adverts showing them in a "Hall of Shame."

The ANR then sued Wilson to reclaim money that had been "improperly used" for "health screening and immunisations of poor children and prenatal care for poor women who are pregnant."(12) Having found an easy source of revenue, the California State government raised cigarette taxes by a further two cents a pack in 1994 to pay for breast cancer care and by another 50 cents in 1998 for 'early childhood development.'

Bringing down the tobacco industry was becoming such a dominant theme in the American anti-smoking crusade that the battle against lung cancer almost seemed to take a back seat. Tobacco control policies were commended as much for the effect they would have on industry profits as the effect they would have on the public's health. "Raising tobacco taxes is our number one strategy to damage the tobacco industry," announced the American Cancer Society in 1997(13). The image of the industry as a demonic entity reinforced the anti-smokers' view of themselves as saviours. Seldom accused of lacking faith in their own righteousness, anti-smoking activists saw their fight more than ever as a battle between good and evil.

The alternative viewpoint - that one could be disgusted by the tobacco industry's behaviour while defending people's right to smoke - was never entertained. The battle-lines were drawn and smokers themselves became irrelevant except as statistics by which both sides could keep score. The industry were murderers, tobacco was evil, smokers were weak-minded slaves, and anti-smokers were their emancipators. To quote Joseph Cherner, of Smoke-free Educational Services:

> "It's the only issue I know of where there aren't two sides - two intelligent sides.
> I have a comic-book mentality - I grew up with comic books -
> and I see this as good versus evil."(14)

The debate over what to do about tobacco was therefore only open to those with fierce anti-smoking views whose opinions differed by the smallest of degrees. The belief in an all-powerful tobacco industry helped the anti-smoking lobby to see themselves as underdog heroes fighting a six-headed beast and, because they were so obviously in the right, any dissenters must be recipients of tobacco money.

Since those who disagreed with their increasingly illiberal agenda numbered in the millions, a grand conspiracy was required. A form of paranoid McCarthyism emerged, dragging in not just cigarette companies and tobacco farmers but legions of politicians, social commentators, restaurant owners, bar owners, hoteliers, journalists, civil rights groups and anyone who had ever worked for the tobacco industry or its suppliers, especially if they happened to be smokers themselves.

Seeing the influence of the industry behind any dissenting voice was nothing new in the history of anti-smoking. During the 1857 *Lancet* controversy, those who wrote to the journal to defend smoking were frequently accused of being in the pay of tobacco companies. Smokers were expected to resist anti-smoking measures because they were addicts and the tobacco industry was expected to resist for obvious financial reasons; the views of both could therefore be dismissed out of hand. It was those who neither smoked nor worked for tobacco companies, but still spoke out in favour of smokers' rights, who were the baffling anomalies and the anti-smokers went to great lengths to impugn their motives, painstakingly searching for their names in the millions of pages of tobacco industry documents now available online.

These names included British writers like Sean Gabb, Tim Luckhurst and Chris Tame. The latter was the founder of the civil rights group, the Libertarian Alliance and had never been a smoker, did not care for smoking and would not allow smoking in his home but was nonetheless director of the smokers' rights group the Freedom Organisation for the Right to Enjoy Smoking Tobacco (FOREST).

In the US, the journalist Jacob Sullum was an eloquent critic of the excesses of the anti-smoking movement and, in 1994, drew attention to the inadequacies of the EPA report on secondhand smoke in an article for *The Wall Street Journal*. Sullum had never received a cent from the tobacco industry but when RJ Reynolds reprinted the article in a newspaper advertisement under the apt heading 'If we said it, you might not believe it,' Sullum was given $5,000 in reprint fees and the anti-smokers were given a stick with which to beat him. Appearing in a television debate with John Banzhaf, the ASH founder attempted to undermine Sullum by announcing: "We also want to tell the folks out there that you're in the pay of the tobacco industry."(15)

When Stanton Glantz* and John Slade put together a compendium of the juiciest excerpts from the Brown & Williamson documents - *The Cigarette Papers* - they attacked Sullum as a tobacco industry stooge on the basis of this $5,000 royalty and, still more tenuously, a $10,000 donation Philip Morris had once given one of his employers. In their narrative, Glantz and Slade recounted a story from the 1950s in which the tobacco industry paid a journalist to write a sympathetic piece and then, breaking free of their chronology, introduced Sullum under the heading 'Using the same technique in the 1990s.' The reader was thereby led to believe that receiving reprint fees for an article written without contact with the tobacco industry was no different from being an industry hired hand, and that questioning the passive smoking theory was no different from disputing the link between smoking and lung cancer (16).

When two journalists wrote an article questioning the validity of the ever-escalating estimates of deaths attributed to smoking, the ANR's Michael Siegel responded by stating: "These authors have strong connections to the tobacco industry." This was simply untrue and after the journalists responded with a thinly veiled threat of legal action, Siegel was forced to apologise and withdraw the accusation (17).

The same tactics were used against many others, including people as transparently untainted by tobacco money as Martha Perske, an illustrator from Connecticut who found that the more she read about passive smoking, the more sceptical she became. Acting as a lone, unpaid

---

*In 'Achieving a Smokefree Society' (1987) Glantz insisted that: "The only significant organized opposition to legislation protecting nonsmokers that has ever appeared is sponsored by the tobacco industry...The primary goal should be to isolate the tobacco companies as the only real opposition and to persuade legislators that if they oppose clean air measures their constituents will perceive them as dupes of the tobacco companies. To this end, keep talking about the tobacco companies and their involvement, even if the specific arrangements they have made are not clear."

researcher, she digested the medical journals and wrote a sharp critique of a paper Siegel himself had written on the subject of secondhand smoke in the workplace (18). Americans for Nonsmokers' Rights responded with an article in the *American Journal of Public Health* which strongly implied that Perske was an industry mole and that "industry documents show that she stayed in close contact with Philip Morris."(19)

None of this was true and ten years later, by which time Siegel had begun to part ways with the hard-liners in the ANR, he spoke out about how the group instinctively reacted to criticism:

"In the 20 years that I was a member of the tobacco control movement,
I was led to believe that there were only two sides to any anti-smoking issue:
our side and the tobacco industry side. Therefore, anyone who disagreed with our
position had to be, in some way, affiliated with the tobacco industry.
I was also taught to respond to their arguments not on any scientific grounds
or on the merit of their arguments, but by simply discrediting
the person by attacking their affiliation with the tobacco companies."(20)

Siegel has since made his peace with Perske and has apologised for the way the ANR belittled and slandered her work. He now accepts that she never had any connection with the tobacco industry and that her work was "tremendously well-researched, meticulous, and precise... I am sorry to have been a part of a movement that treated her in the way that it did."(21)

A kind of philanthropy

Already flushed with wealth as a result of the Master Settlement Agreement, the anti-smokers' rags to riches story was completed when the manufacturers of nicotine replacement drugs began offering their own contributions. General Robert Johnson, the entrepreneur behind the pharmaceutical giant Johnson & Johnson, had died in 1968 leaving a legacy of $1.2 billion to be used for good causes through the aegis of the Robert Wood Johnson Foundation (RWJF). This philanthropic body received the lion's share of its income from Johnson & Johnson, and in the early 1990s, it began donating heavily to the anti-smoking cause.

RWJF was not wholly without a financial motive for pouring hundreds of millions of dollars into the campaign to create a smoke-free world. The nicotine patch had been developed in the 1980s at Duke University, the seat of learning named after the tobacco tycoon Buck Duke. It appeared in commercial form as *Nicotrol*, manufactured by Pfizer and Pharmacia, and marketed by Johnson & Johnson. As its principle benefactor, what was good for Johnson & Johnson was good for RWJF and vice versa. Smoking bans, the demonisation of the tobacco industry and higher cigarette prices were manifestly very good for any seller of alternative sources of nicotine.

In 1991, the FDA approved the sale of nicotine patches on prescription, thereby putting them on the market for the first time. Coincidentally, and also for the first time, the benevolent RWJF began funding anti-smoking projects on a grand scale, including a $10 million grant to fund a campaign to raise the price of cigarettes (22).

In 1996, the FDA approved the over-the-counter sale of nicotine patches and before the year was out, RWJF had announced the opening of the Center for Tobacco-Free Kids, which it would go on to fund to the tune of $84 million. Endowed with a name that strongly implied a remit of educating minors and reducing juvenile smoking - causes few would argue with - much of its money was immediately funnelled into organisations that were building a case for draconian laws to prevent consenting adults from smoking. A $60,000 grant to the Centre for Tobacco Free Kids, for example, trickled down to Project Rolling Thunder, a scheme run by Arizonans Concerned About Smoking to campaign for total indoor smoking bans. By 2005, RWJF was giving the Tobacco Free Kids Action Fund over $200,000 for "legal support for intervention in the Department of Justice tobacco suit" and Minnesota's Tobacco Law Center was provided with $250,000 for "legal technical assistance to the tobacco control community." (23)

Other projects were more obscure but not a stone went unturned. Stanton Glantz's stomping ground at the University of California was given $48,243 for the sole purpose of analysing smoking behaviour "among female nurses." The Lesbian Community Cancer Project was given $50,000 to pay for "lesbian, gay, bisexual and transgender advocates for a smoke-free Chicago" and a further $50,000 was awarded to promote "smoke-free workplace policies among Latino-owned businesses" in Seattle (24).

As smoke-free laws swept through America, Johnson & Johnson's competitors began to make generous, tax-deductible contributions to the anti-smoking cause and, by the end of the decade, Glaxo Wellcome, Pfizer and Pharmacia - the makers and/or distributors of rival smoking-cessation drugs like *Nicoderm*, *Zyban* and *Nicorette* - were all fully paid-up members of the World Health Organisation's Tobacco Free Initiative. Glaxo paid the American Cancer Society $1,000,000 a year for the use of the ACS logo on their nicotine replacement drugs and when the Canadian Cancer Society produced *One Step at a Time*, a booklet of stop-smoking tips (25), it was *Nicorette* manufacturer Pfizer who paid the bills.

When Pfizer and the recently merged GlaxoSmithKline helped finance the Smokefree Europe conference they both chose not to put up advertising boards to promote themselves (26). This was rather odd behaviour considering that they had both paid large sums to sponsor the event, but perhaps the creation of a rally to fight the suppliers of 'conventional nicotine products' was reward in itself. Glaxo and Pfizer also part-funded the Institute for Global Tobacco Control and when the 11th World Conference on Tobacco came to Chicago in 2000, RWJF - having paid $4,000,000 towards the event - was listed alongside the American Cancer Society and the American Medical Association as one of the three hosts. Glaxo Wellcome, Pharmacia and SmithKline Beecham all contributed as patrons.

The anti-smokers had found themselves a powerful new ally.

CHAPTER TEN

'Do not let them fool you'

The 1990s had seen the most draconian anti-tobacco policies since the days of the Anti-Cigarette League and yet the US smoking rate stubbornly refused to recede. At the start of the decade, 25.5% of the US population smoked and David Krogh, writing in 1991, predicted that this would fall to 22% by the end of the millennium. In fact, despite all the smoking bans, tax hikes and anti-smoking commercials, the smoking rate rose to 28%. The surge in teen smoking was particularly dramatic. Between 1991 and 1997, the smoking rate for high school students rose from 27.5% to 36.4% (2). Far from reviewing its policies of denormalisation, segregation and stigmatisation, the anti-smoking lobby called for more of the same.

It had been hoped that the millions spent educating children about the dangers of cigarettes would be enough to virtually eliminate teenage smoking and ultimately bring about a smoke-free world. The educated classes had been the first to give up smoking and there was an assumption that if the rest of society had access to accurate information about the risks of smoking, mass abstinence would ensue. And indeed millions of smokers had quit. Per capita cigarette consumption in the US and much of Europe was halved between 1950 and 1970 (2) but while education had a powerful effect on smoking behaviour, it had not eliminated the habit, and it did not seem likely that it ever would.

Ignorance was no longer an excuse. A 1974 study found that 99.2% of 7-8 year olds believed smoking caused cancer, rising to 100% for the 10-11 age group, and three quarters of them believed cigarettes to be addictive (3). By 1990, these youngsters were in their mid-twenties and many had become parents themselves, and yet smoking prevalence was at 25.5% and rising.

It was no longer tenable to argue that people smoked because they did not understand the risks. An assessment by the economist W. Kip Viscusi found that the public had responded to thirty years of anti-smoking messages by hugely overestimating the risks of tobacco use. The scientific consensus was that around 5-10% of lifelong smokers would die of lung cancer but the American public believed, on average, that 38% of smokers would suffer that fate. While smokers tended to give a lower estimate (31%) than nonsmokers (42%), both groups had an exaggerated perception of the risks (4).

This was not so surprising. State-funded public health campaigns often lead people to believe that they are at greater risk than they really are. The UK's AIDS awareness campaign, for example, created a panic about HIV in heterosexuals that was grossly disproportionate to the actual threat (there were only 171 such cases in 15 years)(5). Similarly, heavy news coverage of dramatic incidents such as aeroplane accidents, terrorist attacks and child murders produce an exaggerated fear of what are, in reality, very rare events. Lung cancer and heart disease are significantly less rare, of course, but with an understanding of how people adapt their behaviour by balancing perceived hazards against perceived benefits, Viscusi estimated that if the public had a true understanding of the hazards of smoking, the smoking rate would *rise* by 7.5%.

For public health campaigners, smoking had no benefits and so there was no trade-off to be made. In any case, they did not consider the indulgence of a few unhealthy pleasures to be worth the possible sacrifice of a few years of existence in old age. Nor did they judge the success of anti-smoking programmes by how well they informed the public about risky decisions. The only criteria was how many people gave up smoking. That over a billion smokers worldwide continued to take what tobacco's enemies emphatically saw as the wrong option seemed incomprehensible, even insane, but health education was only one tool and if it was insufficient to build a smoke-free society, there were other options available.

"We may have gotten down to the hard core of smokers," said John Banzhaf in 1994, when the *New York Times* reported that the decline in smoking had bottomed out. "Others who smoked but were not addicted, or had mild addictions, may all have quit by now. And the only people left are those who are addicted so heavily that it will take much more than education to allow them to quit."(6) Having tried the carrot, the anti-smokers would now use the stick.

Getting serious

The shift from persuasion to coercion was resonant of America's 19th century crusade against alcohol. Long before Carry Nation and Lucy Page Gaston were born, there existed a temperance movement which successfully campaigned for sobriety using nothing more than moral suasion. It came about in the 1820s, when Americans were drinking an average of 7 gallons of pure alcohol a year. Through a combination of education and evangelism, the temperance movement helped to reduce per capita consumption to 3 gallons in the space of just ten years. By 1850, this had dropped to 2 gallons - around the same as US consumption today. It was a spectacular example of a popular reform movement moderating the habits of a nation and it was achieved without the passage of a single law. But success bred militancy. Having started by campaigning against hard liquor, the temperance crusaders began to rail against all forms of alcohol and petitioned lawmakers for total prohibition. Maine was the first state do go 'dry' in 1851 and it was followed a year later by a further 13 states. These included Minnesota, New York, Massachusetts, Connecticut and Ohio and several other East Coast states (7).

That all of these states would also be first off the mark to ban smoking in public places in the next century is not the only parallel between the two crusades. Just as alcohol consumption dropped dramatically between 1830 and 1850, smoking prevalence in the US halved between 1950 and 1970, at a time when there were no smoking bans, no 'denormalisation' programmes, indeed no anti-smoking laws of any kind other than the late introduction of a rather tame warning label on cigarette packs. Militant anti-smoking groups emerged only *after* this unprecedented fall in tobacco consumption had taken place but once they arrived, the political lobbying began and the educational programmes took a back seat. An absolutist mentality developed which dictated that the battle be fought until the last smoker threw away his cigarettes. Prohibition became the ultimate aim.

In the late 1990s, traditional methods of tobacco control were shed in favour of more aggressive tactics. Simon Chapman of ASH (Australia) argued that stop-smoking clinics should be closed down [8] and Stanton Glantz even recommended that efforts to stop young people buying cigarettes be abandoned [9] along with plans to prosecute minors caught in possession of tobacco, albeit on the somewhat predictable premise that: "The real problem is the cigarette companies."[10] In their place came further smoking bans and the whole-hearted adoption of the denormalisation campaign. Anti-smoking advertising completed its transition into anti-*smoker* advertising when it began portraying smokers as smelly, unattractive inadequates with slogans like 'If you smoke, you stink.'

This, said the anti-smokers, was the most effective way of reducing teen smoking. Adults did not always agree. When hundreds of advertisements were put up in the state of Ohio showing a smoker next to the slogan 'Welcome to LOSERVILLE. Population: YOU,' objections came less from smokers than from the local tourist industry which felt that visitors might be put off since the most prominent billboard was positioned outside the local airport.

In New York, an advert showed a smouldering cigarette alongside the words 'If you can smell it, it may be killing you.' On a Californian billboard, a woman responded to the familiar request "Mind if I smoke?" with the words "Care if I die?" Such campaigns served mainly to cement the passive smoking theory in the minds of the public and, in contrast to earlier quit-smoking adverts, were not really aimed at smokers at all. Demonising the tobacco industry and accusing smokers of manslaughter did little to persuade smokers to give up and Stanton Glantz readily admitted that their function was to "enlist" nonsmokers in the cause [11].

With all eyes on California, far reaching anti-smoking legislation was being pencilled in by governments around the world. The Californian smoking ban may have been swung more by emotion than science but two of the largest studies ever carried out into secondhand smoke were expected to produce the killer proof that would end debate on the passive smoking issue for good.

The World Health Organisation passive smoking study

The World Health Organisation commissioned France's International Agency for Research on Cancer (IARC) to carry out a huge Europe-wide study of the effects of passive smoking. It was eagerly awaited, according to the International Epidemiology Institute, "because of the size of the study, the special attempts to minimise misclassification of cigarette smoking status and the ability to control for various potential confounding factors."[12] With 1,008 female lung cancer cases to interview, the sample group was twice as large as in any study to date and no one was in any doubt about the importance of the report, including tobacco executives who made plans to challenge it in the event that it condemned secondhand smoke as a hazard. They considered this to be the most likely outcome after finding out that the IARC's director was a "'fervent antismoker' who believe[d] that 'passive smoking is more dangerous than active smoking.'"[13]

By March 1998 the study had been completed and written up but it remained unreleased, and speculation arose that the results did not support the WHO's view of secondhand smoke as a genuine health threat. This suspicion was heightened when The *Sunday Telegraph* found a summary of the results buried in an internal WHO report. On March 8, the newspaper published an article revealing that the IARC had found no statistically significant elevation in risk for those exposed to secondhand smoke as adults and found a statistically significant *reduction* in risk for those exposed in childhood. Carrying the headline 'Passive smoking doesn't cause cancer - official,' the article not only reported the lack of association but, referring to the data on childhood exposure, suggested that passive smoking "might even have a protective effect." This sent anti-smoking groups into a frenzy but what was good for the goose was good for the gander. For years, they had used weak, non-significant associations to 'prove' the passive smoking theory but were now left in the position of having to dismiss a statistically significant risk reduction of 22% for children while promoting a smaller and statistically insignificant risk elevation of 11% for the wives of smokers (14).

The usual personal insults were dished out to The *Sunday Telegraph* journalists who had reported the story. The British Medical Association labelled them "mesmerised hacks" while an apoplectic ASH (UK) called them "dupes of the tobacco industry."(15) ASH filed complaints with the Press Complaints Commission about both the article and the accompanying editorial (titled 'Setback for Nanny'). Neither complaint was upheld.

The WHO then intervened itself, issuing a press release headlined 'Passive smoking does cause lung cancer. Do not let them fool you.' despite the fact that its flagship study had shown no such thing. Stanton Glantz searched for tobacco industry involvement but, finding none, rather desperately lamented the fact that people focused on the lower confidence interval when they could focus on the higher one, and implied that the whole concept of statistical significance was some sort of tobacco industry trick.

The medical journals were more circumspect. *The Lancet* accepted that the study provided evidence of a link between secondhand smoke and lung cancer risk which was "tenuous at best" (16) but fell back on the earlier pronouncements of the Environmental Protection Agency and Surgeon General. Suddenly one of the most thorough studies ever carried out into Environmental Tobacco Smoke (ETS) was "too small to show statistically significant differences" and "underpowered."(17)

If it did nothing else, the IARC study ended all talk of ETS posing any more than a very modest risk to nonsmokers. It seemed a long time since Hirayama had speculated about secondhand smoke doubling nonsmokers' chance of getting lung cancer. For the time being, the anti-smokers were put on the back foot and instead of predicting evidence of higher and higher risks from ETS, they worked to protect the credibility of lower, insignificant and/or meta-analysed figures of under 1.30. Even in this, they referred back to smaller studies which had not made "special attempts" to minimise smoker misclassification nor had the "ability to control" for confounding factors.

Britain's own version of the EPA report, conducted by the Scientific Committee On Tobacco or Health (SCOTH), came out a week later and diverted attention away from the World Health Organisation's embarrassment. Timed to coincide with National No Smoking Day, the report was never likely to contain many surprises. A similar endeavour had recently been carried out in Australia where secondhand smoke was officially denounced as a major cause of lung cancer on the basis that it killed 11 nonsmokers a year (in a country of 19,000,000 people) (18).

A dress rehearsal for the British version had been performed in the pages of the *British Medical Journal* a year earlier. Under the stewardship of Professor Nicholas Wald, the journal had collated the evidence to date and concluded that secondhand smoke exposure resulted in a 1.26 (26%) increased risk of lung cancer. After reading that report, the Swedish toxicologist Dr Robert Nilsson suggested that the *BMJ* must be "innocent of epidemiology" to have published it, but with the Wald meta-analysis forming the basis of the SCOTH report there was little doubt that the committee would reach similar conclusions. Sure enough, it announced that passive exposure to tobacco smoke increased lung cancer risk by 24% and heart disease risk by 25% (relative risks of 1.24 and 1.25, respectively). The SCOTH report inspired some newspapers to tell their readers that 300 Britons were dying each year as a result of passive smoking (19) and so gave anti-smokers something to smile about after the shock of the IARC study. But there was more trouble in store.

Enstrom & Kabat

The IARC study had been the largest retrospective study of nonsmokers with lung cancer ever conducted. One of the largest prospective studies had been running for decades. Commissioned by the American Cancer Society in 1959, the Cancer Prevention Study was originally designed to study the effect of tobacco on smokers, but it also held data about secondhand smoke exposure and it included a huge sample group of never-smokers married to smokers. Amongst them were 35,561 nonsmoking women from California and it was they who provided the raw data for Dr James Enstrom and Dr Geoffrey Kabat to analyse. The project was also funded by the Tobacco-Related Disease Research Program (TRDRP), another Californian anti-smoking organisation paid for with Prop 99 money.

By 1997 virtually all the data was in but, again, the indications were that this would be a less than ringing endorsement of the passive smoking theory. Faced with the prospect of funding a study which exonerated secondhand smoke, the TRDRP suddenly withdrew its money, the ACS withdrew its support and Enstrom and Kabat were forced to seek alternative funding. With the word out on what their research was likely to reveal, no one within the medical community wanted to be associated with it and, in desperation, James Enstrom accepted a grant from the tobacco industry funded Center for Indoor Air Research to finance the final years' work. The report, published in the *British Medical Journal* in 2003, found no increase in lung cancer or coronary heart disease risk (with statistically insignificant negative associations of 0.75 and 0.94 respectively).

The American Cancer Society and anti-smoking groups around the world reacted with horror. The report was due to be published in Britain on March 17 and, as was its standard practice, the *BMJ* issued an embargoed press release which prevented comments being made about the article before one minute past midnight on March 16. The ACS set about preparing a press release to undermine the report, to be circulated as soon as the embargo ended. This statement seems to have been passed to Stanton Glantz who forwarded it to his supporters by e-mail and, by the evening of March 15, he had arranged a press conference to, as he put it in his e-mail, "debunk" the paper. James Repace was enlisted to give his support and the event took place in Miami at 11 am the following morning.

Inevitably, it was the funding from the tobacco industry which gave them their best chance of rubbishing the study in the eyes of the public. Never mind that the funding had covered a fraction of the study's 39 years or that, for all practical purposes, the research had been completed before the Center for Indoor Air Research became involved. Never mind either that the scientists had only been forced into asking around for money because organisations with an agenda of eliminating smoking had tried to pull the plug.

Both researchers were respected epidemiologists whose integrity had never before been questioned. Geoffrey Kabat had assisted in the production of the EPA's 1992 report on secondhand smoke, hardly a pro-tobacco publication, and James Enstrom had produced several papers that had convincingly condemned smoking as a major health hazard as far back as 1975, as well as helping to write the 1983 Surgeon General's report. No one from the tobacco control movement was able to show how Enstrom and Kabat were supposed to have twisted the data. In addition to the question 'how?' was the question 'why?' If, as was being strongly implied, Enstrom and Kabat were mercenaries, why did they not tailor their conclusions to meet the agenda of the ACS or the TRDRP when those organisations were paying the bills? And pay the bills they did. The ACS provided 90% of the funding while the TRDRP and the tobacco industry provided just 5% each.

Stanton Glantz described the paper as "tobacco industry funded," called Enstrom "a damn fool" and said that "the science that the UCLA study did was crap."(20) Both scientists were dubbed "tobacco industry consultants" by the ACS, and ASH accused them of "deliberately downplaying the findings to suit their tobacco paymasters." Michael Thun, the ACS's head of epidemiology, called the paper "fatally flawed" and "not reliable or informative."

Details to back up these allegations were thin on the ground. In lieu of any serious flaws in the paper, Thun employed a spoiler argument, recently used by Glantz to undermine the IARC study (21). There was, he claimed, no such thing as a reliable control group since everybody was subject to a "considerable amount of environmental smoke before the late 1990s when Californian public places became smoke-free."(22) As a result, since no one was free from exposure, it was impossible to differentiate between one group and another. There was effectively no control group because even those not married to smokers were breathing in so much smoke from other sources. It was an extraordinary piece of reasoning that could equally be applied to Hirayama's 1981 study and, indeed, to every study of its kind ever undertaken. In his eagerness to discredit Enstrom and Kabat, Thun risked throwing the baby out with the bath water. By his logic, no study had ever been legitimately carried out since the supposed omnipresence of ETS made it impossible to categorise anyone as unexposed (23).

The whole controversy made for a lively debate in the letters pages of the *BMJ* but the study's supposed "fatal flaws" remained elusive. For many, the veracity of the study was not the issue. One correspondent urged the *BMJ* to print a "retraction" simply because "unless it is retracted by the *BMJ* the tobacco industry will use it to promote their vigorous opposition to antismoking legislation."(24) On the *BMJ* website, things turned positively vicious. This message board entry was not untypical:

> "Thanks for turning back the clock on public health decades or more.
> We don't need this kind of negligence from what used to be a professional medical
> publication. I seriously wonder who got paid off at the BMJ
> to publish this utter garbage." (25)

Under fire for having had the temerity to publish the study, *BMJ* editor Richard Smith went to the unprecedented lengths of publishing its pre-publication history and peer review procedure. In the following week's issue he wrote that although the journal was "passionately anti-tobacco" it was not "anti-science," adding that he found it "disturbing that so many people and organisations referred to the flaws in the study without specifying what they were. Indeed, this debate was much more remarkable for its passion than its precision."(26)

Enstrom and Kabat vigorously defended themselves in the pages of the *BMJ* the following week. They called Michael Thun's attack on them "character assassination of the worst kind" and reasserted their unimpeachable track record which had led to the ACS funding them time and again to carry out smoking research. Three years later, still under attack from the anti-smokers, Dr Enstrom formed the Scientific Integrity Institute to put 'junk science' under the spotlight, and published a lengthy rebuttal to his critics that read, in part:

> "It is very disturbing that a major health organisation like the ACS made false
> and misleading statements in a press release about our study before even
> reading our full paper and then cooperated with Glantz in distributing these
> defamatory statements on a wide scale basis in violation of the strict *BMJ* press
> embargo policy. It is very disturbing that our study continues to be condemned,
> even though we have presented extensive evidence to refute the
> unsubstantiated claim that our paper is "fatally flawed."
> In addition, it is reprehensible that the ACS and Glantz have continued their
> campaigns to discredit us and "silence" honest research when this research is entirely
> valid. These actions must be kept in mind when evaluating the honesty and integrity
> of the ACS and Glantz…Hopefully, epidemiology can continue as a field in
> which all legitimate research findings can be published and objectively evaluated,
> including those findings considered to be controversial. However, this will happen
> only if advocacy organizations like the ACS and activists like Glantz refrain
> from unethically smearing honest scientists and putting out false and
> misleading statements about their research."(27)

As a parting shot, the American Cancer Society changed its
funding policy in the wake of the study, refusing to grant money to any
researcher who had ever received a cent from the tobacco industry or any
of its associated organisations. This left Enstrom and Kabat out in the
cold, along with many other impartial scientists who had accepted
money from the industry in some form or other in the previous fifty
years. It did not affect anti-smoking campaigners-turned-researchers
because they had always avoided (or never been offered) tobacco industry
grants and, thanks to the anti-smoking industry's own millions, they did
not need them anyway. This lock-out echoed the policy of a growing
number of medical journals which refused to publish any study that was
felt to be tainted by tobacco money (though not the *BMJ*, which viewed
it as a form of censorship). The net effect was that the number of people
entitled to participate in the passive smoking debate shrank still further
and a clear warning was sent to those who might be tempted to ask
whether the emperor was wearing any clothes in the future.

The hastily arranged Miami press conference was an indication of how worried the anti-smoking groups were that the Enstrom & Kabat study would cast doubt in the public's mind about the passive smoking peril. As Enstrom has recalled (above), the counter-attack began before the paper was even published and the volley of press releases and interviews from the tobacco control lobby ensured that news reports were weighted towards assurances that the passive smoking threat was very real. The story received some coverage for a day or two but very few newspapers referred to it in more than one article or revisited the topic later. Some, including the *New York Times*, did not report it at all and where it was covered, the study's findings were tempered with shovel-loads of anti-smoking reaction. The *Sacramento Bee*, for example, wrote: "A new study downplaying the effects of second hand smoke on the health of smokers' spouses is being condemned even before it has appeared in print."(28) The rebuttal, rather than the report, became the story.

But the Enstrom & Kabat study did not "downplay" the risks of secondhand smoke. It explicitly showed them to be a convenient illusion and in so doing was in line with the IARC report and three of the largest recent studies of spousal exposure. Nyberg (1998), Zhong (1999) and Kreuzer (2001) found relative risks of 0.94, 1.1 and 0.96 respectively, all of which were as close to 1.0 (ie. no raised risk) as one could reasonably expect (29).

In Europe, a further three papers reported the findings of long running studies of airline cabin staff. Begun in 1960, they covered the period when smoking was allowed on European aircraft and the health of tens of thousands of air hostesses and stewards was monitored. All of them confirmed that cabin crew had a lower rate of cancer than the general population and that lung cancer, in particular, was significantly less common (30). Meanwhile, America's Occupational Safety & Health Administration, the government agency which - unlike the EPA - had the authority to regulate indoor air quality, found itself unable to condemn secondhand smoke using normal scientific criteria. OSHA already had limits on dangerous toxins and air contaminants, including all the major suspects in tobacco smoke, and after years of investigation concluded that "in normal situations, exposures would not exceed these permissible exposure limits."(31)

By 2007, 64 studies of nonsmoking wives married to smokers had been conducted. Only nine showed a statistically significant positive association with lung cancer, three showed a statistically significant negative association and the remaining 52 supported the null hypothesis. The ten largest studies - all of which involved sample groups of at least 200 lung cancer cases - showed an average relative risk of just 1.06 (see the Appendix). For those who had eyes to see, the passive smoking theory had unravelled.

The Helena Miracle

While anti-smokers made unsupported and unwarranted attacks on epidemiology that went against their preconceptions, their own science was plumbing new depths. In 2003, three researchers declared that secondhand smoke in bars and restaurants might be responsible for not just some but *most* heart attacks. At a tobacco control conference in Chicago, they announced that their study of hospital admissions in the little town of Helena, Montana found that incidence of myocardial infarction (heart attacks) fell by "nearly 60%" in the six months following a ban on smoking in public places. The unavoidable conclusion, as publicised in a worldwide press release by Americans for Nonsmokers' Rights, was that reducing exposure to secondhand smoke immediately saved lives. Released on April 1, one would have been forgiven for mistaking it for an April Fool's joke. If true, this would make secondhand smoke in hospitality venues the *principle* cause of heart attacks in America, and governments who banned smoking in bars and restaurants would have gone more than halfway towards eliminating heart attacks as a cause of human mortality.

The glaring problem was that *active* smoking was not responsible for anything close to 60% of heart attacks - it was said to be to responsible for 17% of heart disease cases - and, regardless of what one thought of the evidence for the passive smoking theory, it was risible to suggest that "nearly 60%" of heart attacks were triggered by secondhand smoke exposure. Not so much questionable as downright impossible, this notion could be dismissed by any layman with a second's thought. Nonetheless, it was picked up by the international media and august news-gathering organisations such as the BBC, *The Guardian* and the *New York Times* singularly failed to ask even the most basic questions of the report. *New Scientist*, to its shame, covered it with the headline 'Public smoking ban slashes heart attacks'(32), a phrase so close to the title of the ANR press release that it is most charitable to assume the journal had not seen the (unpublished) study and instead took the ANR's claim on trust.

It was another twelve months before it was published by the *British Medical Journal* and by the time it was, the supposed decline in cardiac admissions had dropped from "nearly 60%" to 40%, a discrepancy that was never explained. The study was so flawed as to be comical. None of the subjects had been asked any questions about their exposure to secondhand smoke, their lifestyles, diet or age. Two-thirds of them turned out to be either current or former smokers. It transpired that the authors of the paper had merely counted heart attack cases in one hospital and ascribed their own explanation for a brief downward trend. The number of heart attacks involved was exceptionally small; there had been an average of seven cases a month prior to the ban and four cases after it.

One vaguely plausible explanation for the drop in heart attack admissions was that the ban, as intended, had caused smokers to give up, cut down or smoke out of town, but the authors did not entertain any of these possibilities. Nor did they consider by far the most obvious interpretation: that the decline was an unrepresentative blip in a small, isolated community. The size of the town (population 66,000) and the tiny number of cases involved inevitably made month-to-month changes appear more pronounced when put into percentage terms.

Two of the researchers were doctors at the town's hospital and, according to the ANR, had been "at the forefront of the smoke-free policy movement in Montana for four years."(33) They had only decided to conduct the study at the tail-end of the period in question and so had presumably already noticed the blip. The other member of the team was none other than Dr Stanton A. Glantz who had publicly declared that his criteria for working on scientific papers was whether they would further his cause (see Chapter 7).

Americans for Nonsmokers' Rights called the study "a landmark," encouraged tobacco control groups around the world to quote the report's findings and awarded the two Helena activists-cum-epidemiologists the inaugural 'Smokefree Advocate of the Year Award.'

It seemed odd that Glantz was spending his time studying an obscure town in Montana when he lived in San Francisco, the city that had practically invented the smoking ban and which had a far larger population. To date he has not used the data from his hometown to carry out a similar study, although two researchers (funded by neither the tobacco industry nor the anti-smoking lobby), found that following the ban on smoking in bars on January 1 1998, Californian hospitals dealt with 6% more cases of myocardial infarction than they had in 1997 (34). By 2001, with the lowest smoking rate in the US and a state-wide smoking ban in place, California still ranked a lowly 33rd in a list of the states with the best record on heart disease (35).

But by seizing on hospital data from little Helena, Stanton Glantz and his colleagues were able to show that smoking bans immediately saved lives. In doing so, they invented a whole new type of epidemiological study and, by announcing it to the world via a press release, discovered an effective means of reaching the public before too many questions could be asked of it. Once again, California's maverick professor had shown himself to be a pioneer.

Smokers need not apply

"We have to treat them like human beings, I suppose," said the general manager of Cincinnati's Westin Hotel, having reluctantly allowed his staff to smoke outside the building in their break-time (36). Just as they had a hundred years earlier, employers played their part in 'discouraging' smoking among the working class at the turn of the millennium. Paternalism was back in fashion and was no longer anything to be ashamed of. "Developed societies *are* paternalistic," insisted tobacco control advocate Nigel Gray, in an article which argued that companies should refuse to employ smokers altogether (37). By 1991, 17% of American companies stated that they preferred not to hire smokers and 2% refused to employ them at all (38). History was repeating itself but employment law had changed since Henry Ford's day. No longer was it acceptable to discriminate on the grounds of race, gender, sexuality or disability. Only discrimination against smokers remained legal under federal law. Said one company president:

> "I'm a firm believer in protecting people from themselves. Employees were given the option of staying with us or leaving because of the new policy. No one left."(39)

Although couched in terms that emphasised the health of nonsmokers, the anti-smoking lobby was well aware that smoking bans on private property would help force, or in their words 'encourage,' some smokers to cut down or quit. In 1989, the Surgeon General remarked that smoking bans "may have the side effect of discouraging tobacco use by reducing opportunities to smoke and changing public attitudes about the social acceptability of smoking" (40). He was surely being disingenuous, treading lightly so as not to be accused of shameless paternalism. For many in the tobacco control movement coercing, stigmatising and inconveniencing smokers to the point where they had little choice but to give up was not so much a "side effect" as the unspoken primary goal. The passive smoking theory merely provided the spoonful of sugar which would help overcome liberal objections. At the 'Revolt Against Tobacco' conference in 1992, Americans for Nonsmokers' Rights spokesman Glenn Barr explained that the movement's aim was to "force [smokers] to do the right thing for themselves" (41) and the medical community was inclined to agree. Lung surgeon William Cahan remarked that: "People who are making decisions for themselves don't always come up with the right answer."(42) It was now up to others to make those decisions for them.

In the 1980s, for the first time in decades, companies were firing employees for smoking off the job. Fortunoff's department store in New York State was one of the first firms to refuse to hire smokers at all.

Challenging this in the courts, a failed applicant - Amy Lipson - lost her case and a company spokesman explained: "We're a health oriented company and we're committed to preserving the health of our employees." He did not elaborate on whether the company would also be refusing to hire people who were overweight, used sun-beds, went skiing, drove motorcycles or drank alcohol, but an important precedent had been set.

A few years later, Janice Borne of Indiana was subjected to a drug test at work and was judged to have failed it when nicotine showed up in her urine sample. She had smoked six cigarettes the previous weekend and was sacked on the spot (43). John Dixon worked at a packaging plant in Leeds, England, until 1998 when he was caught lighting a cigarette in his car after work and was fired (44).

Discrimination took many forms. Smoking employees at a South Wales interior design firm were paid £1 an hour less than nonsmokers, Thurrock Council proposed making smokers work an extra two and a half hours a week and Stockport City Council was only stopped from marking smokers' ID cards with a red dot when a union official complained of discrimination (45). In 1999, the smokers' rights group FOREST counted over 300 job ads that suggested smokers would be discriminated against and the words "smokers need not apply" were appearing in situations vacant advertisements all over the UK, perfectly legally.

Sophie Blinham was fired within 15 minutes of starting her job at Dataflow Communications when her bosses found out she smoked. As she was not smoking on the job she believed she had been unfairly dismissed and assumed she would have the same rights as someone discriminated against for engaging in any other legal activity in her own time. Blinham felt her case was particularly strong since the firm had advertised for 'healthy' staff and had therefore already breached Britain's tough anti-disability laws. She was wrong. Blinham took the company to court in 2005 but lost her case after the judge ruled that disability legislation would have only applied had Blinham been 'unhealthy' and that the Disability Discrimination Act specifically excluded nicotine addiction as a disability. A spokesman for the victorious firm told the press that they didn't want people coming into the building "smelling of smoke." Smokers did not, he said, present "a good image." (46)

Bar humbug

Anti-smoking activity was entering an era of absurdity and America was in a league of its own, constantly pushing the boundaries of how far the crusade could go. The US Postal Service commemorated the legendary bluesman Robert Johnson by issuing a stamp in his honour. Finding that the only extant photograph of Johnson showed him smoking a cigarette, they did what the Nazis had done with Stalin's pipe and airbrushed it from his mouth. Paul McCartney's cigarette was airbrushed from the Beatles' iconic *Abbey Road* album cover when it was turned into a poster in the US and the British tourist board followed suit in 1998, airbrushing a cigar from a photograph of Victorian engineering genius Isambard Kingdom Brunel (47).

Tobacco Control, the British Medical Association's international journal dedicated to anti-smoking advocacy, argued that Franklin D Roosevelt's distinctive cigarette holder should be expunged from commemorative images and even claimed that FDR would have approved of such historical revisionism. Roosevelt was a paraplegic who died of a brain haemorrage but *Tobacco Control* insisted that it was cigarettes that killed him (48).

The story of the death row inmate being denied his last cigarette on health grounds sounds too good a joke to be true but it was not apocryphal. Gary Lee Davis, executed in Colorado in 1997, was, like others on death row, legally protected from the passive smoke that could shorten his life. Those who dispensed justice were soon subject to the same rules as those who were incarcerated. In an unexpected twist, lawyers representing Phillip Elmore, a man sentenced to death for a murder in Ohio, appealed the verdict on the basis that the jury had rushed to judgment because the judge had refused their requests to be allowed to smoke whilst deliberating (49).

In March 2003, New York City banned smoking in bars, restaurants and even under parasols, a law that owed less to the weight of scientific evidence on passive smoke than it did the crusade of a few wealthy individuals. Joe Cherner earned a fortune as a Wall Street trader before devoting his energy to the anti-smoking campaign as the founder of Smoke-Free Educational Services and the Coalition for a Smoke-Free City. As a gay man with two adopted children, Cherner was a great advocate of tolerance except where tobacco was involved. He spent much of his time in the south of France, reportedly only allowed his family to speak French at home (50) and was described by The *New York Post* as "the world's most annoying human" and an "anti-smoking nazi."(51) He worked tirelessly to make New York smoke-free and had sufficient money and influence to bend the ear of the city's new mayor, Michael Bloomberg.

Bloomberg was a billionaire businessman who had turned his back on a 60-a-day cigarette habit and become an ardent anti-smoker, so he needed little persuasion from Cherner and his friends. A life-long Democrat, he had avoided the competitive selection process of that party by running on a Republican ticket and, having spent $73,000,000 on his electoral campaign, secured a narrow victory in 2002. Upon taking office Bloomberg passed a number of zero tolerance laws in the name of combatting crime and protecting public health, of which the most infamous was his far-reaching smoking ban. Not only was it an offence to smoke in any indoor setting but Bloomberg made it a crime to display an ashtray in public and those who went outside to smoke were liable to be booked for 'loitering outside a business.'

The New York ban was opposed by the tobacco industry, a number of journalists, a small band of libertarians and, above all, the hospitality and bar industry. Health groups insisted that banning smoking would be good for business. Their argument was, in essence, that there was an inherent market failure which only comprehensive legislation could correct. Those in the trade were not convinced and a year after the New York ban took effect, numerous studies showed that the ban had a negative impact on bars and restaurants. Anti-smoking groups dismissed them as tobacco industry propaganda since some of them had been part-funded by the industry. For good measure, they cast doubt on figures coming from the hospitality industry, assuming that their opposition to the ban signified pro-smoking sentiment. If one used the same presumption of bias to dismiss reports paid for by anti-tobacco organisations there was little evidence left to go on.

One report with which the anti-smokers could find no tobacco ties came from Ridgewood Economic Associates. The Ridgewood report showed that the law had cost New York City bars $37,000,000 in revenue and that associated industries (eg. suppliers to bars) lost a further $34,500,000. In total, they reported, 2,650 jobs had been lost as a direct result of the ban in its first year (52), a dramatic downturn for an industry that had previously been booming. On the other hand, Mayor Bloomberg reported that bar and restaurant tax receipts had leapt by 8.7% and that 2,800 jobs (after seasonal adjustment) had been created. The Campaign for Tobacco-Free Kids claimed the ban resulted in growth of 12% in the sector. Who to believe?

Finding the truth amongst all the figures cited in this controversy was no easy task and was muddied further by the World Trade Centre attacks. Throughout 2002, with a significant part of downtown Manhattan in rubble, New York's economy was in an unusually troubled period. Bloomberg's predecessor, Rudolph Giuliani, estimated that business was damaged to the tune of $50 billion by the 9/11 atrocities. Any reasonable economic projection would have predicted the city's trade to improve significantly in 2003 regardless of anti-smoking legislation, but such an improvement was far from obvious.

Some of the discrepancies between the reports mentioned above may be explained by such factors as Ridgewood only examining bars while Bloomberg included restaurants, many of which, like McDonald's, were already smoke-free before the ban took effect. They could also be partly explained by changes to the tax system and the effects of inflation (positive views of the ban always focused on tax receipts rather than sales). Then again, they may be explained by bias. The anti-smokers' favoured method was to carry out surveys asking if people would go out more if there was a smoking ban, a notoriously unreliable method which amounted to little more than asking people if they liked smoking. On the other hand, the tobacco industry tended to ask bar owners if they expected trade to go down and was equally unsound. There were too many partisan interests involved, and too many contradictory figures, to be sure of how much damage - if any - was done to the New York economy by Bloomberg's law.

The picture was also murky in California. Bar takings rose in the years following the ban, but this coincided with a general upturn in the economy and bar revenue in the state rose at a slower rate than in the rest of the country. Stanton Glantz had no doubt that the ban was good for bars and no doubt either that those who questioned it were connected with the tobacco industry. With the help of a grant from the Robert Wood Johnson Foundation he founded TobaccoScam, an organisation which presented the idea that smoke-free laws damaged businesses as a lie propagated by cigarette companies. TobaccoScam launched a long-running advertising campaigning using photographs of pretty barmaids and waitresses to persuade the public that, as the tagline went, 'Big Tobacco is lying again.' The TobaccoScam slogan represented the by-now distinctive anti-smoking argument of 'The tobacco industry says it, so it cannot be true,' an effective approach which acted as a convenient substitute for evidence.

One further tale is worth telling for the light it shines on the influence of vested interests. In 2006, two Minnesotan anti-smoking groups, the Association of Nonsmokers and ClearWay Minnesota, invited the press to relay the results of their study of air quality in the newly smoke-free bars of the city of St. Paul. Air samples had been taken before and after the ban and, in the interests of fairness, they monitored the same bars, on the same day of the week and at the same time, counting the number of patrons therein. With unbridled glee, they reported a 93% fall in particulate levels since the ban came into effect. Having duly reported this story under the headline 'Smoking Ban Clears Air in Bars, Study Says', St. Paul's *Pioneer Press* requested the raw data for review. At this point the anti-smokers suddenly became cagey and it took a request under the Minnesota Data Practices Act and an intervention from the Minnesota Department of Administration for them to hand over the full results. The reason for their reticence became clear when the data was studied. It showed 38% fewer people in the bars after the ban than had been present before.

James L. Repace inadvertently showed a similar effect in the same year. A man of finite talents, he had again been wandering around pubs measuring how much smoke was in the air, this time being paid to do so with another RWJF grant. So excited was he with the findings - which proved the less than earth-shattering fact that there was less smoke around after the smoking ban than before - that he failed to comment on the fact that the pub had attracted an average of over 100 customers before the ban but just 71 a year later (53).

In March 2004, the Republic of Ireland became the first country in the modern age to ban smoking in all its bars and restaurants. This time, the downturn in pub revenue was so unmistakable that it became very difficult for anti-smoking groups to pretend otherwise. The ban had been sold to the Irish pub industry on the basis that it would fill their establishments with nonsmokers who had previously avoided them. Nonsmokers consistently told pollsters that they would indeed go out more often if a ban was brought in but, alas, it was easier for them to agree with someone holding a clipboard than it was to spend enough money in Ireland's pubs to make up for the departing smokers.

Within three months, the Vintners' Association of Ireland reported that business was down by 15% in urban areas and 25% in rural areas. A year after the ban was enforced, the Centre for Economics and Business Research found that overall trade in bars, clubs and pubs had fallen 10.7%; this at a time when the country was experiencing sustained economic growth and where GDP was rising at 7% a year (54).

Evidence of a severe drop-off in trade was so strong in Ireland that anti-smoking groups retreated to a position of declaring the damage was not *too* bad. *Tobacco Control* magazine claimed that trade had fallen by 5.8% but maintained that the ban was a "runaway success"(55). Naomi King of ASH gave an unsupported figure of a 3.5% fall in pub revenue and insisted that "we have figures showing that it's been a huge success and everybody is happy with it."(56)

Every disease is a smoking related disease

It was a peculiar feature of the passive smoking story that when, in the first years of the new millennium, the evidence against passive smoking was at a low ebb, public belief in it was at its highest. In Britain, ASH and the British Medical Association (BMA) continued to preach the gospel of passive smoking in a bid to ratchet up the battle against tobacco. Hopes that a study of thousands would provide a clear indictment of secondhand smoke had been dashed, but since public opinion was broadly sympathetic to the passive smoking theory, there was nothing to be gained from opening up a debate. In the absence of satisfactory evidence, the movement adopted a policy of repetition: Passive smoking was a killer and the case was closed. With neither the time nor inclination to delve into the scientific data, this was enough to persuade much of the press and large swaths of the public that the case against secondhand smoke was proven. Lazy or sympathetic newspaper editors published full page ASH press releases as news stories and, by the middle of the decade, British newspapers regularly stated that 1,000 people were dying in the UK each year as a result of secondhand smoke.

The movement did not retreat an inch in the weight of recent evidence and added cot death and asthma to the list of diseases supposedly caused by secondhand smoke, ignoring the fact there was no geographical or historical correlation between smoking prevalence and incidence of either illness. Indeed, the recent upsurge in asthma was occurring at a time when there was less smoke in the air than ever before and cot death was rare in countries like Russia and Hong Kong where smoking was most prevalent (57). Such common sense observations were not enough to deter the anti-smoking industry from touting mathematical and theoretical death counts which showed passive smoking to be wreaking ever-greater carnage.

In the United States, ASH claimed that 3,000 children a year were dying from Sudden Infant Death Syndrome (SIDS) as a direct result of passive smoking. This was a low blow. Cot death charities had spent years trying to help parents not feel guilty about a syndrome whose cause remained a mystery, and those involved in SIDS support groups could see with their own eyes that their members were not predominantly smokers. ASH's message that parents were responsible for killing their offspring was an unwelcome one and the Sudden Infant Death Syndrome Alliance sent Banzhaf a strongly worded letter criticising his "use of misleading data and terminology when linking Sudden Infant Death Syndrome to your cause," adding:

"The sensational heading for one of your recent Internet reports [07/30] "Smoking Parents Are Killing Their Infants" has gone too far. The fact is, researchers still do not know what causes SIDS...Insensitive generalisations about SIDS broadcast through print or the electronic media serve only to perpetuate the public's misconceptions... Your literature states that smoking 'kills more than 2,000 infants each year from SIDS.' Any published figures are sheer speculation, or guesses, not grounded in actual experimentation...we respectfully request that you adjust your message as far as SIDS is concerned. While we support your cause, we can not do so at the expense of the tens of thousands of families we represent. Thank you for your consideration of our concerns. A copy of our latest information brochure is enclosed. We welcome your reply."(58)

Banzhaf did not reply and ASH continued to quote the statistic.

The real holy grail for the anti-smoking lobby was finding a link between secondhand smoke and breast cancer. Despite the dramatic rise of lung cancer in the 20th century, breast cancer continued to be by far the most common form of cancer in the US. For those who liked to extrapolate tiny relative risks over vast populations, finding any association with secondhand smoke would be an invaluable public relations tool. It was somewhat infuriating, then, that despite numerous attempts, no consistent or convincing link had ever been made with active, let alone passive, smoking.

A 1994 paper published in the *British Journal of Cancer* found no link between breast cancer and first or secondhand smoke (59), nor did a massive assessment of 53 studies that encompassed 55,515 breast cancer patients in the *British Journal of Cancer* (60). The Centers for Disease Control, the American Cancer Society, the IARC, the *Australian Medical*

Journal, the *British Medical Journal* and the US Surgeon General all agreed that there was no link. Geographical and historical spread of cigarette consumption showed no correlation between breast cancer prevalence and smoking, and while lung cancer rates in women began rising in the US from the mid-1960s, breast cancer rates were unaffected by the post-war surge in female smoking.

In any other field of research, this would surely have been enough to lay the matter to rest but, unhappy with the idea that there were still some diseases that had not been associated with passive smoking, the Californian Environmental Protection Agency (Cal-EPA) conducted a meta-analysis of 15 studies. This was its second attempt. The first, in 1997, failed to find any link. The second, released in 2004, showed a small but statistically significant 1.40 (1.17-1.68) relative risk for a selected subset of nonsmoking women exposed to cigarette smoke. This result only applied to young women; the middle-aged and elderly remained mysteriously unaffected.

As with the infamous 1992 EPA report, Cal-EPA cherry-picked the evidence. None of the five cohort studies backed up its hypothesis and the case-control studies that did were based on breast cancer victims filling out questionnaires in the most anti-smoking state in America and were therefore wide open to recall bias. A large cohort study of 1,150 cases found a relative risk of 0.93 but was said to have arrived too late to be considered in the meta-analysis (61). Had it been included, the overall risk ratio would have landed at 1.01.

Instead, and for the benefit of the media, the Cal-EPA gathered together the five studies that best supported the ETS theory and meta-analysed this mini-group to come up with a figure of 1.90. This made passive smoking more dangerous than smoking itself, which was no great surprise since smoking was not a genuine risk factor for breast cancer either and the Cal-EPA was effectively comparing two null hypotheses. If the Cal-EPA proved anything, it was how easy statistical associations could be conjured out of nothing.

Rather than questioning the validity of the report, Banzhaf issued a credulous ASH press release entitled 'Secondhand tobacco smoke more dangerous than smoking itself - implications for women especially frightening.'(62) Stanton Glantz described the link with breast cancer as "the most important scientific development in the last 10 years" and called those who disputed the findings "religious fanatics."(63) But the American Cancer Society, which seldom worried about overstating the dangers of secondhand smoke, declined to back the meta-analysis and its director, Michael Thun, politely remarked that the "lack of an association with active smoking weighs heavily against the possibility." Incensed by what he saw as a betrayal by the ACS, Stanton Glantz all but accused the organisation of siding with the tobacco industry and blamed "pro-tobacco forces" for casting doubt on the reliability of Cal-EPA's efforts (64). His TobaccoScam organisation wasted no time in producing a poster of three pretty waitresses telling the public that passive smoking doubled their chance of contracting breast cancer.

While secondhand smoke was being fingered as the cause of virtually any malady that might affect the human body, teams of eager epidemiologists put together statistics to implicate smoking in the few diseases that had not yet been prefixed with the words "smoking-related." Historically, anti-smokers had reeled off long lists of diseases supposedly caused by the demon weed based on little more than a hunch and a burning desire to scare the public off the habit. The modern anti-smoking movement was no different.

A distinct lack of plausible biological mechanisms did not stop smoking being 'linked to' diabetes, skin cancer, lower back pain, colon cancer, cervical cancer, depression, prostate cancer, brain damage, dementia, obesity, hair loss and low IQ (65-68). One could believe the associations to be unsound or one could believe that major killers had been discovered; killers that had not aroused the least suspicion until the end of the millennium, by which time individual epidemiological studies based on lifestyle questionnaires came to be taken at face value however unlikely their conclusions.

One 'epidemic' that had gone curiously unnoticed for centuries was given a great deal of attention by the media. The opportunity to link smoking with male impotence was too good to pass up and it was announced that 120,000 British men between 30 and 49 were suffering from erectile dysfunction as a direct result of smoking. In the late 1990s and early 2000s, several sniggering advertising campaigns were launched on both sides of the Atlantic with the intention of shaming men into quitting and convincing women that nonsmokers made better lovers. Men who smoked, they claimed, were 50% more likely to be impotent than those who did not. Again, this was hardly supported by empirical evidence and would have been news to the young men of the 1940s who defied their prodigious consumption of cigarettes to create a baby boom.

When one delved a little deeper, this statistic turned out to be entirely based on a mid-1980s survey of Vietnam veterans which apparently showed that a few more smokers than nonsmokers were impotent. The total number of impotent smokers in the study numbered just 74 and the inherent risks of extrapolating from such small numbers - particularly when they come from just one study - were well known to responsible epidemiologists. The estimate of 120,000 men came not from the original researchers but from ASH (UK), who did some quick sums - in reality, wild extrapolations - which converted the findings of one small, twenty year old study onto the population of the UK for the purposes of a press release. ASH also claimed that "though full or partial recovery is possible, this assumption must be regarded as optimistic." This was a perverse statement since the study had actually shown that former smokers were *less likely* to be impotent than nonsmokers. ASH could have reminded the public that self-reported ailments from surveys provided shaky evidence at best and that smokers, as David Krogh found, are less likely to lie to scientists, less concerned about what people think of them and are "more honest than nonsmokers in the view of themselves that they present to others"(69); all characteristics that have particular relevance when embarrassing illnesses are under scrutiny.

Even AIDS was reclassified as a smoking-related disease. Andrew Furber, a doctor working in Sheffield, South Yorkshire, put together a meta-analysis with the help of Google which showed that smokers were more likely to contract the HIV virus (70). This in itself was hardly a shock. Furber admitted that smokers tended to be risk-takers and - although he did not broach the subject - smoking is twice as common amongst gay men than it is amongst straight men (71). Such subtleties were lost on the media ('Smokers at greater risk of HIV' declared the

BBC) and Dr Furber insisted that a biological explanation was likely.

As a further lesson in how statistics can be bent to fit any purpose, some AIDS activists interpreted the findings in quite the opposite way. "People with AIDS have increased lung cancer risk and it's not all due to smoking," reported the journal *AIDS*, which told its readers that having AIDS made an individual more susceptible to lung cancer, even as it accepted that 80% of those with HIV smoke cigarettes (72).

All of this was like saying that bird-songs made the sun came up in the morning. The compulsion to confuse cause with effect led ASH to trumpet the supposed power of cigarettes to cause young people to use marijuana, not floss daily and engage in other "risky teenage behaviour" (73). A report in the journal *Addiction* showed that those who had boyfriends or girlfriends early in life were more likely to become smokers (74). While such associations may well exist, the question remains: 'So what?' As discussed in Chapter 3, smokers do not always behave like nonsmokers. Is there anything to be added by conducting expensive epidemiological studies to prove that smokers are less likely to join a gym or are more likely to try cannabis? All that is left is a pile of associations that are of no use to doctors and are too obvious be to of interest to sociologists. Absurdly, such findings have been used by anti-smokers, including ASH, to 'prove' that tobacco somehow twists smokers' brains and changes their behaviour.

This thinking reached its nadir when the world's press reported that smoking makes people kill themselves. Three British researchers published a study which showed smokers to be more than twice as likely to commit suicide than nonsmokers (75). Again, this was no surprise; those suffering from depression often turned to tobacco. The twist here was the study was written with tongue firmly planted in cheek. The whole point of the paper was to illustrate the challenges facing epidemiologists, and to highlight the danger of putting the cart before the horse when making conclusions from statistics. It was designed more as satire than advocacy.

But irony can be a foreign language in the arena of public health and it was not long before another team published a similar study and claimed that smoking really did make people commit suicide. They even cited the earlier paper as supporting evidence. The original authors responded in the letters page of the *American Journal of Epidemiology* to remind readers that their study had also shown that smokers were twice as likely to be murdered but that "unless health promoters have moved onto a direct action phase, during which they shoot smokers, this association is unlikely to be causal."

Their critique of anti-smoking research that ignores other aspects of smokers' lifestyles bears repeating:

"We live in a world in which associations are more common than lack of associations, and the former are only worth drawing attention to if they increase our understanding of why the world is the way it is. The 'independent' association between smoking and suicide is about as interesting as the equally strong 'independent' association in which never wearing a seatbelt apparently increases the risk of dying of all-cause or respiratory disease mortality.
These findings merely show for the thousandth time that smokers are different to nonsmokers and that people who wear seatbelts are different from people who don't wear seatbelts."(76)

These words represented an oasis of reason in a field of science which seemed intent on presenting tobacco as the source of all mortality, but they fell on deaf ears. The Robert Wood Johnson Foundation and the state-funded Centers for Disease Control immediately paid for more research to be carried out into the smoking-suicide connection.

CHAPTER ELEVEN

'How do you sleep at night Mr Blair?'

"No one is seriously talking about a complete ban on smoking in pubs and restaurants," said Clive Bates, the director of ASH (UK) in 1998, "This is a scare-mongering story by a tobacco industry front group."(1)

Bates was responding to the Fair Cigarette Tax Campaign (which was indeed funded by the tobacco industry) and a survey that showed 35% of smokers would stop drinking in their local pub if smoking was banned. Bates was right to accuse the industry of scare-mongering. No one in Britain, including those working for ASH, saw a ban on smoking in pubs as a realistic proposition in the 1990s.

Even when neighbouring Ireland went smoke-free in 2003, the idea of such a law being passed in England seemed unthinkable. As late as June 2005, public health minister Caroline Flint was rebutting claims that the government was contemplating a total ban on smoking in pubs, calling them "false speculation, anonymous briefings... I don't know where the stories came from."(2) And yet, eight months after the minister said these words, a law was passed which banned smoking in every pub, bar, restaurant, office, bus-stop and train station in England.

The campaign began in 2004, when the British Medical Association nailed its colours to the mast by publishing *Towards Smoke-Free Public Places*, a document which committed it to fighting for a ban on smoking in every enclosed space outside the home. By this time, the BMA was publishing the *Tobacco Control* journal, a quarterly publication that acted as a home for the glut of anti-smoking studies and opinion pieces which could not be squeezed into the regular medical journals. Meanwhile, the BMA's flagship publication, the *British Medical Journal*, had begun to abandon all appearances of neutrality and was becoming an influential proponent of tough anti-smoking and anti-smoker legislation.

The *BMJ*'s rival medical journal, *The Lancet*, was still more outspoken. In 2003, it published an editorial entitled 'How do you sleep at night Mr Blair?' in which it was claimed that 1,000 Britons died as a result of secondhand smoke every year. In a radical move, *The Lancet* demanded the government ban tobacco from sale altogether. This produced a wave of publicity and something of a debate in the press, in the context of which a mere ban in public places almost seemed a compromise. This was very probably the whole point of the article. As the following week's letters page indicated, the medical community was not yet ready to push for total prohibition (3).

The medical journals would go on to play a crucial role in clearing the way for a comprehensive smoking ban in Britain. Their editors were aware that they had the potential to mould public opinion, thanks to a symbiotic relationship with the mainstream media who, in turn, were conscious of their readers' insatiable appetite for health-related news stories; the more alarming the better. Transient health scares based on flimsy epidemiological evidence had been indispensable newspaper fodder for years. Anyone who doubted that the esteemed medical journals courted the press when a story had the potential to tickle a wider audience, could do worse than to read the following description of how the *Journal of the American Medical Association* (JAMA) announced a study to the US media:

> '..the American Medical Association press office deluged 2,500 media outlets around the world with press packets, e-mails, faxes and, for broadcasters, tantalising chunks of ready-to-air film footage trumpeting the finds of the story.' (4)

This is from the *New York Times* in 1998, when *JAMA* was edited by Dr George Lundberg, who had just published a half-finished study which purported to show that eating fish halved the risk of cardiac death. When confronted with the glaring flaws in the research, Lundberg casually replied: "People are told that eating fish once a week is not a bad thing. What harm could it do?"(5) His nonchalance about publishing bad science for a supposed good cause was shared by the editors of several other journals when it came to contentious issues like passive smoking.

Dr Lundberg took over at *JAMA* in 1982 and oversaw the publication of a number of questionable passive smoking studies, including one which apparently demonstrated that passive smoking caused hearing loss in nonsmokers at a rate that exceeded hearing loss in smokers. In 1999, Lundberg's penchant for creating, rather than merely reporting, the story was his undoing when Steven Milloy's junkscience.com exposed him for publishing a report which claimed that "60 percent of those surveyed do not define oral sex as having had sex" the week before Bill Clinton was due to appear before the US Senate over the Monica Lewinsky affair. This piece of blatant political interference, combined with the fact that the report was actually an eight year old survey of college students, cost Lundberg his job.

It was not the only example of an editor of a medical journal publishing a 'scientific' report which could mould public opinion at a sensitive time. When legislation was at stake, this amounted to little short of political lobbying. To take one example relevant to our topic we might go back to 1980, shortly before the Californian electorate was due to vote on Proposition 10 - the statewide bill that would have banned smoking in many public places. The *New England Journal of Medicine* picked this moment in time to publish the White and Froeb study, the first ever undertaken on passive smoking in the workplace. This study suggested that the effect on the pulmonary function of nonsmokers in a smoking office was comparable to that of a light smoker. This contradicted evidence from clinical trials on ETS and most subsequent studies have not supported their conclusion. The *NEJM* must surely must have known what effect publication would have on the California vote, just as they must have known that one of the authors was a member of a Californian anti-smoking group, was actively campaigning for Prop 10 and was so extreme in his opposition to tobacco that he had called for smoking parents to "not be allowed within 50 yards" of their children during school baseball games (6).

With the British media gleefully reporting that everything from salmon to toast caused cancer, the medical community was granted a powerful platform for furthering the anti-smoking campaign through new passive smoking studies. The *British Medical Journal* began a deluge of ETS studies with the explicit political purpose of banning smoking in all so-called 'public places.'

Dr Richard Smith - the BMJ editor who had been abused for publishing the Enstrom and Kabat study - resigned in 2004 after thirteen years at the helm. His anti-smoking credentials had been impeccable. He described the *BMJ* as "passionately anti-tobacco" and resigned as professor of medical journalism at Nottingham University when the institution accepted a grant from British American Tobacco. But Smith did not have a closed mind about passive smoking and the *BMJ* lost an intelligent and independent voice when he departed. Brother of the comedian Arthur Smith, he had brought an air of humourous scepticism towards studies with weak associations and those with ties to the pharmaceutical industry. One spoof article published during his reign discussed HARLOT Plc, whose name stood for 'How to Achieve positive Results without actually Lying to Overcome the Truth.'

After resigning as editor, Smith criticised the way medical journals prostituted themselves to pharmaceutical companies and organisations with vested interests, revealing that "three out of four authors in medical journals have some conflicting interests."[7] Smith went on to write a book - *The Trouble with Medical Journals* - in which he used his experiences at the magazine to frame an argument against partisan groups intruding on the world of science. Since he left the *BMJ*, the magazine has not published any studies on passive smoking which might cast doubt on the legitimacy of the passive smoking theory.

The media assault in support of the proposed smoking ban began in earnest with the release of a report on secondhand smoke as a cause of coronary heart disease (CHD) and stroke (Whincup et al., 2004)[8]. Whincup and his team measured cotinine levels in blood samples taken from 7,735 men in the late 1970s and monitored the subjects for CHD and stroke twenty years later. Cotinine is a by-product of tobacco and is found at much higher levels in smokers than in nonsmokers and the authors therefore used it as a biomarker for ETS exposure.

The authors divided the subjects into five categories: non-exposed nonsmokers, exposed nonsmokers, smokers and those exposed to small, medium and large quantities of ETS. They did so on the basis of cotinine readings - none of the subjects were asked about their exposure to tobacco smoke. Active smoking, on the other hand, was self-reported and a suspiciously high percentage (99%) of former smokers claimed never to have smoked again since the 1970s. Whincup concluded that those heavily exposed to secondhand smoke had a 50-60% increased risk of CHD but found no increase in risk of stroke.

The study appeared to offer solid evidence that secondhand smoke was linked to heart disease until it was noticed that the group deemed to be most heavily exposed to ETS also happened to be the most overweight, did the least physical exercise, had the highest proportion of heavy drinkers, the lowest proportion of nondrinkers, the highest proportion of former smokers, the highest proportion of manual workers, highest proportion of Northerners and were the most likely to be occasional smokers. The actual smokers, who were the least overweight of all the groups, were paragons of health by comparison, and actually had fewer cases of CHD than the passive smokers. Furthermore, the final risk ratios of 1.54-1.67 were peculiarly high; too close to the 1.7 risk of heart disease for active smokers found in previous studies. Were we to believe that people who passively inhaled the equivalent of a few cigarettes a year had a risk of CHD that was not much different to that of a 20-a-day smoker?

It was one of the most obviously flawed studies to date on secondhand smoke but the *BMJ* released it twice; first online on 30 June 2004 and then four weeks later in print, with the attendant media fanfare generated on each occasion. Before even being published on the internet, it had been passed to the BBC, who featured the story on its website under the headline: 'Passive smoke risk "even greater"' and told the public that the problem was "twice as bad as previously feared."(9)

Critics ripped it to shreds on the *BMJ*'s website. Dr Gio Gori called it "unqualified nonsense" and suggested that "if our best journals are given to publish opinion pieces they should be presented as such."

Those few who defended it predictably accused the critics of being tobacco industry stooges ("For which tobacco company do YOU work?") or left messages like this:

> "Those still fighting smoke-free air (to which EVERYONE has a RIGHT) are either
> the tobacco people or their "mouthpieces", brain-damaged from
> tobacco smoke and/or just PLAIN STUPID!
> Tobacco is terrorism, pure and simple. This lethal drug kills 5,000,000 users and
> hundreds of thousands more INNOCENT people around the world every year.
> TOBACCO AND TOBACCO SMOKE SHOULD BE BANNED IMMEDIATELY."
> (Capital letters in the original)

Academic pygmies

Many in the medical profession knew that the evidence on passive smoking had been grossly distorted but few could summon up the courage or enthusiasm to speak out. Those who did tended to be retired and had little to lose from being called puppets of the tobacco industry or foolish old cranks. Sir Richard Doll, who had done as much as anyone to prove the link between smoking and cancer, found that his reputation gave him no protection from the rage of anti-smokers when he told a radio station that "the effects of other people smoking in my presence is so small it doesn't worry me." The outcry was so overwhelming that the 90-year old was later compelled to point out that he was only "speaking personally."

Dr Ken Denson, of the Thame Thrombosis and Haemostasis Research Foundation, was in his late seventies and too old to worry about his career when he talked about the "academic pygmies who jump on the anti-smoking bandwagon":

> "I simply do not know where they conjure up their statistics.
> The statistics for passive smoking, in particular, would not be published
> or even considered in any other scientific discipline."(10)

Certainly, the medical community displayed a far greater degree of scepticism towards weak associations when smoking was not the issue. In 1994, a spokesman for the US National Cancer Institute (NCI) dismissed a cancer risk of 1.3 to 1.5, saying:

> "In epidemiological research, relative risks of less than 2 are considered small and usually difficult to interpret. Such increases may be due to chance, statistical bias or effects of confounding factors that are sometimes not evident." (11)

This was undoubtedly true. Why, then, had the National Cancer Institute been campaigning for years against secondhand smoke, when the risks struggled to reach even weak associations of this order? The simple answer is that the above quote was not made in relation to secondhand smoke but in response to a study which had shown a 30% increase in breast cancer risk for women who had had an abortion. It was not the first study to suggest a link - pro-choice groups called it "yet another anti-abortion scare tactic"(12) - but the medical community wasted no time in debunking it.

When, two years later, a meta-analysis purported to show a similar association between abortion and breast cancer, doctors and scientists lined up to attack it. Dr Lynn Rosenberg, an epidemiologist at Boston University School of Medicine, said:

> "A relative risk of 1.3 (that is, a 30 percent increase in risk) is in epidemiological terms virtually indistinguishable from a risk of 1.0 (that is, no increase in risk). Even if the finding is true, it has no meaning for the individual woman because the change in risk is so minuscule as to be not worth considering." (13)

This was, almost to the letter, what many had been saying about the association between secondhand smoke and lung cancer for years. But when critics of the passive smoking theory made the same point, they were accused of nit-picking, downplaying or worse. Why the double standard?

There was a political dimension to the breast cancer story. Pro-life groups were using this kind of research to bolster their campaign against abortion. The medical community, which was broadly pro-choice, was quick to point out that relative risks of less than 2.0 were generally meaningless. They were less forthcoming (and less pro-choice) when the issue related to tobacco.

This was not a lone example. In 1988, a study found that women who drank alcohol had a 40% increased risk of developing breast cancer. This was in line with findings from several other papers but was dismissed in a *JAMA* article entitled 'Breast cancer and alcohol consumption: A study in weak associations' which pointed out that a relative risk of 1.4 did not differ "significantly from 1.0."(14)

In 1980, the World Health Organisation's IARC institute said: "Relative risks of less than 2.0 may readily reflect some bias or confounding factor, those over 5.0 are unlikely to do so."(15) Ten years later, the Environmental Protection Agency refused to define electromagnetic fields as carcinogenic "largely because the relative risks...have seldom exceeded 3.0."(16) *The Lancet* was very sceptical about a study which found mobile phone users to be three times more likely to suffer from uveal melanoma than controls (3.0; 95% 1.4-6.3)(17), despite the relative risk being reasonably strong and statistically significant. Such scepticism may have been well-founded but it was wholly absent when the WHO and the EPA used far weaker associations of 1.16 and 1.19 as 'conclusive' proof that passive smoking caused lung cancer.

By 2005, the British Medical Association and ASH had settled on a figure for lung cancer risk from passive smoking of 1.24 - based on the SCOTH meta-analysis - and they considered this to be a proven and serious threat to public health. And yet, the medical community remained extremely ambivalent to other health scares which reported similar or greater risks to health. To take three pertinent examples from just one month of the same year:

- A *BMJ* study showed that the heart attack risk for people taking ibuprofen was 1.24 but was dismissed by health professionals. The Royal Pharmaceutical Society pointed out that "this type of study is fraught with difficulties."(18) The BBC echoed medical opinion by saying - as it had never done of the identical 1.24 ETS statistic - that "this translates to a low actual risk."(19) BBC Radio 2's Dr Sarah Jarvis replied to a concerned listener by pointing out that people take small risks every day, adding that neither government nor doctors should try to "wrap people up in cotton wool" and that a 24% increase in risk was very different from a 24% *overall* risk (a common misunderstanding).

- A study of 7,504 men aged 45-69 concluded that those who drank a glass or two of milk a day had an increased risk of 2.3 of developing Parkinson's Disease. A spokesman for the Parkinson's Disease Society downplayed the finding, saying: "Research is still at a very early stage and further work needs to be carried out." The BBC (correctly) noted that the overall risk remained "low."(20)

- Another *BMJ* study reported that children living within 200 metres of an electricity pylon had a 70% increased risk of leukaemia. Although this research was supported by several previous studies, the medical community was quick to talk down the danger. Cancer Research UK, the Health Protection Agency and Leukaemia Research all issued statements to warn that confounding factors could well have been responsible. The *BMJ*'s correspondent from Australia, former MOP-UP leader and anti-smoking activist Simon Chapman, had seen it all before. In 2001 he had penned an article portraying those who worried about pylons as Pythonesque figures of fun and scoffed at a report which seemed to show a doubling of risk to children who lived near them.

Chapman pointed out that, even if the risk was real, it only represented one child dying every two years and that the actual risk of leukaemia for those exposed increased from 1 in 1,400 to 1 in 700 and that these were not bad odds. He complained that the report had inspired newspapers to "talk dramatically about a doubling of risk" and, blind to irony, even lamented the fact that headlines were being taken away from such serious issues as children dying from "asthma and lower respiratory illnesses caused by passive smoking."(21) For context, the official report on passive smoking in his native Australia had found a 1.08 risk for the former and 1.13 risk for the latter (and even then, only for children under 18 months). By contrast, children living near pylons had, according to the *BMJ* report, an increased risk of 1.70. All the same, Chapman was confident he knew which was the more trivial.

Smoking bans in pubs

The publicans of Britain were broadly resistant to any legislation that would require their customers to smoke off their premises. As in Ireland, pro-ban campaigners assured them that nonsmokers would come out of the woodwork to boost their takings, but the question remained why, if the market for nonsmoking pubs was so big, did such pubs not already exist in greater numbers? If smoking was such a turn-off to the three quarters of the population who did not smoke, then it must follow that any establishment which bucked the trend and banned smoking of its own accord would benefit from a huge competitive advantage. Unlike the USA, Britain had never legislated for smoke-free places anywhere; the majority of theatres, cinemas, airlines and offices had done so voluntarily, often in response to public demand. Pubs, in the main, had not. Why? What did state-funded health groups know about the pub business that landlords did not?

When pubs had gone it alone as smoke-free establishments, the results had frequently been disastrous, despite their obvious command of a niche market. Harry Halkett had to close his pub in Elgin, Scotland two months after his self-imposed smoking ban drove away 85% of his customers. The Junction Pub in Kent banned smoking in June 2004 but reversed the decision six months later after selling "thousands of pints fewer."(22) Paddy Mulligans, a city centre pub in Lancaster, made the front page of the local newspaper when it went smoke-free in 2005 but within weeks had a huge sign hanging from its frontage exclaiming, in bright orange letters, "SMOKERS WELCOME." Leeds University was forced to reverse its smoking ban in some of its bars after takings fell by £26,000 in thirteen days. Anecdotal evidence perhaps, but nonetheless worrying for the pub trade.

Anti-smokers refused to accept that this was the reality, at least in public. Dominic Hughes reversed the smoking ban in his pub - the first in Wales to go smoke-free - after trying to make the policy work for nearly two years. In the end, he reluctantly admitted that it was not financially viable. The spokeswoman for the All-Wales Smoking Cessation Service, however, was having none of it. She said she hoped he would reconsider and even did the sums for him: "Only 26% of the population smokes" she explained, "so over 70% of people are nonsmokers."(23)

As the smoking debate heated up in England at the end of 2004, the Scottish National Assembly proposed a total ban on smoking in pubs, clubs and restaurants. The following month, Professor David Hole* of Glasgow University estimated that secondhand smoke was killing 865 Scots a year, including 355 stroke victims; a figure that came to be widely quoted. By early 2005 it became a question of when, not if, a ban would become law and the Scottish government's 'public consultation exercise' was little more than a distraction. A FOREST survey found that 66% of Scots wanted pubs to retain smoking sections and a Populus survey showed 75% felt smokers should be able to smoke in public so long as they did not inconvenience others. Health Minister Andy Kerr's curt response was: "We are not running government by opinion poll." (24)

The news coming from Ireland was not encouraging for Scotland's pub and hospitality industry. Irish pubs had continued to suffer; in 2005, over 430 of them closed down, the largest number of closures in the nation's history (25). It was not so much that smokers were boycotting pubs - though some did - as spending less time and money in them. The Centre for Economics and Business Research said the ban had cost Irish pubs £80,000,000 in its first seven months. The Licensed Vintners Association said that draught beer sales in Dublin had fallen 13% since the ban came into effect and that 2,000 workers - the very people the ban was meant to protect - had lost their jobs.

By now, the Irish pub industry was, in its own words, "pleading" with the government to provide some form of compromise. "We were told nonsmokers would flock into the pubs. We knew this would not happen and it did not happen," said the Vintner's Federation of Ireland.

---

*Author of an influential, but unreliable, passive smoking study (Hole, 1989) - see Chapter 7

By the end of 2006, over 1,000 pubs in rural areas alone had shut their doors for good (26).

Licensees naturally feared a similar effect in Scotland, where the weather, and drinking culture, was closer to Ireland's than California's. The Publican Party was formed to fight the ban but in the face of health groups promising the greatest health reform in a generation, Scottish politicians overwhelmingly voted for the bill which was came into effect in March 2006.

In the meantime, the English government blew hot and cold on the idea of jumping on the smoke-free bandwagon. It had already done much to support the anti-smoking cause by continuing the British tradition of large annual tax rises on tobacco products. Cigarette advertising had been restricted to such an extent that *Silk Cut* and *Benson & Hedges* were promoted with advertisements which were cryptic to the point of incomprehensibility. They disappeared entirely when Blair's government banned tobacco advertising and sponsorship in 1999; only Formula One was excluded, after its boss Bernie Eccleston donated £1,000,000 to the Labour party (27).

The government had, however, specifically promised not to introduce a blanket ban. In November 2004, it issued a White Paper which proposed a ban on smoking in all workplaces, including restaurants, and in some pubs and bars. The only exception would be pubs which did not sell food. "When the legislation is on the statute book," said public health minister Caroline Flint, "we will have 99% of workplaces smoke free." Flint admitted that "there are people in the medical profession who would prefer an outright ban" but - referring to the government's consultation with the public - "it was clear that people felt government should act but that there should be exceptions, as smoking is legal."(28)

Although intended as a reasonable compromise, the government's proposal was a ludicrous and unworkable fudge which only served to make a complete ban inevitable. Banning smoking in establishments which served food may have been a response to the 'nuisance factor' of dealing with smoke while eating - something smokers and nonsmokers alike sometimes complained about - but the law was framed in terms of protecting workers from the perils of secondhand smoke, not protecting customers from a minor nuisance.

Once the ban was portrayed as a health and safety measure, ASH and the BMA could justifiably attack the government for being inconsistent; protecting some bar workers while excluding others. Offering compromises before slamming the door shut on 'loopholes' had long been a tactic of the anti-smoking lobby but, in this instance, the government was doing their work for them by mooting an illogical and indefensible law from the outset. Scenting blood, the pro-ban lobby played on the discrepancy and with the Prime Minister insisting he had no 'reverse gear,' a total ban became the only realistic outcome.

The 'confidence trick'

Throughout 2005, anti-tobacconists, health groups and the medical establishment kept the smoking ban issue on the front pages, taking turns to issue press releases which created the impression that secondhand smoke was a serious and mounting problem that required immediate, uncompromising action.

ASH called this the "swarm effect" and, from the outset, it was they who led the coalition. In an illuminating interview given after the government passed the law, two of the group's senior staff admitted that all the "major health and medical organisations" had agreed to sing, and sing loudly, from the same hymn sheet in the run up to the vote. Through it all, they revealed, organisations like the Royal College of Physicians and Cancer Research had worked in accordance with a "strategy originally drafted by ASH."(29) ASH admitted that they often had doubts about their chance of success and did not know whether the law would be passed until the last moment. The possibility of banning smoking in pubs had, after all, seemed crazy until very recently. Whatever their misgivings, ASH activists resolved to portray the law as inevitable. "Campaigning of this kind," they said, "is literally a confidence trick."(30)

The first objective was to counter the argument that those who spent time in pubs were aware that smoking was permitted and entered them of their free will. This was done by focusing entirely on the employees and framing the case in terms of their health and safety. Having now agreed that decades of passive smoke exposure raised the nonsmokers' lifetime lung cancer risk by 24%, the anti-smoking groups asserted that bar staff were being 'forced' to work in a criminally unsafe environment.

Even in the era of health and safety, there was no legal compulsion to provide completely risk-free workplaces for all. To use Jacob Sullum's analogy, a man has the right not to be punched in the face every time he goes to work but not if he is a boxer (31). And boxers are not alone in putting themselves at risk of physical pain and even death for their livelihoods. Soldiers, policemen, racing drivers, stuntmen, test-pilots and firemen are obvious examples, but no one talks about people being 'forced' to become firemen or policemen. (To be fair, the British Medical Association has been campaigning for boxing to be banned since 1982 so it can at least claim a degree of consistency on that issue.) In the case of bar-work, the supposed harm was so slight as to more analogous to 'forcing' staff to work outdoors, where they might be exposed to ultraviolet light and, therefore, a risk of skin cancer.

But the safety of workers was not an unpopular cause to base the campaign around and changing the public's frame of reference was certainly important. The Department of Health had recently conducted a survey which found 86% of the public were in favour of workplace restrictions but only one in five were in favour of complete smoking bans in pubs (32). An Office of National Statistics survey found that 67% of the public were against a total ban. Public opinion on this issue had barely changed since the 1960s. When given a choice between smoking areas and total indoor smoking bans, one poll after another showed that only 15% to 30% favoured a total ban, roughly the same percentage of people who wanted the sale of tobacco to be made completely illegal. Only when pollsters gave their interviewees a straight choice between allowing smoking everywhere and banning it everywhere did the public give majority support to the latter option. Unsurprisingly, this was precisely how the pro-ban groups framed the question when they commissioned their own surveys during their campaign.

The *BMJ* studies

With a vote due in the House of Commons in the spring of 2005, the *BMJ* published a new passive smoking study in its February 5 edition and combined it with an editorial that concluded with an explicit appeal to governments everywhere: "Eliminating exposure to secondhand smoke is a public health priority not just for European countries but for the rest of the world as well."(33) The study (Vineis, 2005) monitored a group of 123,479 people for ten years and found a statistically insignificant risk of 1.34 for lung cancer and 1.30 for all respiratory diseases. A careful reading showed even these low associations to be deceptive. It transpired that more than a third of the subjects were former smokers and, when they were excluded, the hazard ratios dropped to 1.05 and 1.02 respectively: effectively zero. What ex-smokers were doing in a passive smoking study of this kind was a mystery but it was no surprise that they skewed the results. The higher prevalence of lung cancer in ex-smokers had been proven beyond doubt. Oddly, the author did not attribute their higher rate of lung cancer to their previous smoking habit but instead suggested that "former smokers might be more susceptible to the effects of environmental tobacco smoke."(34)

Two months later, in April, the BMJ published the first study on passive smoking in pubs. This timely paper (Jamrozik, 2005) was pure extrapolation. Konrad Jamrozik was an extreme anti-smoking advocate who compared sceptics of the passive smoking theory to medieval anti-Semites who believed that Jews ate Christian babies, and stated that smoking should be undertaken "only by consenting adults in private."(35) Drawing on conclusions made by Ichiro Kawachi (the author of the February 5 editorial), Jamrozik assumed a relative risk for nonsmokers exposed to secondhand smoke of 1.24 for lung cancer and 1.20 for heart disease. He then tripled these figures on the basis that nonsmoking bar staff supposedly had three times as much cotinine in their saliva as nonsmokers married to smokers, thereby turning negligible relative risks into more substantial ones; 1.73, 1.61 and 2.52 for lung cancer, heart disease and stroke respectively.

Herein lay the problem. Once trebled, the heart disease risk for nonsmoking bar-workers came in line with the known heart disease risk for regular smokers, even though it was biologically implausible that secondhand smoke exposure could damage the heart as much as smoking. The risk ratio Jamrozik arrived at for stroke was still more improbable. His figure of 2.52 was substantially higher than that seen in smokers and was completely out of kilter with Whincup's study, published the previous year, which had found no association at all between secondhand smoke and stroke.

Jamrozik's calculations were based on cotinine readings and yet only a few weeks earlier the *BMJ* had stressed that "cotinine is not associated with lung cancer or other diseases" and that "previous studies have stressed the limitations of cotinine as a biomarker of exposure."[36] His hypothesis rested on a previous study which had shown nonsmokers married to smokers to have a cotinine level of 1.2 ng/ml, while bar-workers had a level of 3.65 ng/ml. Jamrozik assumed this threefold increase in cotinine must result in a threefold increase in risk of disease for the bar-workers. What he did not mention was that cotinine levels in nonsmokers, whether they worked in a bar or not, were a tiny fraction of those found in smokers. Pack-a-day smokers consistently showed levels of at least 300 ng/ml, and often a much more than that [37].

Jamrozik multiplied the nonsmoking wives' supposed relative risk of 1.20 for heart disease to arrive at a relative risk of 1.61 for bar-workers. The folly of this approach was writ large if one applied the same kind of mathematics to smokers. Smokers had cotinine levels 250 times higher than those of the nonsmoking wives and should, by Jamrozik's logic, be 250 times more likely to develop heart disease. This would mean that they had a heart disease risk of 50.0, making them 5,000% - or fifty times - more likely to die of a heart attack than nonsmokers. This would make them nothing short of walking time-bombs liable to drop dead at any minute but in reality, smoking raises the risk of heart disease by about 70%, 4,930% away from what would be calculated using Jamrozik's model [38].

Conversely, one could just as easily use the same logic to show that, since bar-workers had one hundredth of the amount of cotinine of smokers, that they had one hundredth of the risk. But this would equate to a raised risk of just 0.7% and could hardly persuade the public that this was a threat worth worrying about. The same rationale, but completely different figures. Jamrozik's mathematical premise was demonstrably wrong. Like others before him, he had ignored the simple truism that the dose makes the poison. By extrapolating rates of disease from very low doses of harmless cotinine, he had overlooked the fact that the doses involved for both nonsmoking wives and bar-workers were, for all practical purposes, negligible.

Should anyone be tempted to question his conclusions, Jamrozik simply stated: "Given that authorities on three continents have concluded that passive smoking causes disease in adults, my calculations have a firm foundation," a reference to the EPA's report and copycat efforts in Britain and Australia (39). He then announced a grand total of 7 deaths per year from ETS-related lung cancer for pub, bar and nightclub workers and 8 deaths per year for hotel and restaurant workers. By adding in other estimates for heart disease and stroke, Jamrozik came to a combined figure of 54 deaths for all bar, pub, club, restaurant, hotel and casino workers each year; a convenient figure for the media since it worked out at about one a week. He then added in the deaths he believed secondhand smoke caused in the home and other workplaces and concluded that: "Adoption of smoke free policies in all workplaces in the United Kingdom might prevent several hundred premature deaths each year."(40)

Jamrozik's study was a gift to the British pro-ban activists and it kept on giving. The BBC was sent an abstract of the paper a year before publication, in May 2004, and reported that 'Smoking at work kills hundreds.' The following March, the corporation used a preliminary copy to report: 'Passive smoke killing thousands', and when, a few weeks later, the paper was finally published, a spokeswoman for the British Heart Foundation declared that the evidence against passive smoking was so strong that there was "no room left for scientific debate."(41) Based on Jamrozik's work, the BMA now gave a figure of 11,000 as their official estimate of passive smoking deaths in the UK, an eleven-fold increase on the figure they had previously touted.

Two years earlier, a few UK newspapers had tentatively given a figure of 300 UK deaths from passive smoking. The Jamrozik study, such as it was, led to a figure of 10,000 being quoted for the remainder of the campaign.

Clearing the air

There was just one obstacle to overcome. A simple alternative to a ban on smoking was to require licensees to provide reasonable ventilation of their indoor areas. In recent years, aware of the threat of having smoking restrictions forced upon it, the pub industry had spent huge sums of money on better ventilation. Powerful air filtration machines had become affordable for most establishments and were popular with smokers and nonsmokers alike. Since even anti-smoking groups accepted that these systems cleared at least 90% of smoke from the air, the already negligible - and quite possibly imaginary - risks from passive smoking would be reduced beyond measure. It was such an obvious, straightforward and practical solution to the problem of smoky pubs that it had the potential to derail the entire pro-ban effort. It was a technological response to an issue that the anti-smokers believed should only be addressed by modifying behaviour and it could not be allowed to stand.

James Repace came to the rescue with a paper titled *Controlling Tobacco Smoke Pollution* which concluded that the threat posed by secondhand smoke was so great that the level of ventilation required to nullify it would need to be of the scale of a "veritable indoor tornado."[42] Published in the obscure house journal of the American Society of Heating, Refrigerating and Air-Conditioning Engineers in 2005, Repace's article plumbed new depths of numerical illiteracy. He claimed that a normal sized bar required 18 air changes per hour and that for every million workers exposed to secondhand smoke in a lifetime, 6,750 would die as a result. Questionable as these numbers undoubtedly were, he then decided, for no discernible reason, that the safe level of ventilation could be calculated by multiplying the two figures together (6,750 x 18) which left him with a figure of 212,500 air changes per hour, or 33 air changes per *second*. A veritable tornado, indeed, powerful enough to blow sense and logic out of the window (43).

Repace reappeared in early 2006 as co-author of an article aimed squarely at the British government, one which set out to show that ventilation systems were useless anyway. The focus was a state of the art air filtration system then being promoted - as the authors were eager to stress - by British American Tobacco. Repace conceded that the unit successfully removed "haze, tobacco-smoke aroma and total perceived smoke" but insisted that it still did not remove secondhand smoke (44). There was not enough room between the lengthy introduction and the blatant political pleading of its conclusion to explain exactly how this could be so, nor how ventilation systems that were able to safely clear toxic gases in scientific laboratories could not do so in public houses.

Valentine's Day

By 2005, the BBC had practically become an active partner in the pro-ban campaign. In January alone it covered 24 items on smoking, often consisting of little more than quotes from pro-ban activists. Nothing, it seemed, was too small be reported. Croydon's Primary Care Trust's claim that a partial ban would hit the poor became a BBC news story, as did the Scottish Assembly's former health secretary's prediction that England would have a complete ban within 10 years. It regularly referred to ASH as a 'charity' which, as a tax-free organisation, was technically true but such a description painted a picture of this pressure group raising money for lung cancer victims by holding jumble sales. In reality, it was far more likely to be holding press conferences. With less than 2% of its revenue coming from voluntary donations, ASH was, to all intents and purposes, just another outpost of government (45). Nonetheless, the BBC disseminated ASH press releases as if they were communiques of urgent international importance and when, for instance, the group urged bar staff to sue their employers if they developed a disease related to passive smoke, the BBC ran it as a headline news story all day.

The main proponent of a compromise in the British cabinet was John Reid, a former Marxist who had given up a heavy smoking habit upon taking the job of health secretary. When he suggested that poor, working class, single mothers had few pleasures in life other than smoking, ASH was outraged and the press pounced on him as if he was in favour of exterminating the proletariat. Politicians had long-since been expected to refer to smoking as an addiction rather than a pleasure and it was not long before Reid was removed from the Department of Health to make way for the more pliant Patricia Hewitt.

With a new vote going before Parliament in February 2006, the *BMJ* used its editorial pulpit to make a final appeal to the government demanding a total ban. Politically, the stars were aligning for the passage of the law. Tony Blair had announced he would soon be leaving office and, unpopular with both the public and the Labour party thanks to the Iraq war, was on the lookout for grand gestures to secure his legacy.

The government's policy had long since become a shambles and, in the end, Blair allowed a free vote in the House of Commons, not because the issue was a matter of conscience but because the party line had changed so many times that no one was quite sure what it was any more. As late as June 2005 the government had maintained that there were "no proposals for a blanket ban"(46) but when the vote came, MPs were only given the choice between including private members clubs in the ban or exempting them. ASH used this to, in their words, "split the opposition,"(47) meeting with the drinks industry and playing on publicans' fears that smokers would join private members clubs *en masse*.

ASH had used the same tactic a year earlier when it turned establishments that served food against 'wet' pubs. It would have been interesting to have been a fly on the wall at these meetings, since ASH still publicly maintained that smoke-free pubs attracted more punters than they drove away. It was a classic example of divide and conquer. Since both parties were aware that a partial ban gave an inherent financial advantage to the establishments which remained exempt, the anti-smokers used the allure of the 'level-playing field' to enlist the support of the rest.

With a free vote on offer, and with an opportunity to be heralded as health saviours for little to no cost, MPs voted for a total smoking ban in enclosed workplaces, including all bars and restaurants, on February

14th 2006, to be implemented in July 2007.

In a shrewd move that guaranteed widespread compliance, publicans were put in charge of policing the ban and the penalty for allowing smoking on their premises was raised from £200 to £2,500. The House of Commons was one of the very few places to be exempt from the law. Prisons also received an exemption, after the head of Her Majesty's prison service delicately pointed out that a smoking ban "would not be wildly popular with a group who are not always charming and pleasant in their behaviour." Indeed. Prisons in Maine, USA had seen a quadrupling in the number of assaults in the five years since they banned smoking and the enforcement of a similar ban in an Oregon jail resulted in a riot. In New York jails, single cigarettes were being sold for $20 (48).

The Daily Telegraph called the ban "the most draconian infringement of personal liberty yet imposed by this Government" (49) while Simon Clark of FOREST, one of the few people on the other side of the argument to be given a voice during the furore, called it "an unnecessary and illiberal piece of legislation." He added that: "MPs have been seduced by an unprecedented campaign of propaganda about the effects of passive smoking for which the evidence is inconclusive. The medical profession should be ashamed of itself."(50) The British Beer and Pub Association said that "hundreds of community pubs will close and people will lose their jobs."(51) This would, in time, prove to be an extremely optimistic forecast.

The anti-smoking groups allowed themselves a brief period of celebration. ASH's director, Deborah Arnott, called the ban "the best news for public health for more than 30 years"(52) and Peter Hollins of the British Heart Foundation called it "the best Valentine's gift."(53) The party lasted only a few days before the anti-smokers got back to serious business, with ASH demanding that the ban be extended to bus-stops and a spokesman for NHS Scotland castigating band-of-the-moment The Arctic Monkeys for using a photograph of a smoker on an album cover (54). Not missing a beat, the Royal College of Physicians called the elimination of smoking in homes the next "public health priority."(63)

Since ASH had publicly stated that its ambitions did not extend to making tobacco completely illegal, the 2006 vote seemed to remove much of its raison d'être. Rarely had a government capitulated so completely to the demands of a pressure group, but ASH, like the Anti-Saloon League and Americans for Nonsmokers' Rights, was never likely to disband even after far exceeding its original goals. Within a year, ASH was campaigning for cigarette machines to be banned, for 'plain' cigarette packaging accompanied with graphic photographs of hospital patients to be added to cigarette packs and for "fuller controls on the portrayal of smoking in broadcast media."(55)

Smoking bans spread around the world

With the ban already in force in Scotland, anti-smokers began a pre-emptive campaign to prove that smoke-free pubs were not only popular but financially beneficial. In June 2006, just three months after the Scottish ban came into force, and before any figures were available, Cancer Research UK issued a press release announcing that the pub trade had not been "hit" by the ban, a claim based on a telephone survey asking 1,000 people if they were in favour of it. The Scottish Licensed Trade Association (SLTA), which predicted the ban would result in a 7% decline in sales, curtly told them to mind their own business and await the evidence. An ASH spokeswoman contributed to the unsubstantiated hearts-and-minds campaign in August, claiming that the ban had been a "great success" and that pubs were benefiting from new customers. The SLTA told her she was talking "premature nonsense."(56)

Away from the rhetoric, early signs were that the effect on trade mirrored that of Ireland. The Commercial Inn in Coldstream on the English border saw its takings fall by 40% after its customers went over to England to drink and smoke. Its landlord, John Grieve, admitted that he was tempted to defy the law, calling it "so unjust - businesses are going to go to the wall and this is what all these people just don't realise."(57) Scotland's Mecca Bingo halls saw revenue fall by 13% in the first 3 months and Carlton Bingo - the country's largest operator - saw profits fall by 62% (58). With the Scots preferring to give up bingo rather than give up smoking, the bingo industry was forced to close down dozens of premises within months of the ban being enforced.

By August, Scottish pubs were reporting an 11% fall in beer sales despite one of the hottest summers in decades (59). MSP Ewan Robson informed the Scottish Assembly about the damage being done to pubs on the border but his concerns were dismissed. Clinging to theory rather than observable fact, the First Minister insisted that the English might come over the border to enjoy smoke-free bars and a spokesman for the Scottish Assembly said he had not met *anyone* who was opposed to the ban (60).

As the summer dragged on, Scottish officials made it clear that they were taking a firm line on lawbreakers. The actor Mel Smith was briefly at the centre of a national news story when he promised to smoke a cigar on stage while portraying Churchill in a play at the Edinburgh festival. The government publicly threatened to close down the venue if he carried out this daring breach of the law and, after teasing the authorities by smoking out of a window, Smith was forced to back down.

In Fife, the local club association reluctantly cancelled the annual children's gala outing that its members traditionally funded with their donations. The club's spokesman blamed a dramatic drop in attendance, particularly from its older members who preferred to stay at home rather than be go outside to smoke. Carolyn Walker, a 'tobacco issues co-ordinator,' was having none of it. She said the whole thing was "rather silly" and reiterated that "the pub and club trade in Scotland has not been affected by the smoking ban."(61)

When the smoking ban was enforced in England on 1 July 2007, the effect on the pub trade was predictably dire. Already struggling with high rents and tight margins, pubs had been closing at a rate of 4 a week in 2006, but in the first year of the smoking ban this rate rose seven-fold - to a staggering 27 a week, or nearly 4 a *day*. In 2008, the rate of closures accelerated still further, to 39 a week; a ten-fold increase on the pre-ban level (62).

Beer sales fell to their lowest level since the Great Depression of the 1930s and headlines like *'Public smoking ban hits pubs' beer sales'*, *'Smoking ban has devastated licensed trade'* and *'Over 1,000 pubs shut since smoking ban'* told much of the story (63). By 2008, the stark contrast between ASH's promise of prosperity and the reality of financial hardship had not gone unnoticed in the national press:

> "Contrary to most predictions before the ban was enforced last summer,
> it has had a devastating effect on pub trade. When the ban came into effect
> one year ago this week, polls were claiming that up to 80 per cent of all
> adults were more likely to visit a pub. But hardly any of that horde of new
> customers has materialised - while regulars have vanished.
> Last July one health insurance giant predicted: 'The ban will enable village and town
> pubs across the UK to play an even more integral role in community life.'
> Today that boast raises a hollow laugh as village
> after village and town after town lose their pubs." (64)

Around the world, other countries were going in the same direction. New Zealand and Norway passed extensive bans in 2004 and Sweden followed suit in June the following year, resulting in a boost in sales of snus, a form of chewing tobacco that was illegal in the rest of Europe. Italy brought in a near-total ban on smoking in bars, cafes and restaurants on the first day of 2005, a ban which *La Republica* reported had been brought about "in a climate of pedantic rows, battles of principle, farewell parties and legal disputes, and amid continuing protests and confusion."(65)

If a ban in Italy came as a surprise, Cuba's ban on smoking was almost unbelievable, although it was made easier once Fidel Castro had quit smoking his famous cigars. In North Korea, another dictator introduced fierce anti-smoking legislation after giving up smoking on doctor's orders. Kim Jong-Il called smokers the "fools of the 21st century" and banned smokers from attending University (66).

In 2005, the tiny kingdom of Bhutan became the first country in modern times to outlaw smoking entirely on the order of its king ("this is progress," commented *The Lancet*, in a glowing report). With fewer than 5% of the population smoking when the law was passed, it was not as dramatic a move as it could have been, but it briefly put this obscure country on the map. Foreign observers who visited Bhutan in the months that followed found teenagers surreptitiously smoking in the streets, old men refusing to change their ways and smugglers making fat profits.

The same year saw nine National Cancer Centres in Asia sign an agreement to work towards the abolition of tobacco. In Thailand, arguably the most anti-smoking nation in Asia, grotesque photos of gangrenous feet and rotting teeth were added to cigarette packs as a warning to smokers and cigarettes were pixelated when they appeared on television, even - bizarrely - in anti-smoking adverts.

Singapore, which had already banned chewing gum, planned to lead the way in this trans-continental endeavour but was having its own smuggling problems due to a succession of heavy cigarette tax rises. The normally law-abiding Singaporeans were driving round the less salubrious parts of town picking up packs of cigarettes worth $11 for less than half that amount. In 2006, Prime Minister Lee Hsien Luong refused to raise cigarette duty again after conceding that to do so would make an already serious black market problem even worse (67).

When the Spanish, the French and the Dutch announced they would be banning smoking in bars and restaurants it signalled, for many, that the battle was truly over.

By 2008, Germany stood alone as the last major Western power to resist the tide of anti-tobacconism just as, in the 1930s, it had been the first to join it. After 1945, the anti-smoking movement was effectively driven underground, particularly in East Germany where it was forced to dress up in socialist, rather than fascist, robes. East German authorities officially encouraged tolerance but the archive of letters written to the Ministry of Health in the 1960s revealed that some citizens looked back fondly on the Nazi efforts to suppress tobacco. "Before the war many offices did not even permit smoking during business hours," wrote one man, "but these days, no matter where you go, all you see is smoke and more smoke...These people can only be reached with commands."(68) Another wrote:

"With regard to our smokers, I don't believe in the velvet power of reason but in the hard power of state measures." (69)

Post-war opposition to tobacco did nothing to stop smoking rates rising swiftly on both sides of the Berlin wall and Germans remained untouched by the reforming spirit sweeping the rest of the world; a direct result of their memories of Hitler's own crusade. But in late 2006, under pressure from the EU and WHO, they relented, creating smoke-free areas in all public places but falling well short of a total ban. When a more wide-reaching ban was enforced in 2008, there was open defiance in German pubs and protests in the streets. The ban was swiftly ruled unconstitutional and was repealed (70).

But the smokefree bandwagon rode on in Belgium, Malta, Portugal, Turkey, parts of Eastern Europe and most of Scandinavia. All of these bans had certain exemptions that were not part of the uncompromising British and Irish legislation (even New York allowed a small number of cigar and cigarette bars to remain in existence). The oddest exemption was to be found in Holland where, mindful of the value of pot-smoking tourists, legislators took the leap of faith that secondhand tobacco smoke was harmful but secondhand marijuana smoke was not. Only pure cannabis was allowed to be smoked in the nation's coffee shops.

"It's absurd," said the chairman of the Dutch Association of Coffee Shops, "In other countries they look to see whether you have marijuana in your cigarette. Here they'll look to see if you've got cigarette in your marijuana." (71)

CHAPTER TWELVE

'Developed societies are paternalistic'

By the time Britain went 'smoke-free' in July 2007, California's state-wide smoking ban was nearing its tenth anniversary and attention inevitably turned to the great outdoors. Stanton Glantz described a ban on smoking in parks as "the next logical step" for his movement. San Francisco was among the first cities to outlaw smoking in parks, a law initiated and supervised by the formidable Michela Alioto-Pier, whose aunt had, in 1993, written the Californian State ordinance that banned smoking indoors. Lacking any evidence that tobacco smoke posed even the slenderest hazard in wide open spaces, Alioto-Pier adopted the language of environmentalism by claiming cigarette butts "leach toxins into our groundwater."(1) She equated allowing people to smoke in parks with giving guns to children and demanded the state pay for a thousand 'No Smoking' signs to be posted around the city's parks. When the Recreation and Park Department failed to provide these aesthetically unappealing and somewhat Orwellian notices she called it "an outrage" and "wholly irresponsible."

Once smoking was banned in parks, the 'next logical step' was to extend the prohibition to streets. In Australia, Dr Ron Borland of the Centre for Tobacco Control compared people smoking in the street with heroin addicts shooting up in back alleys and called for the creation of "safe ingesting rooms" where smokers could be sent to keep them away from normal people. As a bonus, he suggested, smokers could be made to pay to use the rooms, as one might pay to use a lavatory in a train station. "It is difficult to justify this ban on public health grounds," he conceded, "but in terms of the annoyance factor, people have to walk through clouds of smoke to get into buildings."(2) What Dr Borland omitted to mention was that insofar as smoking outside was a problem at all, it was one which had been largely created by people like himself. That smokers would congregate outdoors after being banished from buildings may have been an unintended consequence of smoking bans but it could hardly have been unforeseen.

In March 2006, it became illegal to smoke not only in parks, buildings and streets in the town of Calabasas, California but to smoke anywhere *near* them. Smoking was prohibited anywhere outdoors at all times unless - as the law stated - "no non-smoker is present and, due to the time of day or other factors, *it is not reasonable to expect another person to arrive.*" (my emphasis)(3)

In Santa Cruz County, it was against the law to possess tobacco products, including chewing tobacco, in public parks. In Belmont, California, it took just one man to complain about smoking in his apartment block for the city's politicians to leap into action. Having been informed by the American Lung Association that "secondhand smokers often end up with more medical problems than smokers"(4) (a highly ambiguous statement), they passed an ordinance banning smoking in the street, in cars and in all private residences other than detached houses. It also became a misdemeanor for any nonsmoker not to inform the authorities if they witnessed anyone smoking outdoors. Encouraged but not satiated, a spokeswoman for the American Lung Association said the law was "a first step"(5) and Councillor Dave Warden candidly told the press: "I would like to make it illegal."(6)

Needless to say, there was no shred of evidence that outdoor 'exposure' carried the least risk to anybody apart from a truly surreal pseudo-study from veteran anti-smoker James Repace into what he called OTS (Outdoor Tobacco Smoke). Repace, outdoing himself once more, concluded that smoke exposure outdoors reached levels "as high or higher" than would be found in indoor areas (7).

John Banzhaf, now the proud owner of a personalised car number-plate reading '5UE 8AST' after his 'Sue the Bastards' catch-phrase, keenly supported the outdoor assault. He had long argued that the children of divorcees should be given to whichever parent did not smoke and he now announced that:

> "Limiting smoking outdoors is the next logical step in the anti-smoking movement.
> It shouldn't be surprising.
> I think the new frontiers in terms of non-smokers' rights are outdoors
> and also protecting children in cars and their own homes." (8)

By this stage, few would have argued with Banzhaf when he said that it was not "surprising" that the endlessly escalating demands of ASH and other like-minded groups had reached the point of wanting to criminalise people who smoked in their "own homes" and "outdoors." The only surprise was that Banzhaf had the nerve to frame the argument in the context of "non-smokers' rights." With smokers forced out of every conceivable building, the nonsmokers' right to clean air appeared to have had its day as a justification for legislation against smokers and was being gradually discarded by other tobacco control groups as they moved into the next phase.

'Big Pharma'

Pharmaceutical interests continued to bankroll the tobacco control enterprise. Once nicotine was isolated from tobacco and placed in the hands of drug companies, it underwent a remarkable image change. Previously viewed as an enslaver and a toxin, the claims now being made for *la diva nicotina* were reminiscent of those made by tobacco's earliest advocates. It was said to be "decidedly good for brains, bowels, blood vessels and even immune systems"(9) as well as being a cure for schizophrenia, depression, Alzheimers, Tourette's Syndrome and ADHD.

After a series of corporate take-overs, the battle for the 'medicinal nicotine' market became a three horse race. Glaxo Wellcome - maker of Zyban - merged with SmithKline Beecham to form GlaxoSmithKline. Pfizer bought out Pharmacia - the manufacturer of *Nicotrol* - and Johnson & Johnson, already the distributors of *Nicotrol* (through its subsidiary McNeil Consumer Products), bought out *Nicoderm*'s manufacturer ALZA. It was now a straight fight between Johnson &

Johnson, Pfizer and GlaxoSmithKline.

The glut of smoking bans had led to a predictable rise in the use of nicotine gum and nicotine patches, often by those who had no intention of quitting but who needed them in the bars, restaurants and workplaces which forbade the use of tobacco products. Advertising their nicotine as 'therapeutic' and 'soothing,' pharmaceutical companies had the anti-smokers to thank for the market shifting in their favour and continued to throw vast sums of money in their direction.

By 2005, the Robert Wood Johnson Foundation (RWFJ) - which owned billions of dollars worth of Johnson & Johnson stock - was funding anti-smoking projects to the tune of around $16,500,000 (10). Washington DC passed a bill banning smoking in all bars and restaurants (and within 25 feet of the same) with the help of a $250,000 grant from RWJF, which donated a further $4,000,000 to promote a similar ordinance in Chicago. By 2009, RWJF had funded anti-smoking projects in the United States to the tune of $450,000,000.

GlaxoSmithKline did not lag behind. Like RWJF, it was an active and generous partner in the WHO's war on 'conventional nicotine' and the company provided unrestricted grants for tobacco control activists to publish studies on anything and everything, from a report that 'proved' the Irish smoking ban was a runaway success to a study that "extinguishes the 'smoking is sexy' myth."(11)

The millions spent by Big Pharma to promote a smoke-free world were dwarfed by the billions being made on 'clean' nicotine products. By 2007, Nicorette and Nicoderm were selling to the tune of $625 million a year and Pfizer's *Chantix* drug was making $883 million worldwide (12). These sales had every chance of at least doubling, and conceivably rising tenfold, if the rest of the world followed America's lead in tackling tobacco use with uncompromising action. In 2003, at an event sponsored by RWJF and GlaxoSmithKline, the WHO launched its Framework Convention on Tobacco Control. This treaty committed its 144 signatories - none of whom consulted their electorate before signing - to increasing the price of cigarettes, killing off tobacco advertising and accelerating the move towards smoke-free places.

The anti-smoking movement's best known figures were well

rewarded by RWJF. Stanton Glantz and James Repace were both given $300,000 as recipients of the foundation's Innovators Award. This was in addition to numerous research grants such as the $399,000 Glantz and UCSF were given for an "educational campaign for restaurant owners on smoke-free restaurants," a campaign that consisted of telling restauranteurs that smoking bans would not damage their business.

Both Stanton Glantz and John Banzhaf argued that doctors who failed to prescribe nicotine replacement drugs to smokers should be prosecuted for malpractice even if the patient did not express any interest in quitting. A landmark paper in *Tobacco Control* recommended that "tobacco availability should become progressively less easy" while 'clean nicotine' should be sold from a wider range of outlets and through vending machines. Tax on tobacco should continue to rise while tax on the medicinal alternatives fall until, in the medium term, they "replace tobacco as the dominant source of the drug... The longer term goal is the virtual elimination of tobacco as it is presently known."(13)

The authors of this article, like many in the movement, viewed state regulation of cigarettes as the immediate priority since it would help in "levelling the playing field" between the cigarette companies and the pharmaceutical industry. The anti-smokers' long-standing preoccupation with state regulation of tobacco products - in America, through the aegis of the Food and Drug Administration - was based on the expectation that government agencies would reduce the amount of nicotine in cigarettes, possibly to zero (this campaign hit the buffers in 2000, when the Supreme Court once again ruled that the FDA had no authority to regulate tobacco) (14).

Although they maintained that low yield cigarettes were as dangerous as full strength varieties, and although they knew that nicotine itself was not a carcinogen, tobacco control lobbyists viewed a reduction in nicotine levels as a priority because the unspoken long term goal was to remove nicotine entirely, thereby effectively banning tobacco. Such a policy would leave pharmaceutical giants as the sole legal purveyors of nicotine. The authors of the *Tobacco Control* paper even suggested that smokers who, in the medium term, "do not obtain adequate nicotine from their reduced nicotine cigarettes" could double up by using 'clean nicotine' products as well. This would create the ideal situation for both parties - smokers could continue to fund the tobacco control industry through cigarette taxes while lining the pockets of the pharmaceutical industry.

That the anti-smoking movement was using money from one supplier of nicotine to put a rival supplier out of business could have raised eye-brows. A glaring conflict of interest? No more than was displayed in the *Tobacco Control* article itself, which was written by eight people, three of whom were (or had been) consultants to the pharmaceutical industry, another of whom had a financial interest in a new nicotine drug and one of whom was a former medical director of GlaxoSmithKline.

SmokeFree Movies

Always at the cutting-edge of anti-smoking efforts, Californians in the 21st century continued to lead the movement in new and bizarre directions. In his book, *Tobacco War*, Stanton Glantz wrote that his rule for "beating the tobacco industry" was: "The battle never ends."(15) He was not joking. Having been given the idea by his friend and fellow health campaigner Dr John Slade*, Glantz approached the Robert Wood Johnson Foundation with the idea of forming a lobby group to censor smoking in films. RWJF agreed to fund the project and SmokeFree Movies was born. SmokeFree Movies campaigned for any film that portrayed smoking to be given an R certificate (similar to the British 15 certificate). This one measure, it claimed, would save 60,000 lives a year.

SmokeFree Movies declared that in just four years, 1,500,000 American teenagers became smokers (or, as Glantz characteristically put it, were "delivered to the tobacco industry") thanks to Hollywood studios allowing smoking to be portrayed on screen. Disney alone, it claimed, gifted the tobacco industry $738,000,000 between 1999 and

---

*Slade had recently died at the age of 52 from a self-inflicted gunshot wound after suffering a stroke.

2004 and "delivered" 70,000 youngsters to its door. Underpinning these terrifying statistics was the new and astonishing premise that half the teenagers who began smoking did so solely because they saw it depicted in a movie, and that those who saw twice as much smoking were twice as likely to become smokers. By this analysis, cigarette use in the movies was the single biggest cause of smoking in America (16).

Glantz's mathematics notwithstanding, the R-rating ruse did seem to rely on a wide-eyed assumption that underage viewers did not have access to films they should not be watching. Even before the age of DVDs and the internet, this would have been a rather innocent view of teenage life. In reality, the SmokeFree Movies campaign depended not on upping the rating on those movies which, as they put it, "exposed" youngsters to smoking, but on pressuring film studios to remove smoking from all but the most grown-up films since an adult rating was known to reduce box office sales. SmokeFree Movies called the R-rating policy: "Reasonable, effective and *inevitable*" (emphasis in the original), but despite vast sums of money being spent, not least on regular full page adverts in *Variety*, the major studios were reluctant to prostitute whatever artistic integrity they might have had to promote the cause of denormalisation.

In 2007, after anti-smoking advocates had carried out a relentless letter-writing campaign, the Motion Picture Association of America (MPAA) caved in to SmokeFree Movies' lobbying and agreed to consider on-screen smoking when classifying films. A weary MPAA pointed out that three quarters of movies that showed "even a fleeting glimpse of smoking" were already receiving R-ratings for other reasons, and gently suggested that the anti-smokers were over-egging their case (17). The MPAA's concession was, inevitably, not good enough for Glantz and SmokeFree Movies who engaged in a fresh bout of letter writing. The American Legacy Foundation, which now estimated that Hollywood films persuaded no fewer than 390,000 teenagers to start smoking every year, called the MPAA's new policy "wholly inadequate" and said it would "cost countless lives."

SmokeFree Movies may one day be remembered as a moderate organisation. Hard-liners in the movement want cigarettes removed from all new movies and have suggested using digital technology to airbrush them out of old ones. If on-screen smoking comes to be seen as the public health threat Glantz claims it is, censorship of films which pre-date the era of tobaccophobia would indeed be the only logical outcome. Why even allow adults to be 'exposed' in this way if lives are at stake? Any film or TV show which depicts smoking would become fair game for censorship.

For the time being, retrospective editing is viewed as an extreme measure but, even here, the anti-smokers have made progress. In August 2006, Turner Broadcasting announced it would be editing smoking scenes out of no fewer than 1,700 Hanna-Barbera cartoons after a single viewer complained about Butch the Dog smoking a cigar in a 1950 Tom and Jerry cartoon.

Smokers' rights

Organised resistance to the anti-smoking movement at the start of the 21st century was patchy, impoverished and very easy to ignore. For all the talk of the tobacco industry's omniscient power, the reality was that it had long-since been outgunned and outfought. If one listened very carefully, the sound of opposition to the anti-smoking crusade could still be heard, but it came less from tobacco executives than from independent groups of smokers who resembled, in many ways, the merry bands of nonsmokers' rights activists of the 1970s. Passionate but penniless, groups like FORCES, Freedom2Choose, Smokers Fighting Discrimination, CLASH and The Smokers Club fought an uphill battle on budgets which ranged from shoe-string to nonexistent.

FORCES (Fight Ordinances and Restrictions to Control and Eliminate Smoking) was formed in 1995 by three gay rights activists in San Francisco who believed that, even as gays were rapidly gaining social dignity, the same was being wrested from people who smoked and they redirected their campaigning zeal to the unpopular cause of smokers' rights.

In New York, CLASH (Citizens Lobbying Against Smoker Harassment) dug in for a long, drawn out 'Can the Ban' campaign to overturn Bloomberg's controversial smoking bylaw. Whereas anti-smoking activists once handed out cards to restaurateurs lamenting the lack of smoke-free sections, CLASH sympathisers now left cards in bars reading:

> "I'm sorry, I'd love to stay for more drinks,
> But not if I can't smoke.
> The law has taken away free choice
> Yours and mine.
> This is how I choose to protest it."(28)

None of these organisations received tobacco industry money and, fearing litigation, anti-smoking groups learned to refer to them as 'apologists,' 'allies' or even 'agents of the brown army' (19) rather than 'front groups.' In contrast with their opponents in public health, the spokesmen for smokers' rights were quite happy to discuss the science behind passive smoking and, tellingly, the FORCES website is, today, the only place on the internet where every one of the secondhand smoke studies can be downloaded.

Some expected anti-smoking legislation to be overturned by reasserting the right of individuals to take risks in their lives. Others believed that proprietors, not politicians, should decide whether smoking took place on their own premises. But FORCES and CLASH predicted that all legal actions that challenged smoking bans based on property rights and assumption of risk were doomed to failure in the era of health and safety. They expected success to arrive only if and when the passive smoking theory was exposed as an "institutional fraud." To this end, FORCES raised funds to launch its own law suit against what it called the "fraudsters" and "con artists" of the public health lobby.

Other opposition was rearing its head. The delegates at the 13th World Conference on Smoking or Health in Washington must have been dismayed to find a group of young men and women standing outside their conference centre sporting 'Smoking Is Healthier Than Fascism' T-shirts and smoking cigars. These people were not stooges of the tobacco industry but activists for Bureaucrash, a chaotic assortment of young people rebelling against what they saw as the spectre of big government.

Too young to remember the anti-smoking movement's hey day of the late 1970s, Bureaucrash retained much of the vigour and humour of GASP and BUGA-UP, combined with a strategy that was more Jackass than Banzhaf. As proponents of what they called 'teensploitation,' they were more likely to throw custard pies than petition the FDA; the highlight of their Washington trip was giving Stanton Glantz the wrong directions down the street.

When the Campaign for Tobacco Free Kids marched to the offices of the Motion Picture Association of America (MPAA) demanding all films depicting smoking be given an R-rating, Bureaucrash formed the spoof pressure group Coalition for Regulating Artistic Products (CRAP), crashed the rally, and demanded the MPAA clamp down on sad films lest they cause suicide through passive depression.

These cheap and cheerful activities contrasted sharply with the professionalisation and wealth of the modern anti-smoking movement. In 1998, James Repace left the EPA to become a full-time 'secondhand smoke consultant' at Repace Associates Inc. By the time smoking was banned in Britain, the UK version of GASP had long-since become a limited company, selling 'No Smoking' signs and other smoke-free paraphernalia. Genuine grass-roots activity on the anti-smokers' side of the camp had become thin on the ground, the more so since its figureheads turned to preaching extremism. When a bill to ban smoking in public places in Austin, Texas was put before the electorate, the American Cancer Society resorted to manufacturing two groups - Onward Austin and Tobacco Free Austin - to masquerade as the "voice of the people."

Smoking bans continued to be brought before lawmakers but while anti-smokers presented them as being inevitable (what ASH (UK) called the 'confidence trick'), they were still as likely to be rejected as passed. New Hampshire, Arkansas, Utah, Maryland, New Hampshire, Louisville, Virginia, North Dakota and Cincinnati all voted against outright smoking bans in public places. Even the residents of California drew a line eventually. In 2006, the Sunshine State's seemingly unquenchable desire to punish smokers hit a brick wall when Prop 86, which would have added $2.60 to a pack of cigarettes, was rejected by the electorate.

When the former 60-a-day European Union health commissioner declared his intention to ban smoking in every public place, office, bar and restaurant on the continent, it appeared that local resistance would soon be futile. The plan was shelved, however, when a smoking ban in the EU Parliament had to be aborted after just 43 days when its own politicians protested by lighting up indiscriminately.

Scattered efforts were made to beat the anti-smokers at the ballot box. When the government of Tasmania outlawed smoking in pubs in January 2006, a 65-year old ex-fisherman named Andy Devine placed an advertisement in his local newspaper reading: "Wanted: Unhappy smokers to form a political party to fight for smokers' and drinkers' rights." Mr Devine received 250 positive replies before telling the press that all he wanted was to "sit inside and have a beer and a smoke like a civilised person."[20] Such small-time initiatives were inevitably doomed to failure as smokers, already in the minority, continued to be reluctant to define themselves, let alone vote, according to their smoking habits.

Diana Reid, a 61 year old grandmother who retired from nursing to open a small coffee shop in Ontario, Canada, was one of a handful of business owners to take a public stand against a smoking ban. Aware that the law was ostensibly created to protect workers, she laid off all her staff, ran everything herself and continued to allow smoking. "I could draw my pension and sit at home," she said, "but I am so mad to be told at my age what is good for me." Though popular with her regular customers, Reid's reasoning did not cut any ice with the authorities who repeatedly raided the premises and convicted her sixteen times for flouting the law before shutting her coffee shop down for good.

In England, a number of publicans openly defied the smoking ban but few were able to sustain their protest and the authorities made examples of those who did. After being found guilty of "failing to prevent smoking" on their own premises, Nick Hogan, landlord of The Swan in Bolton, was fined £11,500 and Tony Blows, owner of the Dog Inn, was fined £12,000.

The most high profile rebel was Hamish Howitt, the nonsmoking landlord of two Blackpool pubs. Howitt put up a sign on his pubs reading: 'Our political conscience will not allow us to put smokers and non-smokers on the street. It's our choice.' Reluctant to make any arrests in the first weeks of the ban, Blackpool Council settled for fining several of his customers but after Howitt called them "weak," "cowardly" and "pathetic," they issued a summons. In November 2007, he became the first English publican to be prosecuted for allowing smoking in an enclosed place and was hit with a fine of £2,500. Vowing to take his case to the European Court of Human Rights, Howitt was prosecuted again six month later and ordered to pay a further £4,000. Determined to fight on, despite being "on the verge of bankruptcy," Howitt announced that he was prepared to go to prison to fight what he called the government's "hate crime." (21)

Most smokers displayed their resistance in a more low key manner. While the anti-smoking lobby saw a war between tobacco control advocates and the tobacco industry, smokers felt they had been punished in roughly equal measure by both and were certainly friends of neither. Having persisted in their habit for centuries despite the threat of fines, slit lips, flogging, exile, excommunication and torture, few would bet against them surviving the vilification, humiliation and extortion that today's anti-smokers set aside for them.

Smoking bans are invariably accompanied with promises that tobacco consumption will fall but, perhaps surprisingly, that is rarely the case. New Zealanders responded to a blanket ban on smoking in enclosed places with two successive rises in cigarette consumption in 2005 and 2006. In Scotland, cigarette sales rose by 5% in the first six months of the ban, an uncharacteristically sharp rise after years of gradual decline. In Ireland, a fall in cigarette sales was loudly celebrated by the anti-smoking lobby in 2004 but was followed by a 3.5% rise in 2005. Having fallen from 33% to 27% between 1998 and 2002, the Irish smoking rate rose above the pre-ban level - to 29% - in 2008 (22).

Millions of smokers have become used to buying their cigarettes abroad or on the internet. Millions more have begun rolling their own. In the US, smokers go to Indian smoke shops or to out-of-state superstores for better prices. With puffs of smoke making wrongdoers easy to catch, open defiance is rare, but 'smoke-easies' - illicit bars where a folded up beer mat doubles as an ashtray - are dotted around New York and California. Non-compliance in Californian bars is estimated to be as high as 60% and this author has visited bars in the state where customers smoke freely on the understanding that it is they, rather than the proprietor, who will pay the fine should they be busted (one bar in rural California had a sign on the wall explicitly stating that this was the arrangement).

"Smoking is worth it. But only just," one female smoker told *Vogue* magazine in 2006, before explaining that she went to fewer parties since more and more of them became smoke-free. How would she respond to smoking bans in bars and restaurants?

"Go out less too, I suppose; certainly enjoy it less," she shudders.

"Spend more time with smokers only because they smoke," she says laughing ruefully.

"I dare say it will come to that."(23)

Some pubgoers found that smoking bans in bars helped, rather than hindered, their social life. "I do quite like the way that no-smoking brings people together," said one, "I've met so many interesting people just through being forced outside onto the kerb."(24) Lasting friendships and relationships were formed out in the cold, as people used their shared exclusion as an excuse to strike up conversation. Within weeks of the smoking ban coming into effect on the Emerald Isle, the Irish invented a word for a new phenomenon - 'smirting' - a combination of smoking and flirting. Smoking bans created a bemused solidarity between smokers, and while their *al fresco* banter was heavy on irony and had a tinge of gallows humour, real anger was as absent as any talk of giving up the habit. The flow of anti-smoking legislation was viewed as frustrating, even absurd, but it was also seen as unstoppable.

Hate

When talking publicly, most professional anti-smokers were keen to emphasise that their beef was with tobacco and not smokers; the sin, not the sinner. And while, for example, Charl Els of Physicians for a Smoke-Free Canada called smoking a "chronic relapsing brain disease" and a "mental illness," and even claimed that "mentally ill persons consume almost 50 per cent of tobacco consumed in North America"(25), he would not openly insult or demean smokers directly. The pamphlets and websites of anti-smoking organisations were always careful not to use adjectives like 'stinking' and 'dirty' when referring to smokers but they were powerless to stop the tongues of their followers. Such words had been the currency of anti-tobacconists for five centuries and, after years of state-funded denormalisation, it was no surprise when the old insults and slurs began to reappear.

Smoking bans were, at best, modestly effective in 'encouraging' people to stop smoking and, at worst, were manifestly counter-productive, but they remained powerful weapons with which to humiliate and ostracise smokers. Simon Chapman, in an article for the *Medical Journal of Australia*, reviewed his three decades as an anti-smoking activist and was proud to say:

> "Today, smokers huddle in doorways and excuse themselves from meetings. To smoke with equanimity is increasingly to wear a badge of immaturity, low education or resigned addiction. Thirty years ago things were very different."(26)

Is there not a hint of perverse glee in this description of the vanquished? The turnaround in the status of smokers happened within a generation and many nonsmokers had vivid memories of having to breathe tobacco smoke in elevators, buses, shops and even hospitals. With the tables turned, and now holding the whip hand, nonsmokers' lingering antipathy towards smokers was allowed to come to the surface. The sight of their one-time tormentors "huddled" and "resigned" provided a frisson of pleasure.

In California, smokers were all-but-officially second class citizens and the nonsmoking majority had become used to dictating terms. This sense of power gave free rein to some of the more unpleasant characteristics that lie in the human psyche, exemplified in an opinion piece from *San Francisco Chronicle* columnist Susan Alexander:

> "You know who they are. They're the people who insist on smoking while they're walking down the street, right next to you and me. Sure, they're angry because they can't light up in stores, theaters, bars and restaurants the way they used to.
>
> And they're annoyed they can't smoke at work anymore.
>
> But hey, street smokers, don't make the rest of us suffer...
>
> Maybe you think that smoking outside is harmless to others. Wrong! If you're within 10 feet of me on a busy sidewalk, or standing near me as I wait for a stoplight to change, I can't avoid inhaling your smoke. And the burning end of your cigarette is more dangerous on the street than off, where you can rest it in an ashtray instead of inches from me...
>
> Listen up, street smokers. Nonsmokers are fed up with you...
>
> So if you don't cut out your lung-damaging, skin-threatening street smoking, we'll organise. We'll form a group called ESS (Eliminate Street Smoking). ESS will create a new morality that makes it unacceptable to smoke in the street.
>
> Then, if necessary we'll lobby for laws banning street smoking."(27)

Notice how the author begins with a conspiratorial whisper to the nonsmoking reader ("You know who they are") before rising to an almost audible scream at smokers, as if shouting at a child ("hey, street smokers," "Wrong!", "listen up, street smokers.") She promises a "new morality" and further laws but it is clear that smokers cannot expect to be consulted about the creation of either. All that is required is the slightest provocation - a few seconds at a stop sign, a lit cigarette within 10 feet of her - and new laws will be passed. Less than 25 years after San Francisco first segregated smokers in public buildings, the tiniest perceived irritation was now sufficient to warrant a further clamp down.

For the first time since the Nazi era it became acceptable to openly describe a group of human beings as 'filthy' or 'dirty' without inviting censure. It was considered a universal truism that kissing a smoker was like kissing an ashtray, and if costing society billions through their own 'slow suicide' was not bad enough, smokers were also happy to endanger the lives of others around them. This was explicitly reinforced on billboards, television and in newspaper columns like the one above. On the internet, anti-smokers could speak still more freely:

> "Smokers never had any respect for others and now they are being left
> out in the cold where they belong."(28)

This frank assessment, posted on a BBC message-board, represented the more civilised end of the online debate. A delve into the murkier depths of the worldwide web unearthed forums specifically designed to play host to the most extreme, violent abuse of "whiny, stinking, anti-social smokers," as the creator of one of them - the self-explanatory filthysmokers.com - put it.

When *The Scotsman* newspaper reported that the smoking ban had led to an increase in pub crawls as smokers restricted themselves to one cigarette between pints, a Canadian reader wrote in approvingly:

> "I like this new custom because it puts smokers where they belong - on their knees and
> cringing and grovelling their way to their next booze fix.
> Perhaps if they stayed in the gutter and drains they would be in their natural habitat." (29)

In contrast with the carefully chosen words of public health officials, the world of the web revealed that 'grass-roots' anti-smokers clearly regarded the *smoker*, rather than the *smoking*, as the villain. To take two relatively eloquent examples:

> "Smokers are the bane of our nation and do nothing but fucking puff
> bullshit smoke in the air so that our kids can breathe it in."(30)

> "Smokers are the scum of the earth and this world would benefit more if all smokers
> were killed...They have been taken in by conglomerate murder companies to buy
> their products and to manipulate the minds of nonsmokers to join their 'Army.'"(31)

Making unpopular decisions

In November 2004, delegates from the World Health Organisation arrived in Malta for a two day conference. By this time, the health lobby had come to view traditional values of individual choice as little more than a hinderance to the notion of 'health for all.' There was no longer any question that public health organisations had the right and the responsibility to change behaviour by force of law rather than by mere advice and education. With this consensus reached, discussions in Malta turned to how their overtly paternalistic agenda could best be presented to politicians, the media and - to a much lesser extent - the public themselves. Since many of their policies remained controversial outside medical circles and were seldom embraced by the very people they were supposed to help, it was apt that the Malta conference was titled *Making Unpopular Decisions in Public Health.* As they breezily admitted: "Launching unpopular decisions is everyday business for top-level policy-makers in public health."(32)

Sandwiched between seminars on how to put a positive spin on closing hospital beds and charging for doctor's appointments, was a discussion of what lessons could be learned from the recent smoking ban campaigns in Ireland, Malta and Norway. The WHO, it was agreed, must be considered central to all decisions made, and lobbyists should "quote the EU directives as often as possible." Freedom of choice was nonchalantly dismissed as "the usual claim" and delegates concluded that "feeling the pulse of public opinion may help but may sometimes mislead a politician...from a public health perspective this compromise may be too great."(33)

There was revealing information about how the campaign to ban smoking in Ireland had been conducted:

"Public opinion surveys were not conducted before the decision was launched
...preparations were made to confront business, with plans for how to do this,
so they did not get too strong."(34)

Furthermore, it was revealed that health lobbyists had been

mobilised in Ireland to get the campaign well underway before the public was made aware that such a law was being considered. Advisors from the US were brought over and legal officers were "available all the time." The Irish public was ignored until the spin doctors had conducted a systematic public relations exercise and businesses were contradicted, silenced or tarred by association with the tobacco industry. This became the template for the campaigns in Scotland, Wales and England.

Also in November 2004, the UK's Department of Health issued a White Paper called *Choosing Health: Making Healthy Choices Easier*. In many ways it was a woolly, touchy-feely document full of New Labour's favourite buzzwords and a near-obsession with the rhetoric of 'choice.' This document sowed the seeds of the smoking ban. In the White Paper, the ban was proposed only for venues which sold food, a move that was explained by Department of Health research which showed that only 20% of the British public supported a total ban. But a partial smoking ban was only one of dozens of measures suggested in *Choosing Health*. It also recommended a broadcast advertising ban for a whole range of food products at times when children were likely to be watching, and greater restrictions on the promotion of alcoholic drinks. Warning labels on food and drink were mooted, and concerns were raised about the presence of smokers in reality TV programmes. It was even recommended that the government issue every British citizen with a pedometer.

Choosing Health was released with some fanfare. Much was made of its central message that a balance be struck between individual responsibility and state interference. Only those who read the Executive Summary (sent to decision makers in the public health community, but not to the media) would have noticed that the document committed Britain to a top-down public health policy the likes of which had not been seen in generations.

Looking back over the past century, the authors noted that "'public health' was often seen as something that was *done* to the population, for their own good, by impersonal and distant forces in Whitehall" (emphasis in original). The authors accepted that the Department of Health may have taken its foot off the pedal for a few decades but, with the NHS no longer constrained by underfunding:

"the time is now right for action...For this White Paper, it is the public who have, for the first time, set the agenda and identified what 'for your own good' means, not Whitehall."(35)

This was a revealing comment. It was highly significant that the authors never questioned the 'for your own good' mentality itself, thereby dispensing with the doctrine of individual liberty that had been dominant in Britain since the fall of Puritanism. The authors only claimed that theirs was a higher form of paternalism because it was the public who had "set the agenda"; as if public health policies dictated by the whims and prejudices of focus groups were any less intrusive or illiberal than those dictated by "impersonal and distant" bureaucrats. They could have saved a great deal of time and ink by simply quoting Oliver Cromwell's order that the English should be given "not what they want, but what is good for them."

The triumph of public health

The Lancet's response to the publication of *Choosing Health* was to congratulate the government for its commitment to ban smoking in 'dry' pubs (interestingly, it did not complain about the exemption for 'wet' pubs at the time), but it urged the state to go much further, particularly with regard to diet and alcohol. The journal approved of the government's plans for clamping down on tobacconists who sold to minors but described its reluctance to prevent 'junk food' retailers from selling their products to children as "defeatist and inconsistent."(36)

The Lancet concluded that the government had "embraced the arguments set out by John Stuart Mill in his essay *On Liberty* in which he argued that the only justification for the state to constrain the actions of an individual were when an individual's actions risked harming others. As long as the individual is an adult, any action that results in harm only to him or herself is not a concern to others."(37) This was a concise and accurate summary of Mill's famous principle, but it was hard to see how it had ever been "embraced" by a government that was proposing the least liberal health policies in modern British history and had created over 3,000 new criminal offences since taking office in 1997 (38).

It was fair to guess that Mill's ideas did not echo around the offices of *The Lancet*. The journal had only recently recommended the outright criminalisation of tobacco and, in countering Mill's philosophy, it cited Karl Marx's belief that societal and economic constraints made free will impossible. This broadly fitted in with the public health claim that people engaged in unhealthy activities due to their own ignorance and because advertisers told them to.

The Lancet shared the view of the country's Chief Medical Officer, Sir Liam Donaldson, who regarded the government's task as being not merely to reduce health 'inequalities' but to *eliminate* them (39). Tasty political talk but impossible in practice. Not only was the notion of everyone sharing a communal pot of health a peculiar fantasy, but even an attempt to eliminate health inequalities would be totally incompatible with allowing people to 'choose healthy options.' If people were free to make healthy choices they must also be free to make unhealthy ones. Even the best informed members of society would surely still take calculated risks with their health (first-hand knowledge of the risks has not stopped smoking being common amongst nurses, for example). Health 'inequalities' are inevitable in a free society.

The very idea that equality of health could be achieved through government action required one to ignore the fact that a person's health is largely the result of genetics and dumb luck. Furthermore, it demanded a highly optimistic view of the effectiveness of state measures. But even if it was a realistic goal, total health equality, like total financial equality, could only be achieved by an all-powerful state, with all the loss of liberty inherent in a totalitarian regime. Since it was unlikely in the extreme that every individual would make identical choices, only by forcibly imposing the lifestyles of those perceived to be the healthiest could this egalitarian scenario even be attempted. Any public doctrine as dogmatic as this would inevitably be at loggerheads with liberal democratic beliefs; *The Lancet*'s invocation of Marx was therefore an appropriate one.

The Lancet editorial claimed that the government had a dilemma because those who complained about rail crashes were the same people who complained about the nanny state. This rather puerile comparison revealed a fundamental misunderstanding of the kind of libertarianism that Mill espoused. Any company that runs a rail service is expected to be competent enough to prevent their trains from crashing. Unless the company is negligent, there is no reason for them to crash, and so there is a reasonable expectation that rail travel is safe. But if the company fails to maintain the track or employs a drunk driver, it is the company that is responsible for the deaths of those who die in the resulting accident. It is precisely because *other people* are *directly harmed* by negligence and incompetence that the company's freedom to neglect the track and employ drunkards is curtailed. There is no comparison between such acts of corporate negligence and allowing an individual to eat french fries or drink wine.

Mill's basic principle has been criticised for various reasons, some valid, and Mill himself made certain exceptions, and yet few critics have been brave enough to dismiss the essence of his argument altogether. It is no coincidence that the world's greatest democracies have embraced his words while the worst tyrannies have ignored them. Mill died in 1873, just before cigarettes became widely popular, and he does not mention tobacco in *On Liberty* at all. We *do* know that one of his last acts as an MP was to support an 1868 Bill in Parliament to designate smoking compartments in trains, a move in keeping with his live-and-let-live philosophy. Since he wrote at length, and disparagingly, about the Temperance and Sunday Observance movements, we can only assume that he ignored the anti-tobacconists because they were a very marginal group and because tobacco was not under any real threat in his lifetime.

We can also only surmise from Mill's writings on other issues how he would have addressed a health hazard like the cigarette. He agreed, for instance, that if someone was about to walk over an unsafe bridge "and there was no time to warn them," an individual would be right to restrain that person. But he added that "when there is not a certainty, but only a danger of mischief, no one but the person himself can judge of the sufficiency of the motive which may prompt him to incur the risk" and that he should be "only warned of the danger."(40)

Mill also believed that any product that bore a threat to health should carry a label warning of the potential risks because "the buyer cannot wish not to know that the thing he possesses has poisonous qualities."(41) This suggests that, had he lived in the 20th century, Mill's involvement in tobacco control would have ended after the appearance of warning labels and stop-smoking adverts. He did not approve of 'sin taxes' since he believed that artificially increasing the price of products to deter purchase was "a measure differing only in degree from their entire prohibition."(42) Speaking specifically of alcohol, he said that the use of taxation to deter purchase was a policy "suited only to a society in which the labouring classes are avowedly treated as children or savages."(43)

For Mill, it was crucial that democracy was always underpinned by the basic principle of self-ownership since, without it, the majority would enshrine its own prejudices and victimise minorities. Unless politicians accommodated the needs and desires of *all* citizens, there was no distinction between democracy and mob rule.

By the early 1990s, Britain's railway companies had banned smoking in all but one carriage of their trains. Since no-one was obliged to travel in this carriage, the system accommodated smokers and nonsmokers alike, just as Mill had intended. Within a few years, however, this final, solitary and isolated smoking carriage was abolished. Explaining its decision, Virgin trains announced that "most of our customers do not smoke and so we have decided to make all our services nonsmoking." This explanation perplexed scholars of logic as much as it pleased the anti-smokers who had lobbied for the ban. It was another small example of the tyranny of the majority in action.

When an Australian council proposed banning smoking in a number of outdoor areas in 2007, the Mayor did not pretend for a minute that smoking in the open air harmed anyone but the smoker. Instead he justified the ban on the basis that nonsmokers were in the majority: "It's only the minority who are disadvantaged," he explained, "Smokers have become marginalised. This is mainstream."(44)

Redefining liberty

Mill's basic principle - that "over himself, over his own body and mind, the individual is sovereign"(45) - does not fit comfortably within the modern public health crusade. And yet, the crusaders are still aware that individual liberty underpins so much of Western democratic thought that they dare not be seen to reject it in its entirety. Instead, they are forced to undermine and redefine it. This is done by changing the definition of freedom and by insisting that 'old' ideas of liberty are no longer sufficient to tackle the unique perils of the modern world (46). This kind of talk should always raise suspicions. One edition of Mill's essay contains an editor's introduction which reminds us:

> "Even those regimes which consistently and flagrantly violate the most elementary precepts of liberty feel obliged to pay lip-service to the idea by claiming for themselves another kind of liberty."(47)

And so the very cornerstone of the concept of liberty - that the *individual* is free to *do* - is perverted and reinterpreted as the freedom of *others* to *prevent*, *protect* and *restrain*.

But liberty is not the freedom to choose one's master, it is the freedom to *be* one's own master, and confusing the two is the oldest and most insidious distortion of the concept of freedom made by those who seek to erode it. The word 'smoke-free' is a fine example. As Mick Hume noted in the pages of *The Times*, this term would not have been out of place in the Newspeak dictionary of Orwell's *1984* (48). Like 'newspeak' or 'doublethink,' 'smoke-free' is formed of two old words and is already losing its hyphen to become simply 'smokefree' in many parts of the world. In its new context, the original meaning of 'free' has been turned on its head. It now indicates that which is forbidden, rather than that which is allowed. In Orwell's dystopia, the word 'freedom' had long since been ditched but the word 'free' survives, albeit in a very different context, as Orwell explained in the book's appendix:

> "The word free still existed in Newspeak, but could only be used in such statements as

'The dog is free from lice' or 'This field is free from weeds.' It could not be used in its old sense of 'politically free' or 'intellectually free', since political and intellectual freedom no longer existed even as concepts." (49)

With this in mind, consider the following statement from the World Health Organisation's Expert Committee on Smoking Control:

"Freedom should be seen not as the freedom of the manufacturer to promote a known health hazard but rather as the freedom and ability of society to implement public health measures." (50)

There is no acknowledgement here of the consumer's freedom to buy and consume tobacco. In fact, the individual is not referred to at all, but notice how the lawmakers of public health have become synonymous with "society"*.

Or consider this proposal from Julian Le Grand, the Chairman of Health England, who wants smokers to be forced to apply for 'smoking licenses':

"Suppose every individual who wanted to buy tobacco had to purchase a permit. And suppose further they had to do this every year. To get a permit would involve filling out a form and supplying a photograph, as well as paying the fee...
You've got to get a form, a complex form - the government's good at complex forms
- you have got to get a photograph. It's a little bit of a problem to actually do it,
so you have got to make a conscious decision every year to opt in to being a smoker." (51)

When Le Grand made this radical suggestion, the smoking ban had been in effect in England for eight months and the government was on the lookout for new policies. Even so, the idea of forcing millions of people to purchase a permit to buy a legal product was exceptionally draconian. Add to that the recommendation that the application form be made unnecessarily complicated (with the none-too-subtle implication

---

*The words are eerily similar to those used by the political philosopher Friedrich Hayek sixty years earlier in *The Road to Serfdom*. Of the supposed liberty offered by "collective freedom" in totalitarian states, Hayek wrote that it "is not the freedom of the members of society but the unlimited freedom of the planner to do with society what he pleases." (p. 162)

that smokers would be too stupid to understand it) and one had the makings of an unashamedly illiberal proposal. And yet, not only did Le Grand refuse to view it as authoritarian, he actually called it an example of "libertarian paternalism" - a oxymoronic piece of Orwellian doublespeak if ever there was one*.

Oddly enough, the international tobacco control community had its own debate about the value of individual liberty in a special edition of *Tobacco Control* magazine in 2005. Written by anti-smoking advocates and funded by the American Legacy Association, the various writers were clearly no more comfortable discussing civil rights than professors of philosophy would be if asked to perform open-heart surgery. One contributor admitted that "the tobacco control community lacks a comprehensive understanding of ethics" and went on to candidly inform his readers that when it came to the battle against smoking "acting ethically may have short term costs."(52)

The whole concept of individual freedom was discussed at one remove, as if it were some obscure disease, and the debate was only ever framed in terms of whether this quirky ideology could be used to further the anti-smoking campaign. Dr Jacobson and Dr Banerjee wrote: "An intriguing strategy that is gaining considerable scholarly attention is the use of human rights rhetoric."(53) There was no sense that the liberty of the individual had any inherent value, nor that it was of great importance to the authors personally (those genuinely dedicated to human rights seldom refer to their beliefs as "rhetoric"). There was, however, a dawning realisation that liberty was important to some people and that, as one contributor put it, it could help "build on the gains already achieved."(54)

Theirs was, of course, a very different idea of liberty to that espoused by Mill. The idea that people smoked out of choice was dismissed with the well-worn claim that tobacco industry machinations made informed choice impossible. Property rights and freedom over one's own body remained subservient to what they called the "right to life," a right that public health would forcibly uphold for individuals who

---

* Orwell defined doublethink as "the power of holding two contradictory beliefs in one's mind simultaneously, and accepting both of them."

were too "weak" or "ignorant" to do so for themselves (55).

Such sophistry has its own internal logic and a superficial appeal. There is no right to smoke in the same way as there is no right to read, dance or play football but just because such activities are not explicitly enshrined in a written constitution does not mean they can be snatched away at will. In a free society, all behaviour is legal unless the state decrees otherwise.

And while we should, of course, value and protect life, there is a gaping chasm between valuing life and forcing citizens to pursue a life free of even the slightest risk. The latter is irreconcilable with free will and a government which criminalises every mode of behaviour that carries a risk is incompatible with a free society, particularly when debased epidemiology can find risk in almost any activity.

But under the precautionary principle, government is obliged to act even when risks are unproven (or hypothetical) and even when the risk is freely taken by a fully informed individual. When state-controlled public health policy reaches this level of intrusion, its proponents can hardly complain when they are called health fascists (predictably enough, one of the authors in the *Tobacco Control* supplement insisted that the term 'health Nazis' was coined by the tobacco industry).

Having decided that paying lip-service to individual rights "may be worthwhile adopting" because they "can lead to specific tactical advantages"(56), Dr J.E.Katz explained how they could be used:

> "Policy could be framed so that smoking would not be permitted in co-occupied places,
> such as offices, sidewalks, and parks, but that appropriately informed adults could,
> with some restrictions, still be entitled to smoke in private."(57)

And this came from one of the writers who was *endorsing* the individual rights argument! One could scarcely ask for a clearer demonstration of the gulf that divides the anti-smoking movement from civil libertarians.

CHAPTER THIRTEEN

'The next logical step'

In the early 1920s, after Prohibition became a reality, one newspaper compared the victorious anti-saloon campaigners to "a soldier of fortune after the peace is signed."(1) Deprived of their flag-ship cause but with their thirst for reform intact, it was widely expected that the reformers would shift their attentions to tobacco, tea and coffee. That is precisely what happened. In 1923, the notorious New York reformer Dr Charles Pease, predicted:

"The prohibition of tobacco will come suddenly, just as prohibition of liquor did.
For years there was waged a consistent campaign against strong drink, and,
while this seemed to make but small inroads at times,
it culminated sharply in national prohibition." (2)

Had the crusaders not been forced to divert their energies towards protecting the ban on alcohol, it is likely they would have succeeded in bringing about further prohibitions. The abolitionists reluctantly abandoned the 'Nicotine Next' crusade but it was an early indication that prohibitionism can be a slippery slope.

Decades later, as the anti-smoking cause found its friends in government, a few voices were raised to warn of a new era of prohibitionism and the spectre of a nanny state. When Joe Califano, having recently given up smoking, announced sweeping anti-smoking legislation in the late 1970s, the tobacco industry spokesman William Dwyer said: "America, beware if Joe Califano ever decides to give up drinking and other pleasurable pursuits."(3) In the 1990s, RJ Reynolds published a newspaper advertisement warning readers: "Today it's smoking. Will high fat foods be next?"

Such warnings were seldom taken seriously, partly because they were so often issued by people who had an obvious financial interest in allowing people to smoke, and partly because it seemed ridiculous to think that anyone would ever equate the 'unique danger' of cigarettes with fatty food or any other "pleasurable pursuit."

By the end of the 1990s, it was becoming difficult to deny that the tobacco industry spokesman had been right and the liberal sceptics had been wrong. Asked what she would do if tobacco miraculously disappeared, Americans for Nonsmokers' Rights vice-president Julia Carol replied that she would "simply move on to other causes."(4) The war on smoking had indeed pathed the way for a new war on "high fat foods" and "other pleasurable pursuits." Joe Califano never did give up drinking but he founded the National Center on Addiction and Substance Abuse in 1992 and became a leading light in the crusade against alcohol and a prominent apologist for Prohibition. The policy objectives of his anti-alcohol campaign were remarkably similar to his tobacco control programme of 1978, focusing as they did on higher taxation, reduced availability and restricted advertising.

But it was not until the first decade of the 21st century that the hunt for 'the new smoking' really gathered pace. By this time, the public health establishment had become set on a programme of legislating to curtail not only tobacco but alcohol, a wide range of foods and various perceived environmental pollutants. In so doing, they believed, the public would be 'encouraged' to correct its behaviour and the battle against cancer and heart disease would be won.

The blind alley

As discussed in Chapter 6, the 'social theory' of disease evolved in the 1970s as a response to medical science's inability to develop effective cures for the new killers of the 20th century. With only the sketchiest understanding of what caused cancer and heart disease, the public health movement relied on epidemiologists who, it was hoped, would identify the hazards to which modern man was unknowingly subjecting himself.

Unfortunately, the whole endeavour was based on assumptions that were, at best, blindly optimistic and, at worst, self-evidently misguided. The vain belief that epidemiologists could answer questions that had eluded the world's greatest scientific minds was just one flaw in this expansive theory. Epidemiology's status as a useful tool in modern medicine sprang from its application in the fields of cigarette smoking, asbestos and Thalidomide, but in all these cases a single, relatively new product had been linked to a specific, relatively rare medical condition (lung cancer, mesothelioma and deformity respectively). These associations were not only biologically plausible but had already been suspected by doctors. Epidemiology was used to provide statistical evidence for existing hypotheses but, by its very nature, was never able to provide a scientific explanation for what it brought to light.

The 'social theory' was plausible only because the upsurge in heart disease and cancer roughly correlated with modernisation and affluence, but this tenuous association was not supported by biological evidence. Indeed, it was biologically *improbable* that the robust human body would be unable to cope with modest changes in either its diet or its environment. Furthermore, the biological agents under examination were not suspect new products like Thalidomide but everyday items like salt, sugar, alcohol and butter which had been consumed by practically the whole of mankind for millennia.

If the project did not seem preposterously ambitious in 1977 it surely does today, for epidemiologists have not alerted the world to a single genuine epidemic from that day to this. As a single, preventable cause of cancer, cigarette smoking was the exception rather than the rule. There was no such simple explanation for heart disease or most other cancers. Genetic susceptibility and - above all - old age remain by far the most significant risk factors for these diseases. The former is not preventable at all and prevention of the latter hardly seems a sound blueprint for public health.

Thirty years of research into the social and environmental causes of cancer did not, therefore, lead to any great strides in public health but it did succeed in yielding forth a slew of bogus health scares which served only to alarm and confuse the public. Richard Doll's 1981 estimate that 70% of cancers were caused by Western eating habits was soon shown to be nonsense. Studies implicating red wine, salmon, toast, electricity pylons, mobile phones, coffee, mineral water, meat, milk, hormone replacement therapy and saccharine as carcinogens were refuted by subsequent research. The idea that tiny levels of 'toxins' were a threat to life ignored the fundamental rule of toxicology that the dose makes the poison. And even if one suspended disbelief and accepted the premise that the majority of cancers were caused by 'toxins' in the diet or environment, three decades of investigation into everything from water fluoridation to passive smoking had failed to unearth any credible evidence to the back it up.

The other premise of public health - that poverty was causally linked to cancer and heart disease - was equally wrong-headed. *Absolute* poverty of the type found in the slums of Dickensian London or modern Calcutta was manifestly linked to poor health but this was not the kind of poverty that concerned Western health theorists. They focused on *relative* poverty and this was defined as any income that was 40% below the national average. To see the glaring flaw in using this as a barometer of health, one only had to consider the fact that - by this yardstick - there are a larger proportion of people living in poverty in Britain (22%) than in India (16%)(5). The theory that the poor would be worst hit by 'diseases of affluence' did, in any case, obviously defy logic and there was no reason to think that one strata of society would become sicker as a result of the rest of society becoming richer.

And yet the belief that modifying diet, habits, income and the environment could bring an end to cancer and heart disease in the West not only persisted but became the dominant health ideology of the age. Why? To quote James Le Fanu, discussing the new public health practitioners:

"Their motivation was simple enough - they had no alternative. By the 1970s, the rigorous epidemiological techniques developed by Sir Austin Bradford Hill had identified only a handful of causes of disease to add to tobacco - a few rare occupational illnesses relating to asbestos exposure and the effects of rubella in pregnancy.

This was quite insufficient to sustain the thesis that social factors caused common illnesses, so others had to be found, and as protagonists had spent their professional lifetimes collecting the incriminating evidence they could scarcely be expected to turn around and admit they might be wrong. This, admittedly, required a certain degree of self-deception, but again there was no alternative."(6)

The 'social theory' persisted for three reasons. Firstly, the public wanted to believe that doctors and scientists had the answer to cancer while those involved in public health could not bear to tell them that they did not. The crisis of confidence that hit medical science in the 1970s had scarcely been noticed by the general population. New drugs continued to appear and new technologies helped to maintain the illusion that the scientific golden age was in full flight. In truth, the creature comforts that reached people's homes in the 1990s were often refined versions of technology developed during the space race and in the early years of the Cold War. The number of genuinely new pharmaceuticals launched each year fell sharply after the 1960s and two of the era's most famous drugs - the contraceptive pill and Viagra - may have been boons for individuals but had little or no benefit for the public health since they were incapable of saving a single life.

Secondly, it did the proponents of the 'social theory' no harm that so many of their findings appeared to provide scientific justification for reformers and protest groups who, in a less secular age, would have appealed to the Almighty. It was popular with the anti-smokers because it supported their belief that tobacco smoke was a health menace to all, and it gained acceptance with the left because it preached that the wealth gap between the rich and the poor was itself a public health issue. The theory that the epidemics of cancer and heart disease were caused, in effect, by industrialisation had an obvious appeal for any number of food faddists, environmentalists, anti-capitalists and technophobes.

Thirdly, the 'social theory' thrived at the highest levels of government because its recommendations provided a justification for a glut of 'sin taxes' which created revenue for the state, increased the government's control over the population and gave politicians an opportunity to portray themselves as life-savers. And so it marched on.

State of emergency

Persuading the public to sacrifice liberty for health rarely proves difficult, even when the health benefits are questionable and the sacrifices are substantial. All that is required is a constant, rumbling state of fear interrupted with regular crescendos of panic. And yet predictions of imminent doom sit uneasily with the indisputable fact that each generation lives longer and in greater health and prosperity than the last.

In 1900, half of all Britons died before the age of 45 and only 12% made it to the age of 75. In 2006, 96% reached the age of 45 and 66% made it to the the age of 75. The figures for the rest of Europe and America are similar.

Today, infectious diseases have been all but wiped out in the Western world. Deaths from heart disease have been falling for decades and the decline has accelerated in the last twenty years. Deaths from stroke have been declining steadily since 1900 despite the steady rise in the consumption of red meat and tobacco. In the 1950s, rates of mortality from circulatory diseases stood at over 600 per 100,000 but are now around a third of that. Rates of stomach cancer - still the third most prevalent form of the disease - have dropped dramatically in the last fifty years all around the world (mainly thanks to the substitution of refrigeration for salting).

The virtual eradication of infectious disease and infant mortality has left most Westerners free to die of the cancers and heart conditions which typically affect those who reach the biblical target of three score years and ten but, as we have seen, these are the very ailments for which doctors have no cure. It is an irony that, as Dr Michael Fitzpatrick noted in *The Tyranny of Health*, "the final triumph of doctors as guardians of public morality comes at a time when they are generally incapable of explaining or curing the major contemporary causes of death and disease."(7) Unable to prolong lives with medical technology, physicians increasingly rely on grim, Malthusian forecasts to provide them with the publicity and funding with which to achieve a forceful modification of behaviour.

Stirring up panic in the face of rising life expectancy and

unprecedented standards of health calls for nothing short of apocalyptic forecasts. Good news, on the other hand, must be downplayed. One might think that the medical community would be encouraged by people living longer but, in the US, reports of rising life expectancy at the start of this century were greeted with cynicism by a public health lobby which had bought into the belief that the human race was heading towards irreversible decline thanks to the unholy trinity of food, alcohol and tobacco. Far from being celebrated as a credit to their profession, these figures were dismissed as a statistical blip. But life expectancy continued to rise every year until it reached 77.6 years in 2003, an all time high that was met with talk of epidemics of heart disease and stroke; talk not dampened by deaths from these diseases also falling in the same year. In 2004, life expectancy rose by a further four months and the health experts expressed their fears about the baby boomer generation whom they regarded as tubby time-bombs with high blood pressure. The International Longevity Center even used the occasion to proclaim - perversely - that, for the first time in history, the next generation would not live as long as their parents.

In Britain, the situation was still more encouraging. The Office of National Statistics predicted that one in five people born in 2007 would live to be 100 years old and the bookmaker William Hill slashed the odds it gave to those who backed themselves to become centenarians. "When we started taking these bets," said a spokesman, "100 years old seemed to be an almost mythical landmark and we were prepared to offer massive odds. But they are starting to cost us a fortune and from now on we are going to push out the age."(8) The 250/1 odds traditionally offered would henceforth only be offered to those prepared to bet on themselves reaching 110.

The perennially record-breaking figures for life expectancy predicted that British females born in 2004 would, on average, live to the ripe old age of 80.4 years. This was several months longer than women in the USA could expect (as American health spokesmen gloomily noted) and was the best prognosis for any generation of women in British history. The *British Medical Journal* quickly acted to dissuade anyone from getting the idea that this might be cause for celebration by emphasising that elderly people's "later years are still spent in poor health."(9) Switching to a new measure of 'healthy life expectancy' the *BMJ* endeavoured to show that far from getting better, the situation had become all the more desperate. The revelation that very old people tended not to be particularly healthy was too much for a spokeswoman for Help The Aged who declared the news to be "appalling."(10)

While the more uplifting forecasts were dismissed and downplayed, dark omens was amplified beyond all reason. vCJD, the human variant of mad cow disease, was predicted to kill half a million people when it appeared in Britain in the mid-1990s. *The Times* reported the words of one "leading scientist" who believed the death count in the UK alone could reach two million. To date, over a decade after its emergence, it has killed fewer than 200 people worldwide.

The respiratory disease SARS was regarded as nothing short of the pale rider when it appeared in 2003 and the BBC gave a platform to public health expert Malcolm Rees who predicted millions of cases in the UK, even though not a single death from the disease had ever been recorded there. Nor would it. Within four months, the global epidemic was declared over with the loss of precisely 774 lives.

The WHO's mystic powers were even less impressive. They forecast that bird flu would kill between 2 million and 7.4 million worldwide. Dr Nabarro of the UN informed the press that it would kill at least 5 million and could go as high as 150 million ("a figure drawn from the work of epidemiologists around the world."(11)). Britain's Chief Medical Officer sought to calm the public's fears by announcing that bird flu would be largely confined to Asia and so would "only" kill around 50,000 Britons. A year on, this 'pandemic' had killed 146 people worldwide, none of them in the UK.

Estimates of smoking-related deaths had always been suspect and became more so after the WHO claimed that tobacco was linked to virtually every disease known to man. Unable to gather actual statistics on worldwide mortality, the WHO simply assumed that half of all smokers would be killed by their habit. In 1990, they estimated that 3 million people worldwide were killed by tobacco. This estimate rose to 3.5 million in 1998 and jumped to 4 million just a year later. Looking to the future, they predicted that the figure would be 8.4 million by 2030. Two years later, they changed their forecast again and stated that, by 2020, 10 million would be dying every year from smoking related diseases.

These numbers were based on the expectation that the number of smokers would rise to 1.6 billion by 2030, from 1.2 billion today. If we suppose this forecast to be correct (and the WHO's track record is hardly awe-inspiring) how will a 33% increase in smoking prevalence result in a 150% rise in tobacco-related mortality?(12) It is not as if cigarette consumption has been rocketing in the last twenty years. Per capita cigarette consumption in North America has been falling for years and although the WHO predicts that smoking-related deaths in Europe will almost double by 2020, it has been falling there as well.

It would take a remarkable surge in the global smoking rate for the WHO's prediction to come to fruition, but despite massive rises in the number of people smoking in China, global cigarette sales have barely shifted since the 1980s. In 1990, 5,419 billion cigarettes were sold. By 2004 this had risen by less than 1.5%, to 5,500 billion and yet the American Cancer Society predicts that "if current trends continue" the world will see 8,000 billion cigarettes sold in 2025 and the WHO predicts that tobacco-related deaths will nearly treble. How? Even if every man, woman and child in China takes up smoking, such a rise in either global cigarette consumption or disease could not occur.

But as frightening as the projections for the 'tobacco holocaust' may be*, the guardians of public health have now found an even greater peril, and it lies in the food we eat.

---

* The ever-dubious US estimates of smoking's 'cost to society' also rocketed skywards, despite falling rates of consumption, from $12 billion (1979), to $50 billion (1983), to $100 billion (1989) and then to $203 billion (2007). Sources: Surgeon General, John Banzhaf, Aaron Leichtman and the Centers for Disease Control. Estimates of deaths caused by passive smoking did not shift downwards despite sweeping smoking restrictions in the US. The same figure of 53,000 - first used in 1991 - was still being used in 2009.

The obesity 'epidemic'

"We are in the midst of an obesity epidemic," declared the British Medical Association in 2006, as it warned that today's children risked becoming the "most obese and unhealthy in history."(13) The WHO predicted that nearly half the world's adult population would be overweight by 2015 (14). In the USA, Dr Julie Gerberding, director of the Centers for Disease Control, called obesity a 'pandemic', claimed it was more serious than the Black Death and requested $6.9 billion from Congress to help tackle it. In a report published in the *Journal of the American Medical Association*, the CDC calculated that obesity killed 400,000 Americans in 2000, up from 300,000 in 1990 (15).

In the UK, the Minister for Public Health, Caroline Flint, announced that a third of British adults would be obese by 2010. A year later, a "landmark study" predicted that no fewer than half of Britons would be obese by 2050. These forecasts were little more than pessimistic guesses but they had the desired effect of mobilising the chattering classes. "Are we turning our children into fat junkies?" asked *The Guardian*, while *The Daily Mail* told its readers that "Obesity is more dangerous than smoking"(16). In *The Sunday Times*, Minette Marrin called obesity a 'plague' and an 'epidemic' and recommended health warnings ("cake can kill") along with a "fat tax" and even the *rationing* of unhealthy food. All this could coincide, she said, with "a public campaign against fattening food, just as there was against smoking, aimed at making everyone ashamed of consuming anything naughty but nice." (17) She was probably unaware that most of these policies had already been pencilled in.

Unlike most other contemporary health scares, the obesity 'crisis' had some grounding in fact. More people were overweight than had been the case fifty or a hundred years earlier and obesity was closely linked to type 2 diabetes and some cancers. The three square meals that had been essential for agricultural and industrial workers of previous generations were too fattening for the office boys and girls of the new millennium.

For those who found themselves getting fatter, there could only be two possible explanations. Either they were eating too much or they were exercising too little. In so far as this required a public health response at all, the most obvious course of action, as Sir Lawrence Gruer wrote in the *BMJ*, was for doctors to tell their patients to "pull yourself together, eat less and exercise more." Alas, he then added that this was advice given only by the "less perceptive health professionals"(18) and instead recommended removing sweets from shop counters, refusing permission to build roads without cycle lanes and adding a warning tag and helpline number to all large-size clothes.

Since the government was physically unable to force people to exercise, it could only hope to control what they ate. There was a good case for consumers to be given more information about what they were eating and how to maintain a healthy diet, but the public health lobby had long viewed education as a soft and largely ineffective approach. They preferred to move straight to legislation.

The anti-smoking campaign had successfully pitted smokers against nonsmokers by persuading the latter that they were being forced to subsidise the former. The anti-obesity movement recommended higher taxes on food for the same reason. Obesity was said to be costing the US $75 billion in medical fees alone and some predicted that, by 2050, "every single adult in the US will be overweight" (including, presumably, the health experts themselves) (19).

In Britain, researchers used WHO data to demonstrate that obesity was costing the NHS £6 billion a year (20); twelve times the previous estimate and four times as much as the often claimed £1.5 billion cost of smoking. A study in the *BMJ* warned that obesity could bankrupt the NHS and, in 2007, another study predicted that, by 2050, obesity would cost the UK £45 billion a year. A tax on foods that were high in salt, sugar and fat was therefore mooted as a way of, at best, reducing consumption and, at the least, forcing the fat to pay their way.

Whether it was fair or not, the 'sin tax' on cigarettes had the virtue of only taking money from 'sinners'. Sin taxes made less sense when everybody had to pay them and, in the case of food, such levies benefitted no one but the treasury. That it would also be ineffectual was amply illustrated when a British study recommended adding VAT to a wide range of food products on the basis that it would save "up to" 3,200 lives a year. This was more than three times the British Medical Association's previous estimate* but it was still a very small figure in a country of 62,000,000 souls. For this negligible gain in public health, the rest of the UK would be compelled to pay £2 billion in extra tax, thereby valuing each of these self-inflicted - and, never forget, completely hypothetical - deaths at £625,000 apiece.

VAT was already levied on chocolate but this did not stop health campaigners calling for further taxation on this most sinful of foods. Dr David Walker warned of a "diabetic time bomb" caused by chocolate and called for an additional tax rise of at least 10 to 20%, saying:

> "With the best of intentions, parents and grandparents will pop a chocolate
> button into a baby's mouth in the first two or three months.
> The baby smiles and everyone is happy.
> But babies and young children are being addicted
> to chocolate before they can even walk." (21)

The doctor's use of the word 'addicted' here was no accident. The chief obstacle facing the anti-obesity crowd was the lingering belief that individuals were responsible for what they put in their mouths. For this, campaigners had a familiar retort. None other than John Banzhaf explicitly called fast food "addictive" with "effects similar to nicotine," (22) and it came as little surprise to find Banzhaf at the sharp end of the battle against obesity. Still pursuing his trademarked brand of legal activism, Banzhaf continued to make pronouncements on tobacco and continued to draw $200,000 a year as ASH's executive director, but he had been spending more and more of his time issuing lawsuits on behalf of people who had been, as he put it, "lured into obesity." (23)

In 2002, Banzhaf wrote an article entitled 'Who should pay for obesity?' in which he made a familiar case against restaurants and food manufacturers on the basis of their cost to society. He called for fat

---

* In 2000, a *BMJ* paper claimed that: "By extending value added tax to the main sources of dietary saturated fat, between 900 and 1000 premature deaths a year might be avoided." (Marshall, BMJ 29.01.00)

people to be charged more for their health insurance, warned that "measures similar to those directed against the costs of smoking may well follow" and that "if - as with the problem of smoking - the government does little to reduce the problem, law suits could be brought." (24)

Indeed they could. Banzhaf's desire to tax the overweight did not deter him from representing them in court. He personally took on the case of Caesar Barber, a morbidly obese man with a serious fast food habit, and helped him become the first person to sue McDonalds for making them fat. Banzhaf lost the case but McDonalds could see which way the wind was blowing. Having fallen victim to hysterical and idiotic lawsuits in the past, the company had already been reduced to cautioning customers that their coffee 'may be hot.' Hated equally by anti-capitalists, vegetarians, environmentalists and the public health lobby, and with the threat of liability suits and government legislation that could restrict its business practices, the burger chain hastily introduced salads and sandwiches into its range in a bizarre attempt to pass itself off as some sort of health food cafe.

Once again, the public were the helpless pawns of big business and the health campaigners were their saviours. Expecting grown men and women to control their appetites and do some exercise was too much to ask, a point that was underlined when Britain's 2007 Foresight report concluded that an expanding waistline was the responsibility of everyone but its owner: "The whole environment is conspiring against people," said one of its authors, "We are putting on weight even when we don't want to, because the forces ranged against us being slim are so powerful."(25) The Foresight committee blamed this on what it called - in all seriousness - "passive obesity," and explained that "the people of the UK are inexorably becoming heavier simply by living in the Britain of today."(26)

If the Foresight report was correct, the solution to the obesity problem lay not in calling individuals to account but in radically changing the 'Britain of today' that had been found to be at fault. The prevailing wisdom was that only a top-down approach would be sufficient to meet the challenges presented by crisps and burgers and that those in government must act, as Foresight's director said, "radically and dramatically." (27)

It was telling that when the celebrity chef Jamie Oliver campaigned against childhood obesity he did so not by appealing to parents (whom he described as "tossers" and "arseholes") but to the highest echelons of government. And he was successful. The government responded to the cook's crusade by setting new rules for school dinners which banned the sale of biscuits, chocolate, sweets and crisps, limited the amount of ketchup that could be made available to pupils and prohibited salt shakers on tables. When the new dietary regime led to the unintended consequence of fewer pupils eating school dinners, health experts simply banned the children from leaving the premises at lunchtime (28).

As had happened in the early days of the anti-cigarette campaign, the battle over diet began by focusing on children and advertising. The Food Standards Agency called for a ban on broadcast advertisements for chocolate bars, crisps and fizzy drinks before the evening watershed in Britain. Margaret Morrissey of the National Confederation of Parent Teacher Associations was unsympathetic to the news that this ban would cost television channels £141,000,000, saying: "If we genuinely wish to improve our children's health and diet then the whole nation has to be prepared to take part in it and sacrifices will have to be made."(29) Exactly what sacrifices the Parents Teachers Associations would be making were not specified but the government capitulated all the same, banning commercials for what they called HFSS (food High in Fat, Salt and Sugar) between six in the morning and nine at night. Campaigners immediately demanded that the ban be extended to programmes that children *might* watch, including soap operas and reality TV shows. In addition, they called for the food industry to be banned from using any form of internet advertising, giving away free samples, running competitions and using cartoon characters or celebrities in their marketing.

In the United States, a special tax on soda was mooted to go alongside the proposed 'Twinkie tax.' New Zealand banned 'sugary' drinks from schools but, as ever, the ban fell short of activists' demands and they called for the removal of all drinks apart from the joyless duo of water and low-fat milk. American anti-fat campaigners followed so closely in the footsteps of the anti-smokers that some demanded the Fairness Doctrine be resurrected to mandate free advertising for healthy foods, just as Banzhaf had done with anti-tobacco advertising in 1968. Michael Pertschuk of the FTC, another veteran anti-smoker, lobbied to have adverts for high-sugar cereals banned by Congress and Michael Jacobson, director of the zealous lobby group The Center for Science in the Public Interest, announced that "it's high time the [restaurant] industry begins to bear some responsibility for its contribution to obesity, heart disease and cancer."(30) He also stated his desire to see tax hikes on butter, whole milk, cheese and meat (31). Jacobson would not personally be affected by such sin taxes since he refuses to eat biscuits, is a committed vegetarian and will not drink coffee, the latter being another product that is coming under attack.

In the case of caffeine, weak epidemiological associations have once again been used to support the preconceptions of those who are naturally suspicious of even the mildest stimulant. Dr Ronald Griffiths of Johns Hopkins University said: "If health risks are well-documented, caffeine could be catapulted in public perceptions from a pleasant habit to a possibly harmful drug of abuse."(32) Griffiths is certainly doing his bit, having already petitioned the Food and Drug Administration to regulate caffeine levels in coffee, tea, chocolate and soda.

One effect of Britain's watershed ban on the advertising of high fat foods was that commercials for cheese, milk and bacon were taken off the air. This was surely not the intention. The targets of the anti-obesity campaign tended to be burgers and pizza rather than pasta and parmesan and, although few dared to admit it, this was largely because the former were produced by hated multinationals and consumed by the working class. In terms of calories, there was little to distinguish bruschetta drizzled in olive oil from bread and dripping and the government's peculiar list of *verboten* foods illustrated how difficult it was to define a 'healthy' food.

In truth, it was really not the type of food being eaten so much as the quantities involved that posed the problem. A sensible public health message would have been to admit that a little of what you fancy does you no harm but that moderation is the key. This was precisely what doctors had been telling their patients since time immemorial. It was, however, too subtle and equivocal for those who imagined themselves to be fighting a 'war' against an 'epidemic.' Their public health revolution required enemies that had to be eradicated and if this meant portraying life-sustaining foods as poisons and salt manufacturers and farmers as 'rogue industries' then so be it.

How much easier it would be if they could demonise and denormalise specific substances and work towards their abolition? In October 2007, the World Cancer Research Fund published an extraordinary report which effectively demolished the idea that all things could be enjoyed in moderation and specifically identified bacon, processed meats, sugary drinks and 'salty foods' as products which should be avoided entirely. The risk of cancer, it seemed, rose with every bite.

This report was a veritable encyclopedia of weak associations and questionable meta-analyses. The authors reviewed 7,000 epidemiological studies covering almost every type of food imaginable and 16 types of cancer. They found no fewer than 60 associations and did not find a single cancer from the larynx to the ovaries that was not either 'probably' or 'convincingly' associated with diet, alcohol or obesity. The survey's chairman, Michael Marmot, suggested that being fat was more dangerous than smoking: "With smoking, we know that if you smoke you increase your risk, but most smokers in the end don't get cancer, so it's not a one-to-one relation. With obesity it is very clear and it is a graded phenomenon. The more overweight you are, the more obese you are, the higher the risk of cancer."[33] This, of course, was sheer nonsense. It was well-known that the risks from smoking increased in proportion to how much one smoked and while it was true that most smokers didn't get cancer, it was also true that most fat people didn't get cancer either. There is never a "one-to-one" relation. That is why it is called 'risk.'

As well as declaring that a range of foods were inherently unsafe, the committee concluded that people should take 30 minutes of vigorous exercise a day, keep to the thin end of the 'healthy' body mass index and "eat mostly foods of plant origin." Even fruit juice did not get a clean bill of health; consumers should limit themselves to no more than one glass a day. If this spartan regime was followed, people could, they said, expect their chances of developing cancer to fall by 30-40%.

Press coverage of the report veered from hysterical exaggeration to weary scepticism. In Britain, it was the threat to the nation's beloved bacon sandwiches that generated the most controversy. This time, it seemed, the architects of public health had finally gone too far. '"Ban Bacon" Say Cancer Experts', exclaimed *The Daily Express*, while *The Daily Mirror* led with 'Bacon Butty Ban to Beat Cancer' (34). The authors responded by insisting that they were only offering advice but this, too, was not wholly accurate. Whilst the report gave guidelines for individuals, it also set targets for government, including reducing per capita red meat consumption to 300g (11 oz) a week, salt consumption to less than 5 grammes a day and halving consumption of sugary drinks "every 10 years." Having spent £4,500,000 producing the report, the British government was unlikely to ignore its recommendations and it was obvious that none of these targets would be achievable without the state flexing its muscles.

One early casualty of this new programme of denormalisation was Peter Jancovic, an award-winning fish and chip shop owner, whose application to open a new restaurant in Berkshire was turned down by the local council because, said one councillor: "In this country we have a huge problem with child obesity and to grant this application would only hinder this."(35) This small assault on Britain's national dish was but one indication that the healthy eating campaign was about much more than issuing friendly advice.

In New York, Mayor Bloomberg banned trans-fats from every one of the city's 24,000 restaurants after a study linked them to a 25% raised risk of heart disease. Those with long memories might have recalled similar claims being made against butter and saturated fats in the 1960s. It had been fears about the link between saturated fat and heart disease that had led to the popularity of the hydrogenated vegetable oils (as used in margarine) of which trans-fats were one variety. Food fashions had since swung back again and while there was little credible reason to believe that trans-fats were worse for the heart than other types of cooking oils, few mourned the disappearance of trans-fats since there were plenty of alternatives.

It is difficult to get worked up about the abolition of a little-known cooking oil. The freedom to eat hydrogenated vegetable oil is a small freedom indeed and it would be churlish to protest its criminalisation at all were it not for the creeping suspicion that it has paved the way for further regulation.

The rationale behind the ban on trans-fats - since copied in California - is intriguing. In 2002, the National Academy of Sciences declared there to be "no safe level" of trans-fat consumption, not because it is hazardous when consumed in moderation but simply because "they are not essential and provide no known health benefit." (36) Trans-fats were therefore unsafe - and had to be banned by law - not because they were necessarily bad for you but because they could not be shown to be good for you. The same could be said of many of the other small pleasures that were now under attack.

The drinking 'epidemic'

"The legislation to ban smoking in public places is very welcome and it is a major step forward," said Dr John Smith, president of the Royal College of Surgeons of Edinburgh, "The logical thing to recognise now is that smoking is very bad for you, but so is alcohol."(37) Having encapsulated the logic of the slippery slope in a nutshell, Smith went on to propose a three drink limit in Scottish pubs, a proposal that was welcomed by his opposite number in England, Professor Ian Gilmore, who told *The Sunday Times*: "Not allowing people to drink more than three drinks in a pub is a wonderful solution if it were practical."(38)

Gilmore was not alone in spotting that such a law would be very difficult to enforce. It was clearly impractical for the state to restrict the number of drinks a person consumed, but it was equally clear that the practitioners of public health would readily embrace such 'wonderful solutions' if only there was a way of policing them. Since there was not, the reformers turned to the stock policies of higher taxation, banning advertising and restricting sale. The last thing they wanted was a liberalisation of the drinking laws but that, rather unexpectedly, is what they got.

Under Tony Blair, the British government exhibited a schizophrenic attitude towards what used to be called vice. Unsure whether to play the part of bossy nanny or trendy uncle, Blair took a hard line on smoking and diet while abolishing betting tax and making cannabis semi-legal. The liberal policies pertaining to gambling and marijuana came in the early years of the New Labour government but, as the years wore on, paternalism and regulation came back into favour. It therefore came as a shock when the government proposed a relaxation of the UK's archaic drinking laws, a move resisted by large sections of the press, the television networks and politicians on both sides of the House, not least Labour's own backbenchers.

Although only a handful of establishments applied for a 24 hour license, it was confidently predicted that Britain would erupt in an orgy of liver-bursting violence and anarchy. That the British were intrinsically, perhaps genetically, incapable of walking past an open pub came to be seen as a universal truism. One judge predicted that the law would create "urban savages" and an 'addiction expert' from the University of Ulster typified the popular view when he said: "Our psyche is not equipped to handle the 24-hour availability of alcohol."(39) Far from allowing the masses to drink after 11 pm, said opponents of the Bill, greater restrictions should be enforced to encourage sobriety. An article in *The Lancet* described alcohol as being "as harmful as smoking" and recommended new tax rises to reduce its consumption.

Just as the pot-bellied suddenly became 'obese' in the terminology of public health, those who liked a drink became 'binge-drinkers'. Like the word 'obesity,' 'binge-drinking' was not an obscure term prior to 2003, but it had traditionally meant a prolonged drinking session, often lasting several days. In the new era of public health, it came to mean the consumption of three or more drinks on the same day; something that had until recently been known simply as 'drinking.'

The public health historian Virginia Berridge went to the trouble of looking for the term 'binge-drinking' in *The Times* and Hansard. She found that, until 2002, there were only a handful of references to it in

The Times and it was never used at all in the House of Commons. Only once the Licensing Act was mooted did it shoot its way into common parlance. In 2005, it appeared on 170 occasions in *The Times* and was spoken 250 times in Parliament (40). By this time, its original meaning had all but disappeared and the British did not even need to get drunk to qualify as binge-drinkers; the official definition encompassed anyone who drank more than twice their recommended daily limit in an evening.

The amount one could 'safely' drink had been falling for years. In the 1960s, Britons were advised to drink no more than a bottle of wine per day. In 1979, the advice for men was to drink no more than 56 units a week (around 4 pints of beer a day). Five years later this was reduced to 36 units and by the end of the 1980s it stood at 21 units, a little over a pint of lager a day (41). In short, the amount of alcohol that could be safely enjoyed was cut by two-thirds in the space of twenty years and for women it was a third lower still (14 units).

No one was quite sure where these limits came from, including, apparently, the doctors who set them. Dr Richard Smith was a member of the committee which came up with the recommendations in 1987 and he remembers "rather vividly" how they were arrived at:

> "David Barker was the epidemiologist on the committee and his line was that
> 'We don't really have any decent data whatsoever.
> It's impossible to say what's safe and what isn't'.
> And other people said, 'Well, that's not much use. If somebody comes to see you
> and says 'What can I safely drink?', you can't say 'Well, we've no evidence.
> Come back in 20 years and we'll let you know'.
> So the feeling was that we ought to come up with something.
> So those limits were really plucked out of the air.
> They weren't really based on any firm evidence at all." (42)

With the criteria for who qualified as a drunk set so low, it was no surprise that Britain found itself in the depths of another public health plague. The *BMJ* described a "worsening epidemic of public drunkenness" (43) and Scottish Health Action on Alcohol Problems declared that "alcohol misuse has now reached epidemic proportions."(44)

What constituted this terrifying epidemic? According to the Office of National Statistics, the number of men drinking more than 4 units a day actually fell from 39% to 35% between 2004 and 2005 (45) and the number of women drinking above government guidelines barely rose - from 8% to 9% - and remained low. Although the BMA chairman claimed that the UK was "one of the heaviest alcohol consuming countries in Europe," the British were firmly mid-table in the drinking league, with twelve European countries having a higher per capita rate of alcohol consumption (46).

Of course, alcohol abuse was not just a health issue, it also had ramifications for social disorder ('drink-fuelled mayhem' being the popular description) but violent crime peaked in 1995 and had dropped by 44% since, even after the offence had been strangely redefined to include 'violence not resulting in injury.'(47) And even if Britain had more than its fair share of idiots who behaved badly when drunk, it was doubtful whether the measures proposed by public health campaigners would have any effect on them. If restricting opening hours and raising prices were the answer to binge-drinking then Britain, with its 11 pm closing time and high rates of alcohol tax, should, by rights, have had some of the most moderate and polite drinkers in the world.

Despite substantial opposition in Parliament and in the media, the Licensing Act was introduced in November 2005 and, contrary to all predictions, failed to bring about the end of British civilisation. Alcohol sales fell by 2% in 2005 and by 3.3% in 2006, the latter figure representing the sharpest drop for fifteen years (48). The biggest fall in consumption was seen in pubs and clubs (49).

As for drink-fuelled mayhem, the last three months of 2005 saw violent crime fall by 21%, in contrast to a 11% rise in the same period in 2004. Disbelieving public health bodies urged the public to wait for more data. The Institute of Alcohol Studies simply refused to accept the news at all, calling the statistics "entirely bogus," and accused the government of "sleight of hand"(50) but crime figures for 2005 and 2006 showed no rise in violent crime or drunken assaults and, for a while, the controversy died down.

By July 2007, however, the political climate had changed. Blair was gone and Gordon Brown had never shown any enthusiasm for the Licensing Act. England's smoking ban had just come into effect and the public health lobby saw alcohol as the next obvious target. New figures from the Office of National Statistics were released that month and, again, they showed no increase in overall violent crime. There was, however, a rise between the hours of 3 am and 6 am. The numbers were small and the rise was more than compensated by a fall in violence at the old closing hours between 11 pm and 2 am, but it was enough for the British press to feel validated in their earlier predictions of anarchy, as was a study published in the BMA's *Emergency Medical Journal* which purportedly showed a trebling in the number of alcohol-related hospital admissions (51). The paper had echoes of the notorious Helena heart attack study, based as it was on data from a single hospital in a single month, but if such a rise was seen around the country it would indeed suggest a serious problem. However, no other hospitals released their own data and the very fact that the national crime statistics showed no rise in drunken violence strongly suggested that the BMA study was erroneous.

Unlike the fears about obesity, which were based on a genuine - if exaggerated - social trend, the panic about 'Booze Britain' came about despite all the facts showing that consumption was going down. To describe it as an 'epidemic' was plainly ridiculous, as Charles Moore observed in *The Telegraph*:

"Doctors, of all people, should use the word epidemic carefully. It is, as the dictionary records, a disease which is 'prevalent among a people at a special time, and produced by some special causes'. Bubonic plague was an epidemic, so is winter vomiting.
The problem with alcohol is almost exactly the opposite: it is endemic.
It takes slightly different forms at different times, but it is with us always." (52)

The facts notwithstanding, there was, by 2007, a general consensus that the UK was in the grip of a binge-drinking epidemic. Still lacking evidence, the Office of National Statistics helpfully announced that henceforth it would assume that all Britons were drinking stronger beverages from larger glasses. This arbitrary decision meant that everyone was now drinking 33% more alcohol than had previously been assumed and 13 million people were now classified as drinking at hazardous levels. This happened to be the same number of people who were smokers and the £1.7 billion that the BMA claimed drinkers were costing the NHS each year was very close to the £1.5 billion that smokers were said to cost the taxpayer. The stakes rose further the following year when the Department of Health announced that alcohol was now costing the NHS £2.7 billion a year (53).

Something had to be done.

One effect of the ONS's decision to assume larger glasses and stronger drinks was that it meant that a woman who drank just one glass of wine a night was consuming significantly more than her weekly limit of 14 units of alcohol. The Department of Health leapt into action to address these 'binge-drinkers' with a £10 million advertising campaign aimed at middle-class, middle-aged ladies. Unable to influence the drinking habits of young thugs and alcoholics, public health campaigners directed their attention towards the mild-mannered people of middle England. Dr Sarah Jarvis, in *The Sunday Times*:

> "Older people think that because they are not vomiting in the street they are not binge drinkers but that is not true. These people share a bottle of wine with their partners every night as well as having gin and tonics before supper." (54)

With "these people" now caught in the cross-fire, the campaign against binge-drinking resembled less of a war against drunken yobs than a crusade to reduce general alcohol consumption to a medicinal level (calls for total abstinence were blocked only by evidence from Richard Doll that showed moderate drinking to be good for the heart). Six weeks after the smoking ban took effect in England, Cheshire's Chief Constable called for a total ban on drinking outdoors. Public health minister Caroline Flint announced that warning labels would be put on all bottles of alcohol and the BMA served up a smorgasbord of policies to tackle the "epidemic of alcohol misuse" including banning happy hours, forcing landlords to stick anti-alcohol posters up in their pubs and putting health warnings on wine lists in restaurants.

Centre stage was the president of the Royal College of Physicians, Ian Gilmore. After declaring himself "blissfully happy" on the day of the smoking ban, Gilmore called for a total ban on alcohol advertising and became chairman of the Alcohol Health Alliance. This newly formed pressure group was a conglomeration of like-minded public health bodies whose members had clearly learnt the lessons from ASH's co-ordinated public relations campaign of 2005-06 and saw that they could achieve more if they spoke with one voice than if they spoke alone (the "swarm effect," as ASH called it). The Alcohol Health Alliance declared that alcohol was worse than drugs and demanded a 10% tax rise on drink which, it claimed, would result in "up to" 30% fewer alcohol-related deaths (55).

The phrase 'passive drinking' had only ever been employed by satirists until Dr Peter Anderson said it with a straight face in a European Commission meeting in 2004. Anderson found it a useful way of paying lip-service to lovers of freedom while planning his assault on the 87% of Europeans who drank alcohol. "You can make the argument that what an individual drinks is up to them," he said, "provided they understand what they are doing and bearing in mind that alcohol is a dependency-producing drug…But when you talk about harm to others then that is a societal concern and justification for doing something about it. I think that is an important argument."(56)

In this one comment, Anderson drew together the familiar themes of addiction, ignorance of risk and cost to society that had been so potent in the hands of anti-smoking campaigners. After consultation with health lobbyists, Anderson drafted a report which concluded that alcohol's cost to society, children and the unborn was 125 billion euros a year - £80 billion at 2004 rates - which, as the authors eagerly noted was "roughly the same value as that found recently for tobacco."(57)

The lengths to which campaigners went to invoke the idea of passive harm was a tribute to the power of the passive smoking theory and the way in which it had transformed smoking from a personal choice to a public menace. It was no surprise that those who were in the thick of the battle over food and drink tried to harness similar terminology, even if the concept had to be stretched wafer thin to do so.

In Britain's Foresight report, 'passive obesity' meant becoming fat accidentally, as a result of societal factors beyond one's control. For the American Obesity Association, it had the same meaning as Anderson's 'passive drinking,' in that the damage was primarily financial. Its spokeswoman Morgan Downey made the link with tobacco explicit: "It's like secondhand smoking, you don't have to be obese to be affected." For MeMe Roth of National Action Against Obesity - an organisation dedicated to "eradicating secondhand obesity"(58) - the term had a still more tenuous definition. Roth advised people against socialising with the overweight in case they came to see obesity as normal and because they were more likely to get dragged into fast food restaurants. It did not really matter how 'passive drinking' or 'passive obesity' was defined. What was important was that those who did not drink or overeat felt personally harmed by those who did.

In all this, the unheard argument that desperately needed to be made was that neither alcohol nor food were legitimate public health issues. The medical estimate of annual British fatalities from obesity in 2007 was 8,500. For alcohol, the figure was 9,000. Even if one ignored the tendency of health organisations to exaggerate such figures for dramatic effect, these death rates were hardly suggestive of a serious problem, let alone an epidemic, except for a tiny minority of chronic alcoholics and morbidly obese individuals who would, in any case, never be deterred by expensive health campaigns or by a few extra pence tax on their burgers or vodka.

It took a peculiar sort of vanity for public health spokesmen to believe that a chronic alcoholic would moderate his drinking as a result of the recommended daily limit going from two pints of beer to one and half. The only people who were likely to respond to such policies were the 'worried well'; those who were at no risk from alcohol-related diseases but whose obedience to government diktats would help the servants of public health hit their targets for overall consumption.

The central premise in the public health campaign against food and drink was that if the general population could be persuaded to make modest changes to its diet and drinking habits, it would somehow, miraculously, bring health benefits to the minority who ate and drank far in excess of what was good for them. The shortcomings of this theory scarcely need to be underlined. It is based on the misguided and patronizing belief that those who eat and drink to excess are blind to the harm they are doing to themselves. Meanwhile, everybody else is lectured, taxed and penalised because they are moderately overweight or get drunk from time to time, despite their lifestyles having practically no detrimental effect on their health.

Those who support and encourage these largely futile campaigns frequently justify them on the basis that they 'send out the right message.' This is the sheerest rhetoric. The 'message' is ignored by the target audience and is irrelevant to those who pay attention. The eagerness of politicians to go along with this nonsense often stems, not from a belief that they will do any practical good, but from a desire to be seen to be doing *something*, preferably with the minimum of effort, about issues which are routinely, if misleadingly, described as public health epidemics. But politicians are no more capable of tackling the underlying psychological causes of morbid obesity or chronic alcoholism than doctors are able to cure cancer. Draconian legislation is embraced by those in government because they feel compelled to act and because they are immersed in a political climate that is as apocalyptic as it is puritanical.

Since most of the laws passed to stem these supposed epidemics are useless, more laws must be passed to paper over the cracks, and a perpetual cycle of criminalisation is set in motion which serves only to bolster the fantasy that politicians are 'getting tough' on the health issue. Every activity must become more intensely regulated, sin taxes must spiral ever upwards, health warnings must become more shocking, advertising must be curtailed and the age at which one can legally purchase certain products must be raised. Above all, no matter how ineffective these policies may be, they can never be relaxed, for to do so would send out the 'wrong message' to the public. The moral panic and media fury that surrounded the Licensing Act amply demonstrated how widely held is the belief in the necessity for creeping regulation. It was a rare example of the Blair government challenging this political orthodoxy. The other notable exception is the subject of our next section.

The gambling 'epidemic'

No war on vice would be complete without a crack-down on gambling but even the most excitable epidemiologists have yet to associate roulette with cancer. It can still be a touching moment when neo-puritan agendas collide. New Zealand's smoking ban hit casinos and pubs hard and gambling revenue in these venues inevitably declined. For the nation's moral reformers, the side effect of less drinking and less gambling in these dens of iniquity was every bit as gratifying as the reduction in secondhand smoke exposure. So keen was Mark Peck, director of New Zealand's Smokefree Coalition, to celebrate this triple whammy that he went off-message and forgot to insist that smoking bans were good for business. "Smokefree bars, clubs and casinos have saved lives by reducing people's exposure to second-hand smoke," he said, "Now it seems there has been another benefit - helping keep money out of pokie machines and in the pockets of families."(59)

Mr Peck, it should be said, was speaking as a straight-forward moralist and was not claiming that abstaining from gambling was an essential part of a healthy lifestyle. Apart from the occasional heart palpitation, gambling clearly does not damage the human body and would, therefore, seem to be outside the remit of the public health movement. But apparently not.

In 2005, the UK government kicked up a storm of outrage by proposing a relaxation of the country's gaming laws. The proposal would have allowed 40 new casinos to be built and the abolition of the 24 hour rule which prevented new members entering the premises on the day they joined. Like the Licensing Act, it was savaged by politicians of all persuasions and was almost unanimously condemned by the press for bringing what they invariably described as 'Las Vegas-style super-casinos' to British shores. After a back-bench revolt, the government beat a hasty retreat and reduced the bill to the point where it allowed just one new 'super-casino' license. Even this was opposed as if the barbarians were at the gates. It was confidently predicted that this solitary casino would drive the British working classes to poverty and ruin, the like of which had not been seen since the days of Hogarth. Police spokesmen who had, only a year earlier, promised urban chaos if the Licensing Act was made law issued the same grim warnings about anti-social behaviour and drunkenness if this last sliver of liberalisation was allowed through.

Professor Jim Orford, a psychology lecturer at Birmingham University, accused the government of being pressured by the "gaming industry" and accused ministers of not giving "sufficient attention to the public health aspects of problem gambling."(60) The *BMJ* waded in with a report, published to coincide with the announcement of which city would get the new casino, and released it early to the press. It became front-page news, with *The Independent on Sunday* warning that "a health time-bomb is ticking and women are most at risk."(61) In this climate of moral outrage, the Conservative party refused to be outdone by its opponents on the left and called for health warnings to be put on adverts for gambling.

As all this chest-beating went on, the National Lottery escaped without a mention. It offered odds that were far worse than any game in a casino and had been launched to much the same dire forecasts in 1994. Back then, the *BMJ* had published an editorial entitled 'Gambling with the nation's health?'(62) which cited the recent suicide of a man who had forgotten to buy his ticket and warned that children might be 'exposed' to the live draw on television. But its main objection was that: "Anything that makes poor people in Britain even poorer, especially if they do not derive benefits in kind, becomes an important public health issue." (63)

In 2007, the *BMJ* published another article - also entitled 'Gambling with the nation's health' (this time without the question mark) - but the best it could manage was the idea that, as the BBC reported it, "gamblers eat badly and their preoccupation means they neglect the early signs of illness."(64)(65)

The *BMJ*'s argument rested on four assumptions. Firstly, that making gambling more readily available would inevitably lead to a rise in 'problem gambling.' Secondly, that this would lead to greater poverty. Thirdly, that poverty leads to ill-health and, finally, that the government was compelled to pass laws to deter, limit and prohibit any activity that puts health at risk, even if that activity is freely entered into.

This was to assume a great deal, and there were plenty of reasons to believe this analysis to be wholly wrong. The 2007 *BMJ* article noted that 2.6% Americans were problem gamblers but failed to mention that the US had such tight gambling laws that many Americans required use of an aeroplane if they wished to visit a casino. In the UK, where betting shops were on every street, fruit machines were in every pub and where most people could easily visit a casino if they were so inclined, just 0.6% were problem gamblers, less than a quarter of the US proportion. Meanwhile the Chinese - arguably the keenest gamblers on earth - lived in a country where all forms of gambling were completely illegal. Availability was clearly no more the agent of gambling than it was of drinking and in neither case was prohibition a viable solution.

The argument against seeing *relative* poverty as a cause of ill-health has been outlined earlier in this chapter and one wonders how many Britons could ever realistically be plunged into the kind of absolute poverty that might result in chronic ill-health and early death. All the towns which applied to become the site of the proposed super-casino were in areas of relative deprivation and they fought hard to win the contract, knowing how many jobs it would create. If the National Lottery can be accused (not unreasonably) of taking money from the poor to spend on the pursuits of the wealthy, it can just as easily be argued that casinos take from the wealthy and give jobs to the poor.

But even if none of this is true - even if gambling really is a pernicious vice with no redeeming features - it is hard to see it as a genuine public health issue. At one time, not so very long ago, public health activists had advised people against drinking contaminated water because it spread cholera and because those who drank it would become ill and/or die. Since the 1970s, they have decided to stop people smoking cigarettes and drinking alcohol because some people *might* become addicted and some of those who did *might* then become ill and die. Now they desire to stop people gambling because a very small number *might* become addicted and *might* lose heavily and *might* become poor and then become...what? Depressed? Malnourished? Alcoholic? Cause and effect has become so tenuous, and there are now so many what-ifs, that if playing blackjack is a public health issue, what isn't?

The *BMJ*'s fears of 1994 were unfounded. The National Lottery quickly became accepted as a harmless, even cherished, feature of British life, not unlike the football pools that came before it. Lottery fever failed to lead to any marked increase in compulsive gambling and despite being exposed to a televised draw twice a week, a generation of children grew up unscathed. Little more was heard of the health perils of gambling until the new casino was proposed and this time the champions of public health triumphed. With Blair gone, it took less than a month for Gordon Brown to announce a review of the Licensing Act, a review of cannabis's Class C status and the abolition of the super-casino.

A real epidemic

While public health officials broadened the definition of the word 'epidemic' until it encompassed almost any popular activity, a real epidemic continued to ravage the world as a direct result of their own misguided efforts.

Malaria has killed more people than any disease in history and has been on the rise worldwide since the early 1970s when, far from coincidentally, activists from groups like the Pesticide Action Network persuaded the Environmental Protection Agency that the mosquito-killing pesticide DDT was carcinogenic to humans and devastating to wildlife. These pressure groups had been heavily influenced by the ideas of Rachel Carson, an environmentalist who studied the effects of DDT on rainbow trout and who concluded that it caused liver cancer in humans. In her book *Silent Spring* (1962), Carson claimed that cancer could reach "practically 100 percent" of the human population if use of the chemical was not stamped out. In addition to being a carcinogen, DDT was accused of lowering sperm counts, causing genetic mutations and decimating wild bird populations. One-time anti-smoking advocate Ralph Nader first stepped into the limelight after he discovered a dead bird in the grounds of Harvard University and became a vociferous campaigner against DDT.

The EPA carried out its own investigation in 1972 and concluded that DDT was harmless to humans but, as converts to the precautionary principle, banned it all the same. The WHO urged unilateral action against the pesticide and, lacking the power to outlaw it worldwide, set the threshold for 'safe' exposure so low that its use was, in practice, impossible (66).

The battle against DDT had almost universal support amongst environmentalists and Western health campaigners. When *Silent Spring* was reissued in 1994, Al Gore penned an introduction which praised the author and the anti-DDT movement she had inspired: "Because Carson's work led to the ban on DDT," he wrote, "it may be that the human species...or at least countless human lives, will be saved because of the words she wrote."(67) Six years later, the United Nations brought 120 countries together to ratify the Treaty on Persistent Organic Pollutants which would bring about a worldwide ban on DDT.

There were only two problems. Firstly, Carson's hypothesis was nonsense. Not only was she wrong but she had been shown to be wrong years before Al Gore celebrated her work, and the WHO's own research proved it (68). Liver problems in the trout Carson had studied were not due to DDT but to fungi. Not a single study ever showed DDT to be carcinogenic to humans and there was no rise in liver cancer cases amongst people - principally farmers - who were most exposed it (69).

Secondly, DDT was, and still is, the cheapest and most effective killer of malaria-carrying mosquitoes. By 1970, it had almost entirely eradicated malaria in Sri Lanka and Bangladesh. In India, DDT reduced the number of annual cases from 10 million to 300,000. This happy trend went into a dramatic and tragic reversal after environmental and health activists embarked on a mission to eliminate DDT.

Carson died of cancer in 1964 and did not live to see the damage her theories caused. The WHO launched a project called Roll Back Malaria, which aimed to cut the death toll from malaria in half by providing bed nets instead of pesticides, but rates of the disease continued to rise. With each year that passed, another two million people died of malaria and those who survived were often left permanently damaged, but Western health groups remained preoccupied with the supposed social and environmental causes of disease. Between 1989 and 1992, when the EPA was putting together its report to show that secondhand smoke caused 3,000 deaths a year, there were ten million deaths from malaria, most of them easily preventable.

In 1996, after international lobbying, South Africa banned DDT and the number of malaria cases rocketed by 1,000% (70). The Centers for Disease Control said nothing about this terrifying rise but did find time to add cigarette smoking to their list of 55 'diseases'. In 2003, when an estimated 400 million people contracted malaria, the WHO put together the Framework Convention on Tobacco Control, an international treaty which stressed the need to "protect all persons from exposure to tobacco smoke" and to increase the size of warning labels on cigarette packs (71).

By 2005, after decades of overwhelming evidence showing that DDT did not cause cancer, even Ralph Nader accepted the urgent need for its re-introduction. Fans of sound science and rational public health policy had a rare reason to cheer in September 2006 when the World Health Organisation partially reversed its opposition to DDT and promoted its domestic use in the Third World. The WHO's U-turn arrived with little fanfare, no apology and no resignations. Dr Arata Kochi, Director of WHO's Global Malaria Programme, simply explained:

> "We must take a position based on the science and the data.
> One of the best tools we have against malaria is indoor residual housing spraying.
> Of the dozen insecticides WHO has approved as safe for house spraying,
> the most effective is DDT" (72)

The EPA, however, continues to oppose the use of DDT and maintains that it is a "probable human carcinogen." Since the agency first labelled it as such, up to fifty million people - most of them children - have died needlessly of malaria.

CHAPTER FOURTEEN

'The scene is set for the final curtain'

From creating nonsmoking sections to banning smoking in the outdoors; the pace of change had been so rapid that it was easy to forget it had all taken place in the space of twenty years. To provide some context, consider the ASH (New Zealand) booklet of 1987 which called for nothing more severe than a smoking ban on all domestic flights, on the basis that they were seldom more than one hour long (1). ASH made no demands of restaurants or airports and did not mention bars at all, only suggesting that nonsmokers tell the waiter that it would be a nice if there was a nonsmoking section. Two years later, the American chat show legend Steve Allen wrote *The Passionate Nonsmokers' Bill of Rights*. This book was one of the most uncompromising anti-smoking tracts of its time and yet it viewed a smoking ban on airlines as "one of the final frontiers of the nonsmokers' rights movement."(2)

Two decades later, total smoking bans in aeroplanes and restaurants were taken for granted. The real 'final frontier' for nonsmokers' right groups remained on the horizon. For some, the fight had only just begun. "We've got to start somewhere," said Georgia State Representative Paul Smith as he proposed criminalising people who smoked in their own cars (3).

Something must be done

A month before the smoking ban was enacted in England, a Department of Health spokesman said: "This isn't about a witch hunt against smokers - it is about promoting healthier and cleaner atmospheres." On the other side of the argument, the smokers' rights group FOREST claimed that "the real agenda is to force people into quitting."(4) By 2008, it was hard to deny that the tobacco industry-funded lobby group had a point.

Any claim that anti-smoking policies were designed only to 'protect' nonsmokers was highly disingenuous. Everyone who worked for the Department of Health was well aware that the government had set them the target of reducing the smoking rate to 21% by 2010. This target had been set in the *Choosing Health* White Paper of 2004 but the clock was running out and reputations were at stake. From Julian Le Grand's plan to force smokers to carry licenses to ASH's proposal to have cigarettes sold under the counter like pornography, everything was fair game in this race against time. The policies that were suggested brought to mind the words of the verbose civil servant Sir Humphrey in *Yes, Prime Minister*:

"Something must be done. This is something, therefore we must do it." (5)

Gruesome pictures of diseased organs were placed on cigarette packs in 2008. Displaying tobacco products in shops was to be banned from 2011. Parents were told that, if they had to smoke, "they must do it not just out of the house but out of sight of their children."(6) Smokers were banned from adopting children. The Royal College of Physicians called for a doubling in the price of cigarettes to £10 a pack (7). There was serious talk of banning smoking in the street and in cars (the 2006 law had already banned it in outdoor stadia and train platforms). A sprightly ASH called all this, and more, the "natural follow-on from the good work started by going smoke-free in 2006."(8) Of the proposed ban in cars, ASH predicted that "in a few years time people will think it's inconceivable that we allowed people to smoke while driving."

As we saw in the last chapter, the UK's sudden endorsement of extreme public health measures did not stop at tobacco. Nowhere in the world was the fabled slippery slope more in evidence than in the British Isles. With a smoking ban now firmly in place, the Mayor of London banned alcohol on public transport; doctors called for pictures of diseased livers and cancerous mouths to be stuck on bottles of alcohol; the police demanded laws to force pub-goers to remain seated while drinking (9); the state-funded pressure group Alcohol Concern said that parents who allowed their children to drink at home should be prosecuted (10); Julian Le Grand called for a "dramatic rise" in the price of drink and proposed banning supermarkets from selling alcohol altogether; and, as if paying homage to SmokeFree Movies, 'a new study' announced that those who saw drinking in films drank twice as much as those who did not (11).

The environmental movement also took a leaf from the anti-smokers' book. The "morally unacceptable" practice of drinking bottled water had to be made "as unfashionable as smoking," according to one government advisor. The Institute for Public Policy Research called for higher air fares to "tackle our addiction to flying" and recommended warnings like 'Flying causes climate change' be placed on holiday advertisements (12). A coalition of global warming protesters chose the first day of England's smoking ban to place adverts in the national press which mimicked those found on cigarette packs, with slogans such as 'Get help to cut down on flying' and 'Flying kills: 160,000 die each year from climate change.' Lest anyone miss the point, they set up a website called flyingsthenewsmoking.com.

Often imitated but never outshone, the anti-smoking groups had no intention of passing on the baton to a new generation of reformers and had no shortage of new policies to pursue. A movement that viewed tens of millions of smokers as child-abusers was never likely to be obstructed by such trifling matters as private property rights or parental sovereignty. In several US states, foster parents were prohibited from smoking in their own homes and plans were afoot to extend these laws to parents and grandparents. When smoking was involved, it seemed, the government had not only the right but the responsibility to put its foot down. Kathleen Dachille of the Legal Resource Center for Tobacco Regulation, Litigation & Advocacy explained:

"There are times when it's appropriate to regulate what people can do in their home. The state is responsible for that child." (13)

Smokers were expected to feel privileged even to be allowed to smoke *outside* their workplaces and were invited to view such small liberties as generous concessions that could, and very probably would, be snatched away when the time came. If some members of the anti-smoking movement had their way, smokers would not have a workplace to go to at all. ASH fully supported discrimination against smokers and urged employers "to save 25% or more on smoking-related costs" by "insisting that their workers not smoke on or off the job."(14) Nigel Gray, a veteran Australian anti-smoking activist and IARC employee, spelt out the next 'logical step' in *Tobacco Control* when he wrote:

> "I have always thought that the ultimate objective is a workplace which is
> both smoke-free and smoker-free." (15)

Some US states had laws prohibiting employers from discriminating against those who smoked but they did not represent any sort of smokers' rights backlash. Smokers were only protected because existing employment laws did not allow discrimination against those who engaged in 'lawful acts' in their own time, a legal obstacle the anti-smokers had yet to overcome. John Slade called these laws "unnecessarily punitive" (on employers) and there are hopes that smokers may yet be exempted from such legislation, as they are in Europe (16).

In 2005, the Michigan health care company Weyco Inc., fired four employees for using tobacco outside of working hours. The firm also has a policy of fining workers $50 a month if their *spouse* smokes or chews tobacco. Clarian Health, a company based in Indianapolis, routinely fines employees if they use tobacco or exceed the company's cholesterol and blood pressure limits. "We're only seeing the beginning of this," said Jeremy Gruber of the National Workrights Institute. "Employers started with smokers. Now they're moving on to the general population." (17)

Those who did not have children and only smoked at home were, in the main, grudgingly tolerated but even this looked like it may be coming to an end. "People are complaining about smoke going from one apartment to another apartment," according to Stanton Glantz. By his assessment, the drift of smoke particles going down corridors and through windows was a real threat to the lives of nonsmoking neighbours because the "level of toxicity in the smoke is very, very high."(18)

That all this amounted to a coercive campaign to eradicate tobacco use amongst consenting adults was becoming obvious to even the most innocent minds and yet the anti-smokers persisted in framing the battle for domestic and outdoor bans in terms of protecting nonsmokers. Fortuitously for them - though hardly coincidentally - the science was "evolving" to suit their new goals.

No safe level

On 27 July 2006, the US Surgeon General Richard H. Carmona carried on the rich tradition of exaggeration and speculation that had characterised his department's pronouncements on passive smoke for 20 years. Since taking office, Carmona had already claimed that smoking caused disease "in nearly every organ of the body" including pneumonia, stomach cancer, leukemia and cataracts, and had gone on the record to say he would like to see tobacco banned by law (19). On the twentieth anniversary of Koop's notorious 1986 report, this self-confessed prohibitionist tackled the subject of secondhand smoke and, having brought in anti-smoking war-horses like Michael Thun and Stanton Glantz to help write it, produced the most outlandish publication yet to emerge from the Office of Public Health.

In keeping with Koop, Carmona saved his tastiest sound-bites for the press conference and, as in 1986, this was because the message he wished to have heard was not supported by the substance of his 700 page volume. "The health effects of secondhand smoke are more pervasive than we previously thought," Carmona announced. "There is NO risk-free level of exposure to secondhand smoke. Let me say that again: There is no risk-free level of exposure to secondhand smoke."(20). According to the Surgeon General (who resigned shortly afterwards) the briefest period - even a few minutes - around smokers could induce heart attacks. Carmona left the press with a simple message to relay to their readers: "Stay away from smokers." Such remarks were overtly aimed at laying the foundations for outdoor smoking bans and what he ominously referred to as "voluntary adherence to policies at home."(21)

The American Medical Association's president-elect Ron Davis called the report "a wake-up call for lawmakers to enact comprehensive clean-air laws that prohibit smoking in all indoor public places."(22) The Campaign for Tobacco-Free Kids said that it "once and for all ends any scientific debate about whether exposure to secondhand smoke is a cause of serious diseases."(23) Carmona's wildest speculations were treated as if they were conservative estimates by the multitude of anti-smoking groups. Americans for Nonsmokers' Rights announced that thirty minutes of exposure to secondhand smoke was enough to give a nonsmoker a heart attack. SmokeFreeOhio went one better by reducing this time to 20 minutes and Stanton Glantz's TobaccoScam declared that 20 minutes exposure was comparable to smoking 20 cigarettes a day.

Minnesota's Association for Nonsmokers beat them all, telling the press that: "Just thirty *seconds* of exposure can make coronary artery function *indistinguishable from smokers*" (my emphasis) (24). This was a whisker away from stating that tobacco smoke killed on contact and yet the idea that brief exposure to cigarette smoke was as dangerous as a lifetime's smoking was somewhere between biologically impossible and certifiably insane. It was official acceptance of James Repace's curious theory that no matter how diluted or how rarely it was encountered, tobacco smoke killed indiscriminately.

With such arrant nonsense being spouted by the nation's most powerful health authority, it was no surprise when politicians and pundits lost contact with reality. "We know that secondhand smoke is worse than first hand smoke," said Pennsylvanian State Representative Peter Daley, in an effort to promote a law banning smoking in cars (something he had been trying to pass since 1988). Proposing similar legislation in California, Senator Deborah Ortiz declared: "Children are effectively smoking a pack and a half a day for every hour they are exposed to smoke in a car" - a miraculous feat of inhalation that could not be matched by the most dedicated chain-smoker (25).

Around the same time, another 'new study' suggested that passive smokers inhaled seven times as much nicotine as smokers and anti-smoking groups claimed that secondhand smoke contained "five times more carbon monoxide" and "twice as much nicotine" as mainstream smoke (26). Anyone reading a newspaper in 2006 could be forgiven for believing that secondhand smoke was not only a cause of lung cancer but was its *chief* cause. When the stop-smoking guru Allen Carr was diagnosed with lung cancer, aged 73, his publicist and business partner strongly suggested that it was passive smoking that had killed him. It seemed to count for nothing that Carr, by his own admission, had smoked 100 cigarettes a day for 33 years (27).

Perhaps the most egregious example of the champions of public health divorcing themselves from science is their assertion that there is "no safe level" of whatever it is they wish to see regulated. Quite simply, and without equivocation, there is a safe level for *everything*. If we take arsenic or benzene as examples, the safe level is very low and it becomes more of an academic distinction than a practical one. Still, both are present in a cup of coffee. In the case of margarine, alcohol, bacon and secondhand smoke, it is misleading to say that they are made up of poisons at all and frankly dishonest to pretend that they are deadly in trace amounts. And yet that is precisely what some health campaigners would have us believe. It is a conceit which defies both science and reason and is served up as a 'noble lie' in the expectation that the public will be frightened into changing their ways for their own good. It is, in a word, propaganda.

The trouble with propaganda is that the truth sometimes gets in the way. When, in 1994, Sir Richard Doll produced an epidemiological study which showed that moderate drinkers lived longer than teetotallers, the WHO was so perturbed by what it saw as its pro-alcohol message that it responded with one of its most outrageous statements yet: "There is no minimum threshold below which alcohol can be consumed without any risk," declared the director of the WHO Programme on Substance Abuse, adding that "the less you drink, the better."(28)

The words were unambiguous. Any health-conscious person would have interpreted them as an instruction not to drink any alcohol at all. But if Doll's research was correct - and it was backed up by plenty of other studies - abstaining from alcohol would make a person more likely to die younger. Increasingly, major health organisations are prepared to issue advice that they know to be untrue in an effort to send out a simple message to the public. As a consequence, moderation has been jettisoned in favour of puritanism and abolitionism, or, to put it in more fashionable terms: zero tolerance.

In 2007, for example, the UK Department of Health told women not to drink any alcohol whatsoever during pregnancy. There was, it said, no known "safe level" of alcohol use for a woman who was pregnant or, bizarrely, was *trying* to get pregnant. In truth, most doctors, along with the Royal College of Midwives, considered the occasional drink to be entirely harmless and accused the government of going over their heads in issuing the warning. Heavy drinking was known to be bad for the unborn child but occasional drinking was not. The fact that there was no consensus on exactly where the line lay between the two was irrelevant and the 'safe level' rhetoric was a distraction.

The Department of Health admitted that it had no evidence for this new zero tolerance approach but had wanted to issue a clear and unequivocal message that would reach those women who were drinking above the *existing* guidelines. These women made up just 9% of the total and, since they had ignored the current advice, there was little reason to believe they would fall into line if the limit was lowered. None of this deterred the government from treating the other 91% like idiots who could not distinguish between moderation and excess.

The real message, which could equally be applied to the 2006 Surgeon General's Report, was that government health agencies could no longer to be trusted to provide accurate medical advice and were now willfully misleading the public in an effort to manipulate behaviour.

It is not truth that matters, but victory

The passive smoking theory was being stretched to breaking point in the bid to ban smoking in parks, streets and in the home. One promising avenue of research was presented by Professor Georg Matt, a psychologist at the University of San Diego. In a paper published in *Tobacco Control*, Matt declared that parents who went outside to smoke still harmed their children when they returned to the house because "90 per cent" of nicotine supposedly clung to surfaces, skin, hair and clothing, which the unfortunate offspring might then touch or inhale. In deadly earnest, Matt called his discovery "thirdhand smoke"(29) and the London *Metro* covered it on its front page with a quote from a doctor which seemed to confirm that the danger was very real: "You can't be too careful with babies and the air they breathe," she said, "even if you think that by smoking outside, at the bottom of the garden, you'll remove all traces."(30) ASH took the hypothesis one step further in a press release titled 'Smoker's Breath is Harmful to Health.' (31)

When it was reported in August 2006, the thirdhand smoke scare seemed to be the archetypal silly season story but, within a month, a UK health authority had banned its employees from smoking out of work, giving two reasons. The first was as old as smoking itself. The smell, they said, "could be offensive." The second was ultra-modern: "Particulate matter from tobacco settles on hair and clothing and may be a particular health risk to children and babies who ingest the toxins."(32)

As an example of junk science, this kind of hokum was tough to beat, but fellow Californian Dr Robert Higginbotham managed to go one better with this bizarre but apparently sincere pronouncement:

"If you smoke in your house at all even if you're not in the same room or *not even at home*, people are still exposed to secondhand smoke. Smoke particles get in the upholstery, rugs and drapes and continue to be re-circulated *for years*."(33) (my emphasis)

Having used the farcical conclusions of the Helena miracle to present secondhand smoke as *the* primary trigger for heart attacks, anti-smoking researchers behaved like ill-disciplined children who had escaped rebuke for one piece of naughtiness and were intent on seeing how far they could go, almost daring the public to call their bluff.

The idea that smoking bans immediately saved lives was an appealing one and although New York, Oregon, Florida, Scotland, Wales, England and California had not seen any significant fall in heart attacks after implementing their own comprehensive smoking bans (34), highly selective hospital admission data from Italy, France, Ireland and parts of the US were used to propagate the idea in the press. The sheer number of studies released persuaded sections of the public that there was no smoke without fire, but every one of them, without a single exception, was flawed to the point of absurdity.

A typical example was the study published in the journal *Preventive Medicine* which claimed that heart attacks fell by 39% in the town of Bowling Green, Ohio. The researchers noted that the number of heart attack admissions had fallen from 36 in 2002 to 22 in 2003; a striking drop and, as far as the report's authors were concerned, a convincing piece of evidence in favour of smoking bans. As ever, the devil was in the detail. Looking at the figures over a period of six years, it was immediately obvious that 2002 had seen an unusually high number of recorded heart attacks:

1999: 35

2000: 24

2001: 24

2002: 36

2003: 22

2004: 26

These figures scarcely require further comment. Quite obviously, there was an unusual peak in 2002 after which the number of admissions returned to average. Such peaks come about by chance, especially when the numbers are small to begin with; there had been a similar one in 1999 (35).

If that was not enough, the smoking ban did not even begin in 2003 but in March 2002. In other words, the peak in heart attack incidence occurred in the very year that secondhand smoke exposure was reduced. It did not take an expert to see the defects in this study and yet the authors concluded that "clean indoor air ordinances lead to a reduction in hospital admissions for coronary heart disease."(36) It was a reflection of the sad state of epidemiology in 2007 that this study not only survived the peer-review process but was published.

The first weeks of 2009 saw the anti-smoking movement's estrangement from rational science turn into a full-blown divorce. Five years after first coining the term, Georg Matt was still no closer to finding any evidence that 'thirdhand smoke' was injurious to health. Left high and dry by science, Professor Matt made the inspired decision to bypass it altogether and simply take his hypothesis to the people. He unearthed a 2005 survey which showed that 65% of Americans believed that "breathing air in a room today where people smoked yesterday can harm the health of infants and children." Taking this to mean that a majority believed in the threat of thirdhand smoke, he used the survey as the basis of a new paper, published in the journal *Pediatrics*, which concluded:

> "Emphasizing that thirdhand smoke harms the health of children may be an important element in encouraging home smoking bans." (37)

The study was, as usual, released to the media in a bite-sized press release and, fortuitously for Matt, the press got the wrong end of the stick. Although thirdhand smoke was almost universally unrecognised even as a concept, journalists feigned shock at the fact that a third of the public were apparently unaware of its dangers. None dared to admit that they, too, were ignorant of a phenomenon which was, it seemed, so well recognised that it warranted a public survey. Headlines such as 'Warning over thirdhand smoke' (BBC), 'A new cigarette hazard' (*New York Times*) and 'Experts warn of dangers of thirdhand smoke' (*Chicago Tribune*) were sufficient to blast the idea into the public consciousness despite the total lack of hard - or even soft - evidence to support it.

Even with science being debased in such a way, there remained a reluctance amongst the scientific community to speak out. When it came to the war on smoking, the dominant ideology was that the ends justified the means, or as Adolf Hitler once put it: "It is not truth that matters, but victory." It took the most risible of the latest claims to stir *New Scientist* into reporting that:

> "...it looks as if anti-smoking campaigners have been distorting the facts to make their case. Some have claimed that a non-smoker exposed to tobacco smoke for just half an hour can permanently increase their risk of heart attack...Some might say, so what?
> If tobacco smoke is harmful, then surely anything that reduces people's exposure to it should be welcomed. Not so.
> Using bad science can never be justified, even in pursuit of noble causes."(38)

For those whose livelihoods depended on funding from public health bodies, challenging this "bad science" required considerable bravery since it meant cutting oneself off forever from millions of anti-smoking dollars and risking personal and professional vilification. When the journal *Epidemiologic Perspectives & Innovations* invited its readers to submit "cases of abuse of epidemiology or epidemiologists by organized political interests" it was shocked by what it received, as the next issue's editorial explained:

> "We expected to discover stories about industry and government, the entities most typically associated with using their power to the detriment of science...
> It turned out that all of the submissions we received about stories that had not previously appeared in the literature involved attacks on epidemiologists or epidemiology by anti-tobacco activists...
> Indeed, in our society today, it is difficult to imagine for-profit corporate entities thinking they could get away with actions like those taken by anti-tobacco activists. There is no doubt that powerful, rich organizations can be a threat to good science, and in the case of tobacco research, it is the multi-billion dollar anti-tobacco industry that currently plays that role." (39)

Criticism of the latest passive smoking claims was, understandably, thin on the ground amongst the tobacco control movement itself, but as the demands became more extreme and the science hit rock bottom, a handful of veteran activists began to express doubts. *Tobacco Control* editor Simon Chapman - hardly a tobacco industry mole - argued against outdoor smoking bans on the basis that they were scientifically unjustifiable and would "risk besmirching tobacco control advocates as the embodiment of intolerant, paternalistic busybodies."(40) Chapman also opposed the smokefree movie policy, believing it would open the door to lunatics of every persuasion:

"By what magic process could the sight of smoking in film be influential while being benign in reality? Doubtless the time is not far away when someone wielding research will call for public smoking to classified alongside indecent exposure as a felony. I would not wish to be associated with such nonsense and believe many others share my concerns that momentum to selectively prune unacceptable health related behaviours from film holds open the door for a conga line of other supplicants using the same reasoning." (41)

The American Council on Science and Health's director, Elizabeth Whelan, criticised the Surgeon General's 2006 report for mixing "facts, speculation and downright hyperbole" (42) and asked the tobacco control movement not to further strain the public's credulity by talking about a few minutes of secondhand smoke exposure knocking people dead. In recent years, Whelan had found herself increasingly adrift from an anti-smoking crusade intent on pushing mean-spirited and irrational extremism. ACSH was formed as a consumer advocacy group and had never focused solely on tobacco. It spent much of its time scrutinising some of the more imaginative health scares unleashed on the public in the era of junk science and this made them uneasy bedfellows with 21st century anti-smoking campaigners.

Whelan had formerly been a proponent of the passive smoking theory but when ACSH reviewed all the available evidence in 1999, she was forced to conclude that the threat to nonsmokers lay somewhere around zero. She was one of the few anti-smoking campaigners to publicly defend the Enstrom and Kabat study and while she approved of the New York smoking ban, she described Mayor Bloomberg's claim that it would save 1,000 lives a year as "patently absurd."(43)

Dr Alan Blum of Doctors Ought to Care criticised the contemporary tobacco control enterprise on somewhat different grounds. He first became involved in the movement in the 1970s, long before it became awash with money, and had never allowed the goal of persuading smokers to quit to be overshadowed by skirmishes with the tobacco industry or by attacks on smokers themselves. Blum expressed concern that the reliance of "perennial grant-receivers" on dollars that were ultimately extracted from cigarette smokers could be counter-productive. "I have yet to meet anyone in tobacco control," he said, "whose job depends on there being a decline in tobacco consumption."(44)

A similar sentiment was put in stronger terms by David Goerlitz. For most of the 1980s, Goerlitz had been RJ Reynolds' 'Winston Man' - the all-action equivalent of the Marlboro cowboy - before breaking ranks and publicly denouncing the tobacco industry for marketing cigarettes to children. His high public profile and insider knowledge made Goerlitz a useful ally of the anti-smoking movement when he began working with the Coalition on Smoking or Health in 1989. Now devoted to the prevention of underage smoking, the former Winston man has spent the last two decades telling his story in schools around the world.

Goerlitz remains passionate about youth prevention and supporting smokers who wish to quit. He is less supportive of high taxes, smoking bans and other policies aimed at adult smokers who have chosen to keep smoking. His approach is to "treat people with dignity and respect. Once you turn on them and dehumanise them and make them feel like lepers you've got yourself a war." (45)

Seeing the movement abandon prevention in favour of what he saw as ineffective and illiberal policies, Goerlitz came to suspect that his own desire to drive down youth smoking rates was not shared by everybody in the movement. In 2009, he spoke out against the "grab-bag of nuts" who were dominating a tobacco control movement which he now viewed as being "criminal and corrupt."

"I can't even guess as to why they've taken this approach in the last 15 years when they had such an opportunity to create a wonderful health issue rather than a rights issue.

It's hateful, arrogant vindictiveness that I think will never, ever put tobacco control
back on the map in a favourable light, even for people like me."

This corruption, says Goerlitz, began with the "unconstitutional" Master Settlement Agreement which effectively gave the government a financial incentive to keep people smoking. Most of the MSA billions were never used to fight tobacco, and those which did were ended up in the hands of "loud-mouthed anti-smokers and wackos." The tobacco control movement has become, says Goerlitz, "constipated" because efforts to educate and inform have been betrayed by "greedy" politicians on one side and "hateful" prohibitionists on the other.

Dr Michael Siegel of Boston University's School of Public Health spent twenty years as a senior member of Americans for Nonsmokers' Rights working alongside Stanton Glantz, and had been employed at both the Centers for Disease Control and the Office of Smoking or Health. For years, he fought for laws banning smoking in public places and restaurants. In 2005, having grown uneasy with the flagrant disregard for scientific methodology amongst large sections of his movement, Siegel began to express reservations. With anti-smoking groups claiming that mere seconds of tobacco exposure could be lethal, Siegel became so concerned that they were trivialising the real hazards of smoking, and were making themselves laughing stocks, that he wrote to several of them, urging them to either provide evidence for their claims or remove them from their literature. In response, his old friend Stanton Glantz sent an e-mail to the hundreds of activists on his mailing list titled simply: 'Please ignore Michael Siegel.'

Siegel now accepts that many anti-smokers have used the issue of 'nonsmokers' rights' to pursue an agenda of persecuting and humiliating smokers and that their true goal is to have tobacco banned entirely:

"When I used to hear smokers' rights groups claim that the anti-smoking movement
was really about prohibition, I thought it was complete crap.
But within the past few months, I'm starting to see that there is an
element of truth to those claims. There is a faction within the tobacco
control movement that I believe is motivated primarily by a hate for smokers

and nothing short of prohibition will ever satisfy this element.
But since anyone who suggests that perhaps we're going down the wrong path
will be censored or attacked, this element will never truly be challenged.
And most scary, this element now seems to be the driving force, or a major driving force,
within the movement. I think, therefore, that it is not inaccurate to state that the anti-
smoking movement is now on a path towards advocating prohibition" (46)

Within months of writing these words, Siegel was proven right. On September 5 2007, New Zealand's branch of ASH became the first major anti-smoking group since Lucy Page Gaston's Anti-Cigarette League to unequivocally call for prohibition. Twenty years after tentatively mooting a partial smoking ban on aeroplanes, the group announced that it was "committed to a ten year countdown towards getting rid of smoked tobacco, and we are calling on politicians to sign up to ending this tragic epidemic." (47)

It had been a long time coming but, finally, the velvet glove of persuasion was discarded to reveal the iron fist of prohibition. In the future, smoking would no longer be a matter for the individual but for the police. Mark Peck of the Smokefree Coalition explained:

"New Zealand has banned tobacco advertising, declared indoor places smokefree,
and committed tens of millions of dollars towards helping smokers quit.
The stage is set for the final curtain.
This is about developing a timed phase-out of smoked tobacco
in a way that is open and transparent."(48)

Halifax hysteria

The anti-smoking movement did not invent junk science, nor was it the first to validate irrational neuroses or demand legislation to pander to the whims of a dogmatic minority. But in each case it laid the way and set the template, and it continues to provide the best indication of where newer campaigns that have also begun with a warning label may lead. The campaign against smoking had been an unarguably noble endeavour for many people, but for others it only represented a lesson in how to ban the things that displeased them.

In Nova Scotia, Canada, hypochondria, mass hysteria and misapplied science combined to produce a parody of the passive smoking terror so bizarre that it belongs in the realms of fiction. It all began in the town of Halifax in the late 1980s when Rose Poirier, an employee of the QEII hospital and an asthma sufferer, found some staff suffering from 'sick building syndrome.' The cause of the problem turned out to be fumes leaking from a faulty dishwasher and was quickly fixed but, in the wake of this incident, several Halifax citizens were put on a course to educate them about a syndrome known as Multiple Chemical Sensitivity (MCS). In it, they were led to believe that they were suffering from 'environmental illness' aggravated by, amongst other things, perfume and aftershave. Consequently Poirier, with the full support of the Nova Scotia Lung Association, introduced a "scent-free policy" in the hospital and banned the wearing of perfumes, lotions and colognes.

MCS spread across Halifax like the proverbial wild fire and soon infected residents in other parts of the province, despite few people quite understanding what it was. The wearing of perfume and after-shave was prohibited by law in public places. Universities banned everything from shaving cream and sunscreen to fabric softener and scented candles. Some employees were even prohibited from using "strong mouth-wash." An 84 year old woman was expelled from Halifax City Hall for wearing cologne, and when a 17 year old schoolboy showed up to class wearing deodorant and hair gel, his 'chemically sensitive' teacher not only sent him home but demanded a criminal prosecution for assault.

Anti-scent policies garnered support from a number of businesses, politicians and the editor of a local newspaper. Most of the townspeople took the sufferers' demands seriously, for fear of appearing (literally) insensitive. As so often happens, the campaign did not end with the ban on scented products. A legal ban on garden pesticides was only narrowly defeated and a hospital receptionist demanded newspapers be banned from her workplace because she believed herself to be allergic to newsprint (49).

Multiple Chemical Sensitivity is, in the view of almost all medical authorities, a phantom syndrome. The American College of Physicians, the World Health Organisation and the American Medical Association have all studied the phenomenon and refuse to recognise it as a *bona fide* medical ailment. "What's taking place in Halifax appears to be collective hysteria over an illness that does not exist," said Dr Ronald House, an epidemiologist from Toronto's St. Michael's Hospital. "The uproar is fascinating from a cultural view...political pandering to a few rather strident activists."(50) Dr House deals with mass psychogenic illnesses and, having treated people with MCS, is certain that the disease exists only in the mind: "From a medical standpoint there is no disease process in [MCS sufferers], and yet they are adamant something is wrong with them. They are not faking. They really do believe they have a problem."(51) Dr Lad Dushenski, a Canadian allergy specialist, said of 'environmental illness': "People who use this term generally use it tongue-in-cheek, or they don't know what they're talking about. It is so broad that it means an allergy to everything or nothing."(52)

Nevertheless, this manifestation of chemophobia spawned a new industry of clinical ecologists and environmental physicians specialising in sick building syndrome and Multiple Chemical Sensitivity. The very fact that the syndrome was so ill-defined and encompassed so many perceived symptoms and irritations meant that vast numbers of people could be diagnosed as sufferers and an endless stream of customers arrived for the experts to treat. One of the leaders in the field, Dr William J. Rea agreed that those who fell victim to MCS "may manifest any symptom in the textbook of medicine."(53) No wonder then, that of 2,000 patients he has examined, 1,996 have been diagnosed with environmental illness.

When examined by scientists, sufferers rarely exhibit the symptoms they claim to have and although some can even appear to have seizure-like symptoms when exposed to fragrance in laboratory conditions, their EEG brain waves do not change in the way one would expect in a real sufferer. This is typical of psychosomatic phobias. Those who believe themselves to be sensitive to mobile phones display the same physical signs of sickness whether the phone they are asked to hold is real or not (54). Similarly, those who believe themselves to be affected by electricity pylons are unable to tell whether the signal is on or off but, when they are told it is on, show an increase in heart rate, begin sweating and say they feel unwell (55). They are not necessarily feigning their distress. They have just learnt to suspect and fear something and honestly believe they are being physically affected by it.

Those with a mild allergy to - or, as is much more common, a strong dislike of - scented products opt to follow a path of self-diagnosis rather than rely on medical science. They point the finger at substances they consider irritating or unnatural, and that often means anything containing 'chemicals.' Most, if not all, of the 'chemicals' cited by MCS activists occur abundantly in nature and the whole movement rests on a morbid fear of the very word. "We don't want a *Silent Spring* brought by cosmetics in Halifax," said one activist (56). In clinical trials, subjects react strongly when told they are smelling a chemical fragrance rather than a natural scent even when they are not, and "industrial chemicals" receive the most violent Pavlovian response. Even some of those who do not claim to have MCS exhibit a similar reaction.

Chemicals, of course, are the building blocks of the universe. They are, as Ian Mabbett, a chemist at the University of Swansea, says "everywhere and everything...To be chemical-free you have to experience a total vacuum greater than that of space."(57) Not an easy proposition but as far as the MCS activists are concerned a ban on scented candles, laundry detergent and Chanel Number 5 is a step in the right direction.

It would be easy to dismiss 'Halifax Hysteria' as a freakish episode of mass frenzy were it not for the adoption of the MCS idea further afield. MCS outbreaks invariably coincide with the launch of public health campaigns drawing attention to the syndrome and their spread becomes a self-fulfilling prophesy. After Halifax, the word about environmental illness moved further afield and the anti-scent movement gathered pace elsewhere in Canada and then in the United States. Wherever MCS activists and specialists went, a new outbreak followed and middle-aged, middle-class women were always peculiarly susceptible. It was only when a state-funded MCS clinic came to town to 'educate' the people of Halifax that hundreds of residents began complaining of watery eyes, coughing and rashes on the skin. As Dr House said: "In essence, the clinic acted as a justification for an illness that did not exist."(58) The whole thing brought to mind the days when a snake-oil salesman would ride into town, generate panic and then depart, leaving behind thousands of delirious residents clutching bottles of worthless medicine.

It is no coincidence that outbreaks of chemical sensitivity are most common in places where fear of secondhand smoke is most intense. In Canada, the Environmental Illness Society reports that 12% of Canadians have the condition, including 2% who are unable to go to go to work because of it. California has taken to the cause with some relish and the State Health Department estimates that 6% of Californians suffer from environmental illness. In Marin County, California, it is - as in Halifax - against the law to smoke within 20 feet of a building or road and there is now a 'voluntary code' against perfumes and aftershaves. Marin County even provided $1,200,000 to create a chemical-free 'Ecology House' for MCS sufferers to live in. Alas, when given this tax-funded safe-house, most of the residents complained that they felt sick and left. In the anti-smoking citadel of Berkeley, California, citizens are warned not to wear perfume and a government newsletter assured residents that those who complain of being assaulted by perfumes "have medical opinion on their side."(59)

The arrival of this new health scare in California resulted in the kind of fantastic exaggeration and zealous anti-industry sentiment that characterised the state's anti-smoking activities. Fragrance and after-shaves, like cigarettes, were deemed to have no value to health and consequently there was no reason *not* to ban them. Many of the symptoms of MCS are identical to those of 'sick building syndrome' which, in turn, are identical to those of secondhand smoke exposure. They include a small degree of physical irritation mixed with various self-reported psychological and psychosomatic symptoms such as rashes, palpitations, tears and coughing.

To the 'sufferer', these symptoms represent something far more serious than a modest discomfort. A minor annoyance becomes a life-threatening menace. Californian activist Julia Kendall, to name but one, is a chip off the old block: "Why should we have brain damage because people are wearing toxic chemicals?"(60) Stanton Glantz's comment that the passive smoking theory "legitimised the concern that people have that they don't like cigarette smoke"(61) is as concise an explanation for the success of the anti-smoking campaign as one could ask for, and MCS likewise validates the prejudices, preconceptions and preferences of those who dislike scented products. As the billboard once proclaimed: 'If you can smell it, it may be killing you!'

The National Foundation for the Chemically Hypersensitive is one of several US groups fighting for the rights of those who believe perfumes to be toxic and deadly. Its founder, Betty Bridges, claims that 5.72 million Americans are allergic to fragrances and that grass-roots movements like hers have struck "fear in the heart of the fragrance industry."(62) Her organisation's stated objective is to re-educate the public about the supposed poisonous effects of perfume with slogans like 'Good sense is no scents.' Their main objective is, somewhat inevitably, to have scented products banned in all public places. Valentine's Day - of all days - has been designated Chemical Awareness Day (the anti-scent equivalent of no-smoking day) and even the World Wildlife Foundation has spoken up on behalf of the fledgling movement, accusing perfume of causing male infertility and damaging the planet (63).

When *Readers Digest* opened up an online debate on the subject, most of the respondents said that the use of perfumes, after-shaves, deodorants and air fresheners should be criminalised in some form or other. One said they were "worse" than secondhand smoke, one blamed them for cot death and another called them a "threat to my life." Some described acute allergic reactions but most objected to the "stink" or found them "disgusting." The consensus was that the government should ban them in public places, particularly in restaurants.

The MCS cause followed in the anti-smokers' footsteps again in 2005 when a big money lawsuit was filed in Detroit by Erin Weber, a chemically sensitive disc jockey, against the radio station that had fired her. Four years earlier, she had sent an e-mail to her employer claiming that a co-worker, Linda Lee, had assaulted her by walking past wearing perfume. "Linda nearly brushed past me and a cloud of perfume trailed behind me," she wrote, adding that "to have brought the perfume with her suggests forward planning. This appears to be a premeditated attack which was entirely unprovoked by me in any way."(64)

Weber had previously taken three months sick leave after air freshener was used in her presence and had already taken the company to the Equal Employment Opportunity Commission, believing herself to be a victim of the glass ceiling. After her e-mail, she was moved to a different shift so she would not have to work alongside Linda Lee but was later sacked. The reluctance of the company to stop her co-workers wearing scent, she believed, lay behind her dismissal. She was duly awarded $10.6 million, including $2 million for 'mental anguish.'(65)

The crusade against perfume rapidly became one more lesson in how a minority can amplify a minor annoyance into a public health panic through the misuse of science and relentless lobbying, aided and abetted by the silent submission of the majority. The parallels with the passive smoking campaign are striking and anti-scent activists revel in the association. According to enforcer and campaigner Karen Robinson:

> "Aromatic chemicals are poisoning people and the planet as much as tobacco or pesticides...many of the chemicals found in smoke and second-hand smoke are the same chemicals that are found in perfume products."(66)

On the last point, Robinson is doubtless correct, but without specifying what those chemicals are, what their toxicity is and what the implications are for health it is a meaningless statement, unless we are to assume that all 'chemicals' (ie. all molecules in the known universe) are dangerous *per se*. Campaigners allege that 90-95% of the ingredients in perfume can be found in petroleum but, again, do not explain why this should be a concern. They claim that fragrances contain up to 5,000 chemicals - upping the ante on the mere 4,000 claimed for cigarettes but still less than the 10,000 'chemicals' found in the average American diet.

A single article in *Natural Life* magazine demonstrates how closely the anti-scent movement sticks to the tried and tested methods of the anti-smokers. It blinds its audience with science:

> "Hexachlorophene acetyl-ethyl tetra- methyl-tetralin, zinc pyridenethione butanol toluene benzal chloride methylene chloride and limonene
> - many of the ingredients currently used by the fragrance industry are hazardous."

It ridicules its users:

> "There's nothing sexy, or healthy, about spraying yourself with toxic chemicals."

It quotes the EPA to justify unlikely statistics:

> "A recent Institute of Medicine study sponsored by the EPA in the United States put fragrances in the same category as second hand smoke as a trigger for asthma in school-age children. Up to 72 percent of asthmatics report their asthma attacks are triggered by fragrance."

It cherry-picks evidence to play on people's natural concern for the well-being of unborn children:

> "At least one study has demonstrated links between heavy perfume exposure during pregnancy and learning disabilities and behaviour disorders in children."

And it claims that it is pointless to switch to a less harmful 'brand,' in this case natural scents:

> "Consumers should beware that 'natural' is not necessarily better, since many so-called natural products – including essential oils – are also allergens and irritants." (67)

The activist group Take Back the Air uses the same rhetoric in its battle against laundry detergent and lawnmower exhaust fumes. But its primary focus is the burning of wood, as its president, Julie Mellum, explained in an article for the *Star Tribune*:

"One big source of air pollution - as deadly as vehicle exhaust, and with many of the same toxicants as cigarette smoke - is wood smoke...

Wood smoke comprises fine particulates, many of which are carcinogenic, such as benzene, toluene, formaldehyde and polyaromatic hydrocarbons.

It is far more concentrated than cigarette smoke and travels much farther, spreading soot and fine particulates directly into our air and our lungs." (68)

By 2007, the divide between irritation and legislation could most easily be bridged by making the assertions that had served the anti-smoking movement so well. At the top of the list was the claim that a malevolent industry was responsible for misleading the people. This was closely followed by the belief that those who indulged were ignorant and addicted. Neither of these notions stood up well when applied to the trivial issue of log-burning but Mellum made them all the same:

"Why, then, do people continue to burn?

First, because they don't know how harmful it is.

Second, because it is strongly promoted by the hearth and home industry.

And third, because burning wood is an addiction."

At this late stage in the book, the reader will surely guess what Mellum's proposed solution is.

"We must urge our City Council members to ban recreational wood burning."

Fear of industry

"We want to destroy the perfume industry," declared anti-scent activist Julia Kendall. Like anti-smokers, her movement blames a money-hungry industry for the popularity of what it views as a worthless product; one that would not be purchased at all were it not for underhand marketing practices and brainwashing. Such an approach helps to depersonalise a conflict between family, friends and colleagues and redraws it as a gallant David and Goliath contest. As aggressive as wanting to destroy an industry might sound, it is far better than saying you want to destroy your neighbour's right to wear deodorant, smoke a cigarette or light a barbeque.

Reformers have not always been anti-industry. A hundred years ago it was industrialists who spear-headed the reform movement and it is with some irony that the Kelloggs company, whose founder was so closely involved with the anti-cigarette leagues, now finds itself one of the main targets of the anti-obesity campaign for using salt in its cereals. But as the 20th century wore on, health activists gradually divorced themselves from their roots in industry. The Edisons, Kelloggs and Fords who helped fund earlier efforts were replaced by individuals employed in the public sector who owed nothing to the world of business, manufacturing or commerce. They were, however, well-connected in political and the media circles. As this new, left-leaning 'knowledge class' took over from the industrial middle-class as pioneers of social change, it became mistrustful of 'industry' and came to view the very word with suspicion.

Today, this suspicion borders on paranoia and is a characteristic of protest movements from anti-smoking to environmentalism. Some vegan groups see the sinister hand of the hitherto unthreatening dairy industry in the most unlikely places, while the food industry ('Big Food'), salt industry, restaurant industry, pharmaceutical industry, casino industry and drinks industry are increasingly regarded as malevolent forces. Reluctant to accept that their fellow citizens might freely choose to adopt lifestyles that are different to their own, activists assume that the money, political influence and advertising campaigns of multi-national corporations have misled those who are less wise than themselves into consuming whichever product it is they currently wish to have banned.

In the 1990s, anti-smoking activists demonised the tobacco industry to such an extent that the public assumed everything they said was a lie. Anti-scent campaigners, deprived of evidence that perfume kills, employ the same trick. The newsletter sent to Berkeley residents, informing them that the chemically sensitive had science on their side, happily accepted that many studies had shown scented products to be harmless, but it used the fact that some of these studies had been paid for by the perfume industry as *de facto* proof that the reverse was true. 'Big Perfume' was, said the authors, a "$5 billion a year industry, so it is not in their best interest to document severe health problems." And it was left at that, with the lingering suspicion that anyone making money out of a product must have something to hide (69).

The presumption of innocence has been turned on its head. Industry denials have become tantamount to confessions. According to *Natural Life* magazine:

> "The entire perfume industry has been built on the premise that natural body odors are offensive and need to be covered up or enhanced with various sweet-smelling chemical compounds. But when asked, many people actually find human scents to be quite compelling." (70)

This is opinion, not science. Some people prefer natural smells. Others do not (which is, of course, why perfumes exist). In Nova Scotia, only those with a preference for natural body odours went to the lengths of forming alliances, seeking out media attention and framing their opinions in terms of life and death. The rest could only watch, bewildered, as they were relieved of another small liberty.

Panic

Suspicion of industry is matched by a fear of 'chemicals' which, though often borne of a fundamental ignorance of science, has nurtured a rampant hypochondria which certain obsessives are happy to exploit.

This knee-jerk fear of the unknown and - it is supposed - 'the unnatural' is not confined to Californians with a fear of cologne. Anti-smoking groups have for years excitably listed some of the 'chemicals' - more accurately known as 'particles' or 'compounds' - found in cigarettes and have helpfully provided examples of nasty sounding products which also contain them, as if the doses involved were in any way comparable.

The list - reprinted by anti-smoking groups the world over - includes "toulene (paint thinner)," "cadmium (batteries)," "ammonia (household cleaner)," plus familiar 'poisons' such as formaldehyde, cyanide and arsenic. While you would not want to eat a handful of any of these, their presence in tobacco can only be measured in parts per *billion* and in fractions of nanograms. One would, for example, have to be in a room with 165,000 cigarettes burning to absorb the same amount of arsenic present in one glass of tap water (71). As hazards to human health, these kinds of doses are not so much negligible as utterly irrelevant, all the more so in the diluted secondhand smoke which is invariably the focus of the groups that produce these 'fact sheets'.

Sadly, politicians and health authorities fail to confront the forces of unreason and frequently encourage them. The precautionary principle reigns supreme and allows shoddy epidemiological studies created by partisan groups to dictate public policy. Well orchestrated health scares do not require a scintilla of solid evidence for them to generate alarm. The result is an almost daily string of baseless health scares which ultimately lead to fear and confusion amongst the public.

In August 2006, to take but one example, the British Skin Foundation recommended that "anyone without a very dark skin should apply factor 15 sunscreen every morning, even if they are going to spend most of the day indoors."(72) Macmillan Cancer Support concurred, advising the use of sunblock every day between April and October. Anyone who lives in, or has ever visited, Britain will be aware of how absurd this advice is. On the very same day, the Institute of Child Health reported that black and Asian people who used sunscreen, or covered their bodies for religious reasons, risked inducing Vitamin D deficiency which "has been linked to some cancers, diabetes, high blood pressure, multiple sclerosis, and rickets."(73) The British were, it seemed, damned if they did and damned if they didn't.

Or take electrosensitivity, a cousin of Multiple Chemical Sensitivity which sees everyday electrical appliances as life-threatening. The main symptoms are the same - rashes, 'tingling,' confusion, fatigue, headache and palpitations - and all are self-reported and unverifiable. Again, most sufferers are middle class women who demand recognition and political action and, again, the medical profession says it is a psychological phenomenon. Electrosensitivity UK is the British support group (there are others in Canada, Sweden and California) and it advises "lining walls with a layer of aluminium foil and hanging special silver-plated curtains over windows" for protection (74). Jill O'Meara of the British government's Health Protection Agency accepted that there was no evidence that electrosensitivity was a *bona fide* medical condition and, as such, had the opportunity to quash the scare. Responsible advice for anyone who lines their walls with tin foil is to seek psychiatric help; instead she spinelessly applied the precautionary principle and issued a warning against buying "cheap and tinny hairdryers."(75)

The appearance of mobile phones and wireless internet (wi-fi) brought electrophobia into the mainstream. The epidemiological evidence against phone masts as a cause of cancer is stronger than that against secondhand smoke but then - it has to be said - most phantom health scares can boast a more impressive body of evidence than that offered to support the passive smoking theory. Around half of the studies into phone masts do indeed show some kind of statistically significant risk. Qualitatively, however, the case remains weak, sketchy and - once again - biologically unlikely. Wi-fi gives off three times as much radiation as phone masts, or so say its critics, but the radiation emitted by wi-fi computers remains 600 times lower than the legal limit, and one would need 100,000 wi-fi enabled laptops to generate the same amount of radiation as a single microwave oven (76). Still, the BBC's *Panorama* produced a show called 'Wi-fi: A Warning Call', the head of the Parents Teachers Association expressed concern that the "non-thermal, pulsing effects of electromagnetic radiation could have a damaging effect upon the developing nervous systems of children" and the chairman of the Health Protection Agency called for an urgent review of wi-fi networks in schools (77).

The eagerness of politicians to endorse and inflame transient health scares is a worrying trend. The appetite for regulation and micromanagement, combined with an exaggerated sense of risk, poses a threat to liberty greater than any threat to health. In the 1980s, Clive Turner, a spokesman for the British tobacco industry, called those involved in the anti-smoking movement "shower adjusters," explaining that: "I think if they could get into your bathroom they would adjust the temperature of the water because they know what is good for you."(78) It was meant as satire. In 2005, with the British government seeing no limit to its reach into the lives of its citizens, the deputy Prime Minister John Prescott announced plans to regulate thermostatic mixing valves to prevent bath-water temperature going over government approved levels. He described this move as "essential."

Prohibition by stealth

The eradication of tobacco has been the ultimate objective of every anti-smoking crusade in history and it is becoming increasingly difficult to pretend that its latest incarnation is any different. And yet prohibition remains a dirty word, with negative connotations born of America's failed experiment with alcohol in the 1920s and, to a lesser extent, today's ineffectual war on drugs. The thirst for prohibition is also tempered by the modern anti-smoking movement's financial dependence on tax revenue from the very product it seeks to destroy. What lies ahead, therefore, will be prohibition with a twist. When, in the early 20th century, the tobacco tycoon Buck Duke protested that he had never sought to create a monopoly, one cynic suggested that all he wanted was "the world with a barbed wire fence around it." One might equally say that today's anti-smoking movement does not desire the prohibition of tobacco, it just wants it to be very difficult to obtain, extremely expensive to purchase and virtually impossible to consume.

So where next? The passive smoking theory is surely coming to the end of its useful life. It is doubtful - though not impossible - that fears of 'thirdhand smoke' will mesmerise even the most lazy-minded politicians into pushing for smoking bans in fields and gardens. It is conceivable that laws 'protecting' workers from secondhand smoke will be extended to wives, husbands, children and friends of smokers in all settings. Anti-smoking groups have gone some way towards portraying parents who smoke as child-abusers and, by the same logic, there is no reason why a married man who smokes should not be viewed as a wife-beater. If smoking is a form of assault, a case could be made for banning smoking in the presence of *any* nonsmoker in public or in private. Domestic smoking bans are, however, unenforceable without the full apparatus of a police state and tobacco's enemies may have to change tack if they wish to maintain their momentum.

ASH has advocated banning smoking outdoors because it sets a bad example to children who might see it as "common adult behaviour."(79) Again citing precedent, ASH claim that alcohol bans on beaches and parks existed "obviously not to prevent drunkenness" but to prevent the impressionable from witnessing people drink (80). Aside from the fact that this is simply untrue - the prevention of drunken and disorderly behaviour is surely the principle reason behind such regulations - ASH is suggesting that individuals who indulge in grown-up and possibly unhealthy habits should be banished to where no one can see them.

This is perhaps the most ominous idea the movement has yet concocted and it is one that carries troubling implications for smokers and nonsmokers alike. To the anti-smokers, preventing children from seeing smokers with their own eyes is just another 'logical step.' If the portrayal of cigarette smoking in movies is to be censored then why not keep real smokers out of sight too? It is the extension of the idea that smoking is an 'epidemic'; that it can literally be transmitted by contact with the afflicted. If smokers are, as Lennox Johnston once said, a "living advertisement for tobacco," then they have no place in a society that prohibits the marketing of tobacco. Hiding them from view - and, above all, from the view of children - sends a powerful message of what is and is not socially acceptable. But if all this appears logical in the context of anti-smoking rhetoric, it is only because that logic has long-since become hopelessly twisted. Smoking is not an epidemic. Smokers do not carry disease. Lung cancer is not contagious. People are not advertisements.

If ASH is right in what it says, then the law should also prevent the eating of pizzas and the drinking of *Coca-Cola* in public, lest children see such unsanctioned behaviour as 'normal.' Such a proposal might seem far-fetched, but the history of anti-smoking shows us that yesterday's satire frequently becomes tomorrow's policy. In 2007, yet another 'seminal study' reported that "when an individual becomes obese, the chances that a friend of theirs will become obese increase by 57 percent."(81) One of its authors, Nicholas Christakis, said: "What we see here is that one person's obesity can influence numerous others to whom he or she is connected both directly and indirectly. In other words, it's not that obese or non-obese people simply find other similar people to hang out with. Rather, there is a direct, causal relationship."(82)

The worldwide media took this to mean that obesity was literally contagious and the findings did seem to support the concept of 'passive obesity.' "What appears to be happening," said Christakis, "is that a person becoming obese most likely causes a change of norms about what counts as an appropriate body size. People come to think that it is okay to be bigger since those around them are bigger, and this sensibility spreads."(83)

The authors did not discuss the implications of their research but if their study is correct, and given that obesity is a public health priority, the segregation of fat people can be the only logical solution. There are still many more consumers of chocolate bars than cigarettes but who would bet against a health movement that portrays 1.2 billion smokers as abnormal from stigmatising, reviling and denormalising those who indulge in other unhealthy pleasures in the future?

New skins, old wine

As the passive smoking theory becomes less useful to its cause, the anti-smoking movement has begun to employ arguments which have nothing to do with health for the first time since the Second World War. Those involved in what are ostensibly health organisations and nonsmokers' rights groups are beginning to pursue objectives that are related to neither health nor nonsmokers.

Recall Michela Alioto-Pier's successful campaign to ban smoking in San Francisco parks on the basis that cigarette butts leached toxins into the groundwater. ASH (Ireland) called for a ban on smoking in cars after suddenly becoming concerned that drivers might be less attentive at the wheel. The American Cancer Society asked motorists to report anyone they saw dropping cigarettes out of their cars, presumably because they were worried about littering.

But since when has the ACS been preoccupied with littering? Since when did ASH trouble itself with road safety? How many other public statements has Ms Alioto-Pier made regarding the quality of groundwater? The answer, of course, is that none of them expressed the slightest interest in any of these topics until they offered a way of clamping down on smokers and, once they have served their purpose, it is safe to predict that they will never mention them again.

For those who see the modern crusade against tobacco as being only and always a question of health, the sudden interest in groundwater, road safety and littering may seem incongruous, but it should not be a surprise. For five centuries, tobacco's enemies used fire safety, Christianity, Islam, public morality, nationalism, racial hygiene, economics, environmentalism, public decency, socialism and fascism as pretexts for the war on smokers. The sole focus on health is a relatively new development, and the focus on the health of nonsmokers an even newer one.

Flexibility has always been one of the movement's strengths. Consider Utah Senator Reed Smoot who, in the 1920s, called for the FDA to regulate tobacco products and put forward a proposal to ban smoking in most federal buildings. As a Mormon leader, his dislike of tobacco ran deep but he argued for smoking bans not on religious grounds but on the pretext of fire safety. When the Senate rejected that argument he went away, only to return later with the same Bill, this time claiming that smoking cost industry and government millions of dollars. Years later, Stanton Glantz told his followers that their war against tobacco "should be framed in the rhetoric of the environment" and *Tobacco Control* recommended its readers endorse "the use of human rights rhetoric." There is always a new skin for old wine. A new angle, a new emphasis, but always the same objective.

Moralists, prohibitionists and other battlers for public decency have traditionally been at the heart of efforts to wipe out smoking. Are we to believe that this element has disappeared? The modern public health movement makes no claims to moral authority and goes out of its way to avoid passing judgement, particularly in sexual matters. Doctors will gladly hand out free condoms to minors and syringes to heroin addicts but they are increasingly unwilling to perform life-saving surgery on smokers. The liberal medical establishment insists that it has no more interest in preaching and moralising than do our politicians. Today's anti-tobacconists deny that they have anything in common with their religious forebears of the 19th century and would be appalled to be compared to their more recent predecessors in Nazi Germany. Smoking, they maintain, is simply a health issue and they are in the business of promoting health.

So what happened to the people who, since Columbus's day, have hated the "stink" of the weed? Have there not always been, as the 19th century newspaper put it, "a good many people with whom the Indian herb does not agree"?(84) Have there not always been those who find habit-forming indulgences and unnecessary pleasures intolerable and, for that reason alone, have tried to stamp them out? And is it a coincidence that the current targets of public health - smoking, of course, but also gluttony, drunkenness and gambling - also happen to have been the targets of finger-wagging scolds in the past?

The idea that a public heath movement based on science and reason has banished the moralising impulse is an illusion. In a secular society, it is unfashionable to judge a man by the measure of his soul, as once we did, but we can instead judge him by the measure of his health. The old religious rules are replaced by a new moral code but both allow ample room for prejudice, and since the new rules claim to be based on absolute (scientific) truth rather than mere religious faith, they can be enforced all the more rigidly. To quote Dr Michael Fitzpatrick:

"In this way, the individual's state of health - as manifested in the state of their body -

provides a sphere in which they can be held to account for their personal behaviour. People may no longer confess their sins to the priest in private, but their state of health provides public testimony to their conformity with the new moral code of healthy living, a code which is in many ways more authoritarian and intrusive than the religious framework it has replaced."(85)

"If health is the new religion," said one critic of the English smoking ban, "the anti-smokers are its Spanish Inquisition."(86) That a prurient morality lives on in the anti-smoking campaign was illustrated when ASH produced a press release to promote a ban on smoking outdoors. It was interesting not because of the objective itself - which was entirely predictable - but for the reasons ASH gave to support it, and the light it shone on the character of the movement in the new millennium.

The pressure group provided no fewer than 16 reasons why smoking should be prohibited in the open air; a rather desperate litany which included the idea that it was "harmful to birds."(87) After quickly exhausting the tenuous implications for the health of nonsmokers (human and avian), ASH declared that it was perfectly acceptable to criminalise activities "simply because they are annoying or irritating even if they do not pose a health hazard." Smoking, they said, was a "repugnant" habit which it put alongside swearing, drinking, gambling and "scanty attire,"(88) none of which were harmful to health but all of which were morally objectionable to those of a certain sensitivity. Smoking, therefore, was added to a list of sins, and what a puritanical list it was.

Here, the moralising impulse at the heart of the public health movement was made explicit. In the years ahead, this prurient element may come to the fore. This would be no bad thing for the standard of public debate. If laws are to be passed on the basis of moral prejudices and personal preferences it is only proper that they be declared as such and not masquerade as 'evidence-based science.'

Since the war on smoking shows no sign of abating, and since similar campaigns on diet and alcohol are well underway, it is perhaps time for those who believe that the state has a right to control the health and habits of its citizens to declare where they draw the line between personal freedom and state control. They might also tell us what their ultimate goal is and what, if any, affiliations they have with drug companies who stand to benefit from their efforts.

Once all the cards have been laid on the table, a more honest and informed debate on the issue of personal liberty versus public health will be possible. For the anti-smokers, the risk of opening themselves up in this way may prove too great. "Acting ethically," as the contributor to *Tobacco Control* wrote, "may have short term costs."(89) Nevertheless, an open admission of paternalism could benefit them in the long term, not least because they would no longer have to rely on implausible health scares, some of which are so patently groundless that they positively invite a popular backlash.

Telling the public that they simply do not like smoking and want it banned is a more frank and credible message than pretending that nonsmokers can be killed by a few seconds of exposure to tobacco smoke or by molecules lingering in upholstery years after the event. They would do well to remind themselves that many of the anti-smoking crusades of the last five hundred years seemed unstoppable just before they collapsed beneath the hubris and hyperbole of their advocates.

Count Corti concluded his 1931 *History of Smoking* with the observation that "the most absolute despots the world has ever seen were powerless to stop the spread of smoking."(90) Pointing to the depleted band of anti-tobacconists of his own day, Corti predicted that any anti-smoking efforts in the future could "result only in a miserable fiasco."(91) To say that times have changed since Corti wrote those words would be to engage in the glibbest of understatements. And yet it would still take a fool to look back at tobacco's long history and predict that the habit will ever be fully stamped out. Today's anti-smoking movement may be influential, wealthy and untouchable but only by avoiding a "miserable fiasco" will it be unique.

Appendix

The evidence for the passive smoking theory

"There is overwhelming evidence, built up over decades, that passive smoking causes lung cancer"

- Vivienne Nathanson, British Medical Association

Glossary of terms

Case-control study

Epidemiological research which surveys a sample group (the cases) and compares them to a healthy sample group (the controls). In this instance, the cases are lung cancer sufferers. When the subject is no longer alive to answer questions, family members may be asked to provide information. Also known as a retrospective study.

Cohort study

Epidemiological research which monitors a group of people (the cohort) over a period of time, usually several years. Typically, they are surveyed at the outset of the study, at its end and sometimes in between. In the field of secondhand smoke research, the cohort are healthy individuals at the outset and are monitored for lung cancer over time. Because they are healthy to begin with, the possibility of *recall bias* is eliminated. For this, and other reasons, cohort studies are considered of greater value than *case-control studies*. Also known as a prospective study.

Confidence interval

The margin of error between the lower and upper end of the relative risk. Shown in brackets after the *relative risk*. In epidemiology, it is standard practice for there to be a confidence of 95% ie. only a one in twenty theoretical chance of the true risk falling outside the upper and lower ends of the interval. In practice, this confidence is often misplaced.

Confounding factor

Any external factor that may influence the results of a study. In the field of lung cancer research, these particularly include age, occupation, income, asbestos exposure, infection, radiation, diet and smoking history.

Data-dredging

A term used to describe the practice of asking subjects about a vast number of lifestyle factors in the hope of finding an association with one or more of them. Data-dredging is one of the reasons why the 95% confidence level is misleading. A researcher may ask his sample group about 100 different lifestyle factors. Chance dictates that 5 statistically significant findings will emerge, even if none of them are a genuine risk. The researcher is, however, free to publish these 5 statistically significant associations. Now consider that there are thousands of multi-factoral studies being conducted at any one time around the world. The sheer volume of findings guarantees that bogus associations will frequently be reported. They will be statistically significant, but far fewer than 95% of them will be real.

Dose-response relationship

If A leads to B, any increase in A should lead to an increase in B. In the case of active smoking, it has been proven that heavier smokers have a greater risk than lighter smokers and that risk increases according to the number of years spent smoking. If secondhand smoke poses a risk to nonsmokers, one would also expect to see a linear relationship between lung cancer risk and length and intensity of exposure. If the reverse happens, it is an *inverse* dose-response relationship.

Null hypothesis

The premise that no relationship exists between A and B.

Null study

Any epidemiological result which does not achieve statistical significance and therefore supports the *null hypothesis*.

Publication bias

There is a well-known, proven tendency for medical and scientific journals to favour publishing epidemiological studies which deliver *statistically significant* results. Although it is not necessarily the case, *null studies* are generally of less interest to their readers and the media. If *null studies* are not published, evidence for the null hypothesis will be under-reported. Publication bias is particularly common when results support the editorial stance or are topical.

Recall bias

In case-control studies, where information is gathered retrospectively through interviews, there is a known tendency for some subjects to exaggerate or downplay their exposure to A as a result of what they have been told about B. In the field of secondhand smoke research, this usually means lung cancer cases overstating their past exposure to tobacco smoke because they see their condition as uniquely related to smoking.

Relative risk

The term relative risk, which has particular pertinence to cohort study computations, is also commonly used in describing risk estimates from lifestyle epidemiology generally. The most common form of risk computation is specifically and properly called an odds ratio yet is more typically referred to as "relative risk" by general definition. The relative risk, however specifically computed, is the headline estimate - or what might be called the best guess - provided by epidemiologists to show the relationship between A and B. The relative risk falls between the low and high ends of the *confidence interval.*

Statistical significance

Meaning that the finding is probably not the result of chance. Significance is attained when the lower and upper confidence limits are both above (or, for negative associations, both below) 1.0. In epidemiology, significance is not an objective measure, as it is in common parlance. It is sometimes mistakenly said all relative risks below 2.0 (or 3.0) are statistically insignificant. This is not true. They may not be considered a substantial or meaningful in practical terms - and they may still be false findings - but they are statistically significant if they meet the test above.

Smoker misclassification

When information about smoking behaviour is self-reported (as is usually the case), there is a known tendency for some smokers to classify themselves as nonsmokers (see chapter 6). Nonsmokers very rarely classify themselves as smokers, however, and this misclassification leads to a muddying of results. Since around 1990, some researchers have tested their subjects for cotinine - which is present at high levels in users of tobacco. This procedure helps to exclude current smokers from the sample group but because cotinine disappears from the body after several weeks, it does not eliminate former smokers. In case-control trials, this can be a significant problem, since many smokers quit their habit when diagnosed with lung cancer.

Wish bias

The researcher's desire to reach a preconceived conclusion can sway the results. The bias may be personal, financial, political or institutional. Wish bias manifests itself in confounding factors being overlooked, alternative explanations ignored, unfavourable data omitted or the study design being skewed to make a positive association more likely.

A brief history of passive smoking

Takeshi Hirayama conducted the first epidemiological research into passive smoking by monitoring the health of nonsmoking women married to smoking husbands and this model remains the gold standard for research of this kind. In the 25 years since Hirayama's paper was published (1981), a further 63 similar reports have been published. Taken together they form a substantial body of evidence which, according to one Surgeon General, is "overwhelming" in supporting the hypothesis that nonsmokers exposed to secondhand smoke are more likely to suffer from lung cancer than those who generally avoid exposure. After reading all of these studies, I have not been able to endorse this interpretation.

There are only three possible outcomes in studies of this kind. The first is that the hypothesis is correct (ie. that passive exposure to tobacco smoke increases lung cancer risk). The second possibility is that there is a negative association (ie. that passive smoking reduces the risk of lung cancer). The third possibility is that there is no association either way; this is known as the 'null hypothesis'.

A relative risk (RR) of 1.0 represents no association either way. An RR below 1.0 represents a negative association and an RR above 1.0 represents a positive association. For example, 0.9 = 10% less risk, 1.35 = 35% greater risk and 2.0 = 100% greater risk.

In the studies listed below, researchers typically compare a group of married, nonsmoking women who have lung cancer (the cases) with a group of married, nonsmoking women who do not (the controls). Questions are asked of both groups regarding exposure to tobacco smoke and, to put it in simple terms, if marriage to a smoker is a more common trait amongst the lung cancer cases than amongst the controls, it might be inferred that marriage to a smoker increases lung cancer risk. If, for example, 60% of the lung cancer cases are married to smokers and only 40% of the controls are married to smokers, it might be inferred that marriage to a smoker increases lung cancer risk by half (RR = 1.5).

Or it might not. In this example, can we be sure that it was the husband's smoking habits that made the difference? Can we be sure that the women were not smokers themselves? What if the women all lived in a city or all worked in the asbestos industry? What if they were older than the controls and therefore had a higher risk of cancer anyway? Are their diets comparable? Did they used to be smokers? All these are confounding factors and need to be identified and avoided. If they are unavoidable, the figures must be adjusted to take them into account.

The numbers involved are crucial if we are to draw any conclusions from a study of this kind. In the example above, the women married to smokers appear to have a relative risk of lung cancer of 1.5; a 50% increase. That is based on 40% of the healthy controls being married to smokers. But what if there were only 5 women in each group? That would mean two of the controls were married to smokers and three were not. Among the cases, this ratio is reversed. Technically, 40% of the controls were married to smokers but the difference between the two groups comes down to one woman in each group saying that she is or is not married to a smoker. The study is vulnerable because of its small size and may not be - indeed, probably *is* not - representative of the population at large. If, on the other hand, 1,000 women are in each group and the percentages remain the same we can say with rather more confidence that marriage to a smoker increases lung cancer risk and that this lies somewhere around 1.5.

Clearly, we must exercise caution before drawing conclusions from small sample groups but as the number of participants increases, the margin for error is reduced and our estimates should become more accurate. As discussed in chapter 7, epidemiologists distinguish between chance results and genuine associations by using a standard of statistical significance. In our example of 5 lung cancer patients, the RR is 1.5 but this does not tell the whole story. The full RR is 1.5 (0.4-5.5) with the figures in brackets being the lower and upper limit. Because of the small number of cases, the confidence interval (or the margin of error) is very wide and we can only surmise that the risk to the nonsmokers falls between a 60% reduction and a six-fold increase - not very useful.

In the second example, there are 500 cases and so the margin of error is much narrower and the RR is 1.5 (1.3-1.7). This tells us that risk is increased by at least 10% and may be as high as 100%. This association is statistically significant because the lower limit of the confidence interval is above one. If it was 1.0 or lower it would not be significant, since the RR includes the null hypothesis and the negative hypothesis. And if an RR is not statistically significant, it tells us nothing. It does not matter whether the headline figure is higher or lower than 1.0, it supports neither the positive or negative hypothesis.

The null hypothesis itself cannot be proven even in the unlikely event of the RR landing exactly on 1.0. However, if enough studies show nonsignificant findings, one might reasonably infer that there is no association to investigate.

Of the epidemiological papers that studied the effect of secondhand smoke on nonsmoking wives, 9 found a statistically significant positive association, 3 found a statistically significant negative association and the remaining 52 found no statistically significant association either way. Some within the tobacco control movement have claimed that the risk from passive smoking is too small to be demonstrated conclusively in small and medium sized studies. Only very large studies, they say, have the statistical power to meet the criteria for significance but these studies are difficult to carry out thanks, in part, to the relative scarcity of lung cancer patients who have never smoked. There is some truth in this, although it is worth pointing to the 12 findings below that have achieved statistical significance (albeit with 3 of them going in the 'wrong' direction).

Since the mid-1980s, it has become clear that early reports from Hirayama and Trichopoulos showing a doubling of lung cancer risk were erroneous and that if a risk exists at all, it falls at a level well below 1.5 and that if risk exists at all, it is realistically imperceptible. In the past twenty years, very few statistically significant associations have come to light and so those who have put their faith in the passive smoking theory have used the nonsignificant findings found in the bulk of studies to make their case. They have claimed that although the majority of epidemiological papers do not show significant associations, the weight of evidence points towards a positive association and that, taken together, they show a risk of around 1.20.

While it is unusual to infer anything from relative risks that do not meet the minimum standard of statistical significance, it has been claimed in this sphere that it is not completely unreasonable to draw conclusions if they all point in the same direction and show a similar relative risk. However, that is not the case here.

Of the 52 statistically insignificant results, 18 (35%) have a relative risk of 1.0 or below and 34 (65%) have a relative risk above 1.0. The best that can therefore be said of this data is that there are a few more studies pointing up than down. This is feeble stuff. No one is claiming that secondhand smoke *protects* people from lung cancer but if the 18 studies that point in that direction are not to be trusted, why trust the 34 that point the opposite way?

If we accept that secondhand smoke causes lung cancer in nonsmoking women because a slim majority of the nonsignificant results lean that way then we must also accept that women who are exposed to secondhand smoke in childhood are less likely to suffer from lung cancer (a majority of the studies regarding passive smoking in childhood have shown a negative correlation).

If the majority of studies showed relative risks that were closely grouped between 1.20 and 1.30 then one might be more inclined to accept the plausibility of the passive smoking hypothesis. Britain's SCOTH committee and anti-smoking groups around the world have now settled on a relative risk for secondhand smoke and lung cancer of 1.24 but not one of the 64 studies below shows a risk of that magnitude. Even if one allows a generous margin of error and settles for any risk between 1.20 and 1.29, there are only five studies that fit the bill.

For every study that shows a statistically significant positive association, there are six that do not. This is hardly overwhelming evidence in support of the passive smoking theory and yet these nine significant associations do exist, compared to 'only' two in the opposite direction. Are they suggestive? The reader should not infer that it is difficult or unusual for a random result to achieve statistical significance. Most, if not all, of the transient health scares that appear in the daily newspapers achieve this minimum scientific criteria. Any epidemiologist who asks questions about enough aspects of their subjects' lifestyle will chance upon plenty of apparent associations and although passive smoking may seem a limited field there is plenty of scope for data-dredging.

A study of one case group can, therefore, produce over a hundred individual risk ratios and the chances of finding a significant association becomes far more likely. In the studies below, patients were asked about everything from the length of their menstrual cycle to whether they owned a black and white television. Findings can be made for those with heavy smoking husbands, light smoking husbands and ex-smoking husbands. Results can be divided by age, occupation, diet and social status. They can be split according to the major types of lung cancer the cases are suffering from (there are four), as well as other cancers, heart disease, stroke and overall mortality. They can be rearranged according to the type of exposure (childhood, adulthood, spousal, mother, father, sibling, social, workplace) and, finally, the risks can be adjusted as the author sees fit in order to account for confounding variables.

There is a natural tendency for epidemiologists to want to show a positive result if only because null studies are of little interest and are less likely to be published. This tendency is particularly strong when the issue relates to secondhand smoke and when the researcher has a personal or financial bias. From the very outset, there was a hope and expectation that passive smoking was indeed linked to lung cancer in nonsmokers. This prevailing bias has led to studies being written up in such a way that emphasised the results that supported the passive smoking theory and ignored the vast majority that did not.

How these results are presented is entirely down to the authors and their interpretation invariably moulds the report's summary and the accompanying press release. They may choose to publish only the results that appear to support the hypothesis or, if they tabulate the rest of the findings, write up their paper in such a way as to stress positive associations and downplay the null findings. If 99 results support the null hypothesis and one supports the a priori hypothesis, it is the single positive association that makes the headlines. The early 1990s studies of Janerich, Brownson and Stockwell are fine examples of this tendency.

What follows is every peer-reviewed study of nonsmoking wives ever published with the editorialising stripped away to reveal the data in its pure form. Doctoral theses and dissertations are not included unless they have subsequently been published in a book or scientific journal. When results have been published more than once (eg. Hirayama, Fontham), the most recent version has been reviewed. Where confounding factors have been accounted for, the adjusted odds ratios have been used.

The studies are listed in order of size, with the studies with the largest sample group listed first. The order of the studies is important since those with the largest sample group are likely to offer the most accurate results. The reader will notice that the higher relative risks appear towards the bottom, where the smallest and least reliable studies lie. If one examines the results from the ten largest studies it is very difficult to view them as anything other than a random assortment of numbers hovering either side of 1.0. In order, they appear: 1.29, 1.11, 0.70, 1.03, 1.53, 1.10, 0.89, 1.10, 0.90 and 0.96. Between them, they give an average relative risk of 1.06 which is so close to a zero risk that if it were not so political, the issue of passive smoking would have been quietly shelved years ago. The smaller studies lift the average slightly higher - as the EPA found to its benefit - but some of these involve just 8 or 9 women and, with apologies to their authors, they are meaningless.

The results of studies that have investigated childhood exposure, workplace exposure, the effect on men or the association with other diseases are no more consistent or compelling than those involving nonsmoking wives and lung cancer (and the reader is encouraged to seek them out) but there are fewer of them and so the studies listed below provide the largest body of evidence regarding the passive smoking theory.

The number of subjects is based on the total number of female lung cancer cases involved in the study. The relative risks are taken from the tabulated evidence given in the original study in most cases. In a small minority of cases, relative risks are not shown in the original papers and in these instances the risks have been calculated from the available data. Statistically nonsignificant risks that exceed 1.0 are marked "(null)" and those that fall below 1.0 are marked "(negative)". Statistically significant findings are marked with an asterisk.

The studies

Fontham (1994) 651 subjects: RR = 1.29* (significant - positive)

As the largest cohort study of its kind, Elizabeth Fontham's 1994 study provides the strongest evidence for a slim association between passive smoking and lung cancer in nonsmokers. In 1991, she released preliminary results, just in time for them to be included in the EPA report and her final paper (1994) produced much the same findings. For those with husbands who smoked cigarettes, cigars or pipe tobacco, relative risk narrowly achieved significance at 1.29 (1.04-1.60).

Exposure in occupational and social settings also showed a significant risk of 1.39 and 1.50 respectively but there was no association with exposure in childhood (0.89). Generally, there was evidence of a dose-response relationship and the results were adjusted for diet, race, age and occupation. Although slight in every instance, the associations were consistently more compelling for adenocarcinoma that for other types of lung cancer. This was surprising since, of the four major types of cancer (the others are small cell, large cell and squamous cell), adenocarcinoma is least associated with smoking.

Boffetta et al (1998) 508 subjects: RR = 1.11 (null)

The World Health Organisation commissioned the International Agency for Research on Cancer to carry out this European study of 650 never-smoking lung cancer patients, of whom 508 were married women. When compared against a control group of 1,008 healthy women, no statistically significant link was found between a husband's smoking habits and lung cancer: RR = 1.11 (0.88-1.39). The only statistically significant finding in the paper was an apparent protective effect from exposure to secondhand smoke during childhood of 0.77 (0.61-0.98).

Wu-Williams (1987) 417 subjects: RR = 0.7* (significant - negative)

By 1987, several papers had provided the unlikely and, to many, unwelcome suggestion that exposure to tobacco smoke actually protected nonsmokers from lung cancer but it was not until the publication of Anna Wu-Williams' study that such an association achieved statistical significance. Wu-Williams was working in UCSF's Department of Preventive Medicine when her study into lung cancer risks for women in China appeared in the *British Journal of Cancer* showing a statistically significant 0.7 (0.6-0.9) negative association between secondhand smoke and lung cancer.

Wang (2000) 407 subjects: RR = 1.03 (null)

This large Chinese study apparently demonstrated that lung cancer risk was doubled by owning a colour TV and trebled by owning a refrigerator but came up empty-handed with regard to secondhand smoke. The RR of 1.03 (0.6-1.7) for passive smoke exposure in adult life was highly supportive of the null hypothesis.

Zaridze (1998) 358 subjects: RR = 1.53* (significant - positive)

This study from Moscow found an association between passive smoking and lung cancer although there was an inverse dose-response relationship; ie. the women's lung cancer risk dropped as the husband's cigarette consumption rose. Risk also fell as the duration of exposure rose. Zaridze's relative risk for women married to smokers was positive and statistically significant (1.53 (1.06-2.21)). Strangely, a similar association was found with marriage to a smoker even when the husband did not smoke in her presence (1.48 (0.86-2.53)) and exposure in childhood or from any other family member yielded statistically nonsignificant negative results of 0.92 and 0.91 respectively.

Zhong (1999) 322 subjects: RR = 1.10 (null)

This large Chinese study sought to find the causes of the recent rise in lung cancer in Shanghai and identified statistically significant associations with low vitamin C consumption, genetic susceptibility, high risk occupations and cooking fumes but not secondhand smoke. After comparing 322 lung cancer cases with 377 controls, the relative risk supported the null hypothesis with an RR of 1.1 (0.8-1.5). The RR for those exposed in childhood was similar, albeit in the other direction, at 0.9 (0.5-1.6).

Wen (2006) 294 subjects: RR = 0.89 (negative)

This Chinese cohort study had a sample group of 64,881 nonsmoking, married women who were interviewed between 1997 and 2004. In direct contrast to Stockwell (1992), it found some evidence that secondhand smoke exposure in the workplace was a risk factor for lung cancer but found no risk when that exposure was in the home. Like Stockwell, the author wrote at length about the positive association while skimming over the more plentiful evidence that showed no link between passive smoking and lung cancer.

The relative risk to a woman exposed to smoke by her husband was 0.89 (0.42-1.92) and the risk from exposure in childhood was 0.21 (0.03-1.61). This very low latter association was compensated by a higher, positive association with workplace exposure of 2.25 (0.95-5.27). None of these results were statistically significant. When all three sources of exposure were taken together, the RR in this sizeable study was effectively zero: 1.03 (0.57-1.87). As is often the case in these studies, there was scant evidence of a dose-response relationship between length or intensity of exposure and risk. Indeed, the wives who had the most exposure had the lowest risk (0.79 (0.48-1.31)).

[The paper does not make it clear exactly how many of the subjects succumbed to lung cancer. However, the author showed that 106 of the lung cancer cases were married to smokers, and that 36% of the wives were married to smokers. The above figure is a calculation based on these two figures.]

Schwartz (1996) 257 subjects: 1.1 (null)

This study of lung cancer patients in Detroit examined various possible causes of the disease but failed to support the passive smoking theory. The sample group included a minority of men and the authors did not provide relative risks for either gender, but the overall figure for people 'exposed in the home' supported the null hypothesis with an RR of 1.1 (0.8-1.6).

Gao (1987) 246 subjects: RR = 0.9 (negative)

Another large Chinese case-control study found no association between lung cancer and exposure to secondhand smoke in adulthood; RR 0.9 (0.6-1.4). There was, however, a dose-response relationship between years spent married to a smoker and increased lung cancer risk (1.1, 1.3 and 1.7 for 20-29 years, 30-39 years and 40+ years). None of the findings achieved statistical significance, except for the relationship with the stir-frying of food (2.6 (1.3-5.0)).

Kreuzer (2000) 234 subjects: RR: 0.96 (negative)

This substantial study from Germany included 234 female lung cancer patients who had never smoked matched against a control group of 535 healthy women. There was no association between lung cancer and secondhand smoke exposure from a spouse (0.96 (0.7-1.33)) or in childhood (0.78 (0.56-1.08)). Both results were negative and neither were statistically significant.

Sun (1996) 230 subjects: RR = 1.16 (null)

This obscure Chinese study reported an association between secondhand smoke and lung cancer for those exposed in childhood and for those exposed both at home and at work but there was no association with smoking by the husband (1.16 (0.86-1.69)). As insignificant as that risk was, it fell still further if the wife was exposed for more than 35 years to 0.86 (0.45-1.65). It is not clear whether the paper was subject to the peer-review process.

Lee (2000) 228 subjects: RR = 2.2* (significant - positive)

This study of lung cancer patients from Taiwan is the only retrospective (case-control) study that fully supports the passive smoking theory. The authors apparently adjusted for all the important confounding factors and there was a linear dose-response relationship. The researchers asked their subjects whether or not their husbands smoked in their presence; those who answered yes were found to have a statistically significant relative risk for lung cancer of 2.2 (1.5-3.1).

Wu (1985) 220 subjects: RR = 1.2 (null)

Anna Wu and her colleagues surveyed 220 female lung cancer patients in Los Angeles between 1981 and 1982. As they reported: "We did not observe any elevated risk associated with passive smoke exposure from either parents (RR=0.6; 95% CI= 0.2,1.7) [or] from spouse(s) (RR=1.2; 95% CI= 0.5,3.3)."

Brownson (1992) 218 subjects: 1.0 (exactly zero)

As discussed in Chapter 7, the authors of this study drew conclusions that were at odds with the statistics they presented. According to Brownson, his study "suggests a small but consistent elevation in the risk of lung cancer in nonsmokers due to passive smoking" before adding: "The proliferation of federal, state, and local regulations that restrict smoking in public places and work sites are well founded." These words formed the basis of the media reports that covered the study and few journalists would have delved further. Had they done so they would have found a relative risk for wives married to smokers of 1.0 (0.8-1.2). For squamous cell carcinoma - the type of lung cancer that was most strongly associated with cigarette smoking - the risk was just 0.5 (0.3-1.3) and when the study was extended to cover 431 female lung cancer patients who recalled exposure from all family members, the relative fell to 0.8 (0.6-1.1).

Hirayama (1984) 200 subjects: RR = 1.45* (significant - positive)

Although sometimes treated as a separate entity, Hirayama's 1984 study was an expanded version of his pioneering paper of 1981 (discussed in Chapter 6). Hirayama's methodology has much to commend it since the time-scale was lengthy and the number of participants fairly large. Furthermore, it was a cohort study and, as such, eliminated recall bias. The sample group of 142,857 women was assembled in 1965 and, by 1979, 427 had contracted lung cancer. 269 were married and, of these, 200 were nonsmokers. Of these, 163 had been married to a smoker or an ex-smoker and it was they who became the focus of Hirayama's research.

The Japanese paper was noteworthy for not only finding a statistically significant association between marriage to a smoker and lung cancer but for showing a dose-response relationship. When their husbands smoked less than a pack a day, the association was 1.45 (1.04-2.02) and when they smoked more than a pack a day, the association rose to 1.91 (1.34-2.71). Both these figures were lower when Hirayama published his final study in 1984 by which time he was now using the lowered confidence interval of 90% to make his estimates, effectively doubling his chances of finding a significant relationship. The overall relative risk was 1.45 (1.02-2.08).

Lam (1987) 199 subjects: RR = 1.65* (significant - positive)

This study from Hong Kong found a positive association of 1.65 (1.16-2.35) between secondhand smoke exposure and lung cancer, based on 199 nonsmoking wives against a control group of 335. As the EPA noted, upon reviewing the study in 1993, confounding factors may have been at work. Lam did not ask questions about diet, air pollution, cooking fumes, occupation, age, class or any other factors that might confound the data. Since the only attempt to tackle smoker misclassification was to ask subjects if they had a history of tobacco use, it is likely that some ex-smokers and smokers were mistakenly classified as nonsmokers. Additionally, there was an inverse dose-response relationship between the amount smoked by the spouse and risk. According to Lam, the women married to the lightest smokers were at greatest risk of lung cancer.

Janerich (1990) 191 subjects: RR = 0.93 (negative)

No fewer than nine authors put their name to this report which strived to draw some evidence against secondhand smoke after Luis Varela had studied the same data and found none (see Chapter 7). Varela had found no association between secondhand smoke and lung cancer and it took a good deal of statistical conjuring for Janerich to suggest otherwise. The most newsworthy finding was a relative risk of 2.07 (1.16-3.68) for the 52 subjects who recalled at least 25 'smoker-years' of exposure to passive smoke in childhood ('smoker years' were calculated by multiplying the years of exposure by the number of smokers in the home) but there was no association with those who had less than 25 'smoker years'. This finding contradicted the weight of evidence that showed childhood exposure to smoke to have no effect on lung cancer risk in later life.

More pertinently, there was a nonsignificant negative risk ratio for the lung cancer patients who had been married to smokers: RR = 0.93 (0.55-1.57).

Wang T. (1996) 181 subjects: RR = 1.11 (null)

Another Chinese study and another study full of null associations. A husband's smoking resulted in a risk ratio of 1.11 (0.65-1.88), exposure in childhood showed 0.91 (0.55-1.49) and workplace exposure showed 0.89 (0.45-1.77). Once again, lung cancer was significantly associated with exposure to cooking oil vapours (3.79 (2.29-6.77)).

McGhee (2005) 179 subjects: RR = 1.38 (null)

This cohort study was published in the *BMJ* in the run up to England's smoking ban and was brief and to the point. It showed a nonsignificant relative risk of 1.38

(0.94-2.04) with lung cancer. Only subjects aged 60 or over were included and there was no adjustment for diet, occupation or air pollution.

Enstrom & Kabat (2003) 177 subjects: RR = 0.97 (negative)

Of the 118,094 Californians who enrolled in the ACS's Cancer Prevention Study in 1959, 25,942 were nonsmoking women married to a smoker and it was they who became the focus of Enstrom and Kabat's prospective study (discussed in Chapter 10). Monitored through to 1998, the authors found no statistical link between passive smoke and lung cancer and the relative risk of 0.97 (0.90-1.05) strongly supported the null hypothesis.

Neuberger (2006) 160 subjects: RR = 0.37* (significant - negative)

160 women with lung cancer from the state of Iowa answered questions about their exposure to various suspected carcinogens, as did 542 controls. As expected, asbestos, urban living and a personal history of lung disease were found to be statistically significant factors but passive exposure to tobacco smoke was not. Only 37% of the cases recalled exposure in adulthood, against 62% of the healthy controls, and this led to a statistically significant *negative* relationship between passive smoking and lung cancer of 0.37 (0.26-0.54).

Garfinkel (1981) 153 subjects: RR = 1.17 (null)

Garfinkel's paper was the first in a series of failed attempts to use the vast American Cancer Society national database to produce evidence for the passive smoking theory (see Enstrom & Kabat and Cardenas). Started by Cuyler Hammond in 1959, this survey was carried out by ACS volunteers across the United States and included 375,000 nonsmoking women. By 1981, 203 of them had contracted lung cancer. 153 had been married, 88 of them to smokers.

Comparing these rates to those expected in wives married to nonsmokers, Garfinkel found no statistically significant relationship between secondhand smoke exposure and any cancer except, perversely, that women married to smokers were less likely to suffer from cancer of the uterus.

The wives were grouped between those whose husbands smoked less than a pack and more than a pack of cigarettes a day. The former had an RR of 1.27 (0.88-1.89), the latter - those more heavily exposed to smoke - had an RR of just 1.10 (0.77-1.61). When the figures were adjusted for confounding factors, the former rose to 1.37 and the latter fell to 1.04. The overall risk ratio was 1.17 (0.85-1.61). None of these figures came close to statistical significance and Garfinkel did not pretend otherwise. His own assessment was that women married to smokers had "very little, if any, increased risk of lung cancer" and that "even if the estimates from this analysis are in error and there was a slight increase in lung cancer trends in nonsmokers, it did not appear to be an important problem."

Cardenas et al. (1997) 150 subjects: RR = 1.2 (null)

The American Cancer Society's million person study also provided the data for this study. When Garfinkel used the database in 1981 (above), he found no association between secondhand smoke and lung cancer, nor did Enstrom & Kabat (2003). The Cardenas study had a slightly smaller sample group of lung cancer patients but it also supported the null hypothesis, albeit with a slightly different RR of 1.2 (0.8-1.6) for women. For men, the RR was 1.0, although this was raised to 1.1 after the authors made adjustments. As with Garfinkel's paper, there was an implausible reverse dose-response relationship between years spent living with a smoker and lung cancer risk. And again, none of the RRs were statistically significant.

Lan (1993) 139 subjects: RR = 1.15 (null)

Another Chinese study and another strong correlation between indoor air pollution and lung cancer. Lung cancer was strongly associated with coal burning with a risk ratio of 7.53 (3.31-17.17) but, alas, there was no association with passive smoking. The crude data showed a risk of 0.84 but after (unexplained) adjustments were made, this rose to 1.15 (0.43-21.82), which, as the very broad confidence interval suggested, was anything but statistically significant.

Garfinkel (1985) 134 subjects: RR = 1.31 (null)

As in his earlier prospective study, Garfinkel's 1985 retrospective study found no significant association between secondhand smoke and lung cancer. The relative risk here was 1.31 (0.94-1.83), although there was a stronger risk ratio for those who were most heavily exposed. Exposure during childhood also supported the null hypothesis with 0.91 (0.74-1.12). Perhaps the most intriguing aspect of the paper was the insight it gave into the misclassification of nonsmokers. Of the 283 female, nonsmoking lung cancer patients enrolled, 113 were later revealed to be smokers and 36 turned out not to have lung cancer.

Sobue (1990) 120 subjects: RR = 0.94 (negative)

This Japanese study surveyed 120 nonsmoking, female lung cancer patients and found no association between marriage to a smoker and lung cancer: RR = 0.94 (0.62-1.40). The only statistically significant associations that came to light in this report were a protective effect if the subject's father smoked - 0.60 (0.4-0.91) - and a link between lung cancer and cooking with wood and straw - 1.90 (1.09-3.30)

Kurahashi (2007) 109 subjects: RR = 1.34 (null)

Another Japanese study and another statistically insignificant positive association: 1.34(0.81-2.21). Co-authors of the study included Liu, Sobue and Inoue, all of whom had previously conducted passive smoking studies with mixed results. 80% of the cases had adenocarcinoma.

Stockwell (1992) 108 subjects: RR = 1.6 (null)

This American study retrospectively interviewed 210 female lung cancer patients, of whom 108 were married. Results were adjusted for age, race and education but not for diet and occupation. The relative risk for spousal exposure was a nonsignificant 1.6 (0.8-3.0). There was no association with exposure in social settings.

Chang-Yeung (2003) 106 subjects: RR = 1.01 (null)

This study examined various possible carcinogens but found few relationships, particularly with regard to passive smoking. Funded by Hong Kong's Anti-Cancer Society, the authors made much of an apparent association between exposure to secondhand smoke and lung cancer in men but the statistical significance disappeared once the figures were adjusted for confounders. No amount of cherry-picking could mask the fact that the relative risk for wives married to smokers was zero: 1.01 (0.47-2.18).

Ko (1997) 105 subjects: RR = 1.3 (null)

This was another study designed to identify why the lung cancer rate was so high amongst nonsmoking women in Asia. 105 female patients were retrospectively surveyed and significant associations were found with low vegetable consumption, frying food and kitchen ventilation but not with secondhand smoke. Relative risk for women married to smokers was a nonsignificant 1.3 (0.7-2.5) and childhood exposure gave a nonsignificant 0.8 (0.4-1.6).

Dalager (1986) 99 subjects: RR = 0.86 (negative)

This paper from the US - co-authored by Elizabeth Fontham - drew together three studies from Texas, Louisiana and New Jersey. The overall lung cancer risk for nonsmokers living with smokers was exactly in line with the null hypothesis with an RR of 1.0 (0.64-1.56). When the figure was adjusted for gender, race, age, asbestos exposure, diet and employment, the RR fell to 0.86 (0.52-1.34). This was based on male and female subjects combined since the authors did not split the findings by gender. In their own assessment of risk to women, the authors excluded the Texas study (which was the largest) and since the New Jersey study only included men, this limited them to the 28 women from Louisiana. Here the authors reported nonsignificant risks of 1.96 (0.82-4.7) for women and 0.93 (0.3-2.9) for men.

Kabat (1984) 97 subjects: RR = 0.79 (negative)

In their study of 749 females with lung cancer, Geoffrey Kabt and Ernst Wynder identified 97 cases who were nonsmokers and found no association between secondhand smoke exposure and their disease either in the home or in the workplace. The authors did not assign relative risks to their statistics but when the EPA assessed the study in 1992, they found the association to be 0.79 (0.25-2.45) ie. a nonsignificant protective effect. The only significant positive association that emerged from the paper was a link with those who "worked in a textile-related job" (3.1 (1.11-8.64)).

Kalandidi (1990) 91 subjects: RR = 2.1* (significant - positive)

Along with the Fontham study, Kalandidi's paper provides perhaps the best evidence of secondhand smoke being a carcinogen to nonsmokers. 91 nonsmoking women with lung cancer were surveyed and a positive association of 2.1 (1.1-4.1) was found. This association did not vary significantly whether adenocarcinoma or other forms of lung cancer were under scrutiny.

Shimizu (1988) 90 subjects: RR = 1.10 (null)

The authors of this Japanese study were quick to emphasise that their statistics showed a four-fold increase in lung cancer risk for those exposed to tobacco smoke by their mother. Closer examination showed that this finding was based on the experiences of just three individuals. More reliable was their finding that "no association was observed between the risk of lung cancer and smoking of husbands or passive smoke exposure at work."

Nyberg (1998) 89 subjects: RR = 0.94 (negative)

Another null study with a slender tendency towards the negative. Using data from a Swedish sample group, a relative risk of 0.94 (0.53-1.67) was found for wives and risks of 0.76 and 0.29 for those exposed to smoke by their father and mother respectively.

Koo (1987) 86 subjects: RR = 1.64 (null)

This retrospective study of 86 female, never-smoking lung cancer cases found a statistically nonsignificant relative risk from a husband's smoking of 1.64 (0.87-3.09). Adjustments were made for age, education and (for some reason) number of children, but more important confounding factors such as diet, pollution and cooking methods went unmentioned. The subjects who had the heaviest smoking husbands, and those who recalled the most frequent exposure, had the lowest lung cancer risks and, as the author reported: "The lack of a dose-response pattern, and an almost consistent drop in the RR at the highest doses of exposure would seem to lend little, or only weak support for the passive smoking linkage with lung cancer."

Chan (1982) 84 subjects: RR = 0.75 (negative)

This retrospective study from Hong Kong focused on 189 female lung cancer cases, of whom 84 were nonsmokers. Of those who were married, 40% recalled being exposed to secondhand smoke. 60% did not. This left a relative risk of 0.75, thereby implying that exposure to tobacco smoke reduced the chances of suffering lung cancer in later life by 25%.

Zatloukal (2003) 84 subjects: RR = 0.43* (significant - negative)

This retrospective study from the Czech Republic had a sample group of 366 female lung cancer cases, of whom 84 were life-long nonsmokers. Various possible causes of lung cancer were investigated, and statistically significant associations were found with high red meat consumption, low fish consumption and a family history of lung disease.

Of the 84 subjects, only 7 had been exposed to secondhand smoke in adulthood (defined as 3 or more hours a day). Zatloukal broke down the results by adenocarcinoma (0.36 (0.11-1.22)) and other types of lung cancer (0.66 (0.22-1.96)), thereby disguising the fact that when the figures were combined to show all lung cancer cases, the negative relationship with secondhand smoke becomes statistically significant: (0.43 (0.19-0.95)).

Wang. S (1996) Up to 83 subjects: RR = 2.5* (significant - positive)

The tabulation of results makes it hard to ascertain how many female, nonsmoking lung cancer patients were married in this study but it is evident that there were no more than 83. The source of exposure is also vague and, critically, the sample group appears to include smokers. The authors gave a risk ratio of 2.5 (1.3-5.1) for women, falling to 1.02 for men. As with Sun (1996), the standard of the peer review process - if any - is unclear.

Du (1996) 75 subjects: RRs = 1.09 (null)

This Chinese study found statistically significant associations between lung cancer and both indoor air pollution and cooking fumes, but once again found no such link with secondhand smoke exposure. A sample group of 75 nonsmoking women was compared to two control groups. Against one group there was a nonsignificant RR of 1.19 (0.66-2.16); against the other the RR was precisely 1.0 - a valuable reminder that picking the right control group is as important as selecting the case group. There was no dose-relationship, indeed the RR for those who lived with a smoker for more than 30 years was below 1.0.

Akiba (1986) 72 subjects: RR = 1.5 (null)

The focus of this Japanese study was 72 female nonsmoking wives of smokers. All the women were, in a unique twist, atom bomb survivors from Hiroshima and Nagasaki.

Although various factors were considered, only those women who actively smoked were found to be at greater risk of lung cancer than those who were unexposed. The lone exception was women from blue collar families who lived with a heavy smoker, but only 6 of the subjects fell into this category.

While these findings were not statistically significant, the authors emphasised that there was a dose-response relationship between the amount smoked by the husbands and the lung cancer risk of the wives. This was true. What was also true was that the risk declined as the years of exposure rose. If the husband smoked for 1-19 years, the risk to the wife was 2.1 (0.7-2.1) but if he smoked for more than 40 years the risk fell dramatically, to 1.3 (0.7-2.3).

Zhou (2000) 72 subjects: RR = 0.94 (negative)

Another Chinese study, this time surveying 72 nonsmoking wives married to smoking husbands with a negative, statistically nonsignificant relative risk of 0.94 (0.41-1.97). Women exposed in childhood also showed an inverse risk of 0.89.

Kabat (1995) 69 subjects: RR = 1.08 (null)

The second in Geoffrey Kabat's trio of studies retrospectively surveyed 69 female nonsmokers with lung cancer and found no association with secondhand smoke exposure.

Vineis (2005) 69 subjects: RR = 0.82 (negative)

A strange one, this. No fewer than 26 people put their name to it and as a prospective study of 123,479 individuals (from 10 European countries), it stood every chance of making a valuable contribution. It spanned seven years and asked questions about diet, physical activity, age and various other confounding factors before falling at the final hurdle by including over 20,000 ex-smokers. Almost every other reputable study had made sure only never-smokers were included and with good reason: some of these women had been smoking for forty years or more before they quit and for many the damage had been done. It was well-known that ex-smokers had a greater risk of lung cancer than never-smokers.

Sure enough, the study showed that ex-smokers died of the disease at a greater rate than never-smokers and yet the authors appeared genuinely bewildered. "The fact that the association is stronger in former smokers is difficult to understand," they wrote, before hazarding the guess that former smokers "are more susceptible to low levels of environmental tobacco smoke."

Ultimately, it had little effect on the outcome of the study. Of the 69 women who contracted lung cancer, only 20 had been exposed to smoke in the home, leaving a risk ratio of 0.82 (0.37-1.82). More surprising was a statistically significant association between childhood exposure and lung cancer; an association that appeared to rise in relation to the level of tobacco exposure. As the authors admitted, this was the first time such an association had emerged from an epidemiological study. After 25 years of searching, it was unlikely to be representative of a genuine phenomenon.

Pershagen (1987) 67 subjects: RR = 1.2 (null)

This cohort study enrolled 27,409 nonsmoking women in Sweden in the early 1960s. When they were followed up in 1984, just 77 of them had contracted lung cancer. There was no significant association with smoke exposure and the risk ratio was 1.2 (0.7-2.1). The authors made much of a stronger association with squamous and small cell carcinoma where the relative risk was 3.3 (1.1-11.4). By contrast, there was a negative RR of 0.8 (0.4-1.5) for all other types of cancer. At the time of publication, this appeared to be a suggestive finding since squamous and small cell carcinomas were strongly associated with smoking and Dalager had recently found a similar association, albeit weaker. If the passive smoking theory were true, it seemed logical that smokers and passive smokers would suffer from the same types of cancer. But subsequent studies (notably Fontham's) have not replicated these findings and adenocarcinoma has been found to be the prevalent form of the disease in nonsmokers.

Brownson (1987) 66 subjects: RR = 1.68 (null)

Ross Brownson's first study into passive smoking retrospectively surveyed female, nonsmoking lung cancer patients in Colorado. He found no association between any form of secondhand smoke exposure and lung cancer. The study was confined to adenocarcinoma, a form of lung cancer least associated with smoking but more closely linked with women, and claimed a statistically nonsignificant relative risk of 1.68 (0.39-2.97) for those exposed to more than three hours of smoke per day (those with less than 3 hours exposure were taken as the controls. Only ten women fell into the case group, however, hence the very wide confidence interval. Other than active smoking, the only statistically significant association with lung cancer was found to be a low income.

Wang F. (1994) 55 subjects: RR = 0.78 (negative)

This Chinese study of 114 women with lung cancer included 55 life-long nonsmokers. Unfortunately, smokers were not excluded from the sample group and so the findings should be treated with caution. The author found a negative association with secondhand smoke in adulthood and a positive association with exposure in childhood, with the latter achieving statistical significance. Since smokers were not excluded, the latter result is most likely due to the known tendency of the offspring of smokers to become smokers themselves.

Joekel (1998) Fewer than 55 subjects: RR = 1.12 (null)

This German study had a sample group of 55 men and women and found no association between passive smoke and lung cancer: 1.12 (0.54-2.32). Results were not broken down by gender.

Geng (1988) 54 subjects: RR = 2.16* (significant - positive)

In 1988, a book published to commemorate the recent 'Smoking and Health' conference provided a dumping ground for a number of studies and theses that did not make it into the mainstream medical journals and which, therefore, did not have to undergo the normal peer-review process. Inoue's study (see below) and Guan-Yi Geng's typewritten paper were two of them. The latter's presentation was amateurish and its origins uncertain but it is included here because (like Wang, 1996) it is a rare example of a study finding a statistically significant association between secondhand smoke and lung cancer.

The data came from Tianjin, a city which, according to the authors, had the highest rate of female smoking prevalence in China and - unsurprisingly - also the highest incidence of female lung cancer. Not enough data was presented to allow much analysis although the author concluded that nonsmoking women married to smokers had a lung cancer risk of 2.16 (1.03-4.53). This narrowly achieved statistical significance and, as with the Hirayama study, a dose-response relationship was evident. Also in line with the Hirayama study, the apparent risk was peculiarly high. The 2.16 risk ratio given here for nonsmokers living with smokers was very close to the 2.61 (1.4-4.6) risk found for (female) smokers living with nonsmokers.

Liu (1991) 54 subjects: RR = 0.77 (negative)

The authors of this Chinese study found that those with a family history of lung disease, and those who cooked with coal, had a significantly increased lung cancer risk but there was no association with passive smoking. The 54 female lung cancer patients had not been exposed to secondhand smoke any more than the 202 controls and their relative risk was 0.77 (0.30-1.96).

Jee (1999) 51 subjects: RR = 1.9 (null)

The relative risk found in this Korean cohort study was not statistically significant but it came close with an RR of 1.9 (1.0-3.5). If this seemed suggestive, the inverse dose-response relationship suggested otherwise. According to this paper, those who lived with a heavy smoker were substantially less likely to suffer lung cancer as those married to a light smoker (2.0 and 1.5 respectively).

Appendix

Shen (1998) 50 subjects: RR = 0.75 (negative)

In keeping with most other studies, this retrospective Chinese study found lung cancer to be strongly associated with a family history of lung disease (4.36) and with exposure to cooking fumes (2.45) but not with passive smoke exposure.

Rapiti (1999) 41 subjects: 1.2 (null)

This study from India threw up a remarkably high relative risk for exposure to ETS in childhood of 12.0 (4.3-32.0), something that has not been supported by any other study. For women who had smoking husbands, however, there was no statistically significant relationship with lung cancer incidence (RR = 1.2 (0.5-2.9)) and there was a negative dose-response relationship; the risk ratio fell below 1.0 for the women who had been most heavily exposed for the longest time.

Trichopoulos (1981) 40 subjects: RR = 2.4* (significant - positive)

This paper (discussed in Chapter 6), surveyed 40 nonsmoking women with lung cancer in an Athens hospital between 1978 and 1980. Trichopoulos found that wives married to husbands who smoked 20 cigarettes or fewer each day had an elevated lung cancer risk of 2.4. This rose to 3.4 for those who had husbands who smoked more than 20 cigarettes a day. Since the study also showed that female smokers had an RR of 2.9, this meant that being married to a heavy smoker was more dangerous than being a heavy smoker. This was a far-fetched idea that Trichopoulos admitted sounded "strange." Nonetheless, the findings were statistically significant and there was a dose-response relationship.

Liu (1993) 38 subjects: 1.72 (null)

Unlike most other Chinese studies, Liu did not find a clear association between cooking fumes or a family history of lung disease with lung cancer. The association with secondhand smoke was unclear. The author split the subjects between those whose husbands smoked less than a pack a day and more than a pack a day. Taken together, there was no significant relationship (1.72 (0.77-7.3)) but there was some evidence of a dose-response relationship; those whose husbands smoked less than a pack had a risk ratio of 0.7 (0.23-2.2) and those living with heavier smokers had a risk ratio of 2.9 (1.2-7.3).

Buffler (1984) 33 subjects: RR = 0.78 (negative)

Conducted on lung cancer patients in Texas, this study found no association between secondhand smoke and lung cancer. The relative risk for the 33 nonsmoking women in the study was 0.78 (0.34-1.81); a result that was both nonsignificant and negative. For men, the findings were even less compelling, with an RR of 0.52 (0.15-1.74).

Lee (1986) 32 subjects: RR = 1.0 (exactly zero)

This English study found a relative risk of 1.0 (0.37-2.71) for 32 nonsmoking wives married to smokers compared to 66 controls. As a small study, it was unexceptional in its format and methodology apart from being funded by the Tobacco Research Council which, in turn, was funded by the tobacco industry.

Inoue (1988) 29 subjects: 2.25 (null)

Co-authored by Takeshi Hirayama, this retrospective study focused on 18 married women with lung cancer and claimed an RR of 2.25 (CI 90%: 0.91-7.10). There were a number of peculiarities, not least the way in which the authors doubled their chances of achieving statistical significance by using the lowered 90% confidence interval. They excluded women from the study if their husband smoked fewer than 5 cigarettes a day on the basis that these men never smoked in the house. This assumption was based on a separate questionnaire of 133 men which showed that those smoking 1 to 3 cigarettes a day never smoked at home. It was odd that the researchers went to the lengths of surveying a group of men who were not involved in the study when they could have simply asked the subjects if their husband smoked at home.

The numbers were very small and although it is slightly unclear from the paper, it seems that the 18 exposed cases were compared with just 2 unexposed cases, thereby making it impossible to draw any conclusions. The numbers were so small that statistical significance eluded the authors despite lowering the confidence interval, and they were not even able to show a strong link between active smoking and lung cancer. Stranger still, their RR for active smoking (1.66 (0.73-3.76)) was lower than that shown for passive smoking. As with Trichopoulos (above), it is hard to take any study seriously when it suggests that being a smoker is a healthier option than marrying one.

These shortcomings, and the probable lack of a peer-review (see Geng above), casts serious doubts over the value of this paper, as does the obvious bias of the authors. Their conclusion was that "smoking at home shud (sic) therefore be restricted strictly in oder (sic) to prevent nonsmoking family members from suffering unnecessarily from lung cancer and other selected diseases."

Kubik (2001) 24 subjects: RR = 1.17 (null)

In this paper from the Czech Republic, smokers were found to be ten times more likely to develop lung cancer, in line with countless previous studies, but of the 24 female, nonsmoking lung cancer cases involved, only 2 had been around a smoker for 3 or more hours a day. The raw data showed a relative risk of 0.91 but, as often happened with these studies, the authors' unexplained adjustments increased the figure slightly, to 1.17, with a very wide confidence interval of 0.2-5.6. For those exposed to tobacco smoke in childhood, the risk was smaller still: 0.85 (0.5-1.5).

Nishino (2001) 24 subjects: RR = 1.8 (null)

This Japanese study examined the possible effect of passive smoking on a huge variety of cancers. After adjustments, the RR for lung cancer was a nonsignificant 1.8 (0.67-4.6). The wide confidence interval was a reflection of the small number of participants; 11 of the women had a husband who smoked, 13 did not, and clearly it was impossible to make any firm conclusions from such a statistic. The limitations of the study are underlined when one considers that the only statistically significant finding was that exposure to secondhand smoke *reduced* breast cancer risk by 42%; RR 0.58 (0.34-0.99)

Johnson (2001) 23 subject: RR = 1.20 (null)

This small, retrospective Canadian study found a slim majority of controls reporting exposure to tobacco smoke in adulthood and a slim majority of the lung cancer cases reporting the same, leaving an insignificant risk ratio of 1.20 (0.5-3.0).

Correa (1983) 22 subjects: RR = 2.07 (null)

This retrospective study identified 22 married, nonsmoking women with lung cancer, of whom 14 recalled exposure to passive smoke. The numbers were small and the authors (including Elizabeth Fontham, in her first foray into this area of research) found a nonsignificant RR of 2.07 (0.81-5.25).

The authors found an association between a parent smoking and the development of lung cancer later in life but this finding was substantially undermined when it became clear that this only applied to those who went on to become smokers themselves and, even then, only for males with a mother who smoked. Women were not affected at all by childhood exposure and, oddly, having a father who smoked had no effect on either gender. The authors admitted that this was "puzzling."

Humble (1987) 20 subjects: RR = 1.8 (null)

The data for this study came from New Mexico and the small numbers involved meant the margin for error was wide. The authors employed a 90% confidence interval, rather than the more conventional 95%, but the findings still fell well short of achieving statistical significance; RR 1.8 (0.6-5.4).

Hole (1989) 9 subjects: RR = 1.37 (null)

This masterpiece of extrapolation is discussed in Chapter 7. As the result of a single additional lung cancer case, the risk from passive smoking rose from zero to 1.37 (0.29-6.61). The extraordinarily broad confidence interval is a fair indicator of how unreliable this finding is.

When the EPA assessed this study, its members increased the supposed risk by arbitrarily excluding three women who had lung cancer but who had not yet died of the disease. It must be assumed that two of these women had been married to nonsmokers, since their exclusion led to the EPA's RR rising to 1.99, with an even wider confidence interval of 0.24-16.72. The exclusion of these lung cancer cases is a further example of the EPA's manipulation of the data to strengthen the case against secondhand smoke.

Notes

Introduction: A unique case?

(1) 'Just can't quit: How far will smoking bans go', Reason.tv, November 2008
(2) 'This proposed smoking ban has some fuming', Maria L. La Ganga, *Los Angeles Times*, 29/1/07
(3) Full page magazine advertisement, RJ Reynolds, June 1994
(4) *Portland Oregonian*, 11/12/1919
(5) 'California Activists' Success Ignites a Not-So-Slow-Burn', John Schwartz, *Washington Post*, May 30, 1994, p. 1

i. 'Joyful news out of the new found world'

(1) S. Gilman & Z. Xun (ed), *Smoke - A Global History of Smoking*, Reaktion books, 2004; p. 9
(2) R. Kluger, *Ashes to Ashes*, Random House, 1997; p.9
(3) Count Corti, *A History of Smoking*, Bracken Books, 1931; p. 41
(4) Ibid. p. 42-43
(5) Ibid. p. 63
(6) Gilman & Xun; p. 10
(7) James Walton (ed), *The Faber Book of Smoking*, Faber, 2000; p. 26-27
(8) Gilda Berger, *Smoking Not Allowed*, Impact books, 1987; p. 37
(9) Gilman & Xun, p. 45
(10) Orpheus Junior, *The Golden Fleece*, 1626, Chapter 15
(11) Walton, p. 29
(12) Ibid. p. 37
(13) Gilman & Xun; p. 16
(14) Tara Parker-Pope, *Cigarettes - Anatomy of an Industry*, The New Press, New York, 2001; p. 141
(15) Walton, p. 30
(16) Despite this law, tobacco continued to be grown in England, even though it was invariably coarse and of low quality. Samuel Pepys described running battles between locals and the authorities over the tobacco crop in the village of Winchcombe. By the 1640s, Parliament had given up trying to suppress homegrown tobacco and levied a tax on it instead.
(17) Jordan Goodman, *Tobacco in History: Cultures of Dependence*, Taylor & Francis, 1994, p. 69 (In 1642, Pope Urban VII censured those who were smoking during Mass - and there must have been many for him to have bothered - but the Vatican, too, would go on to form its own tobacco monopoly and ban anti-smoking literature.)
(18) Walton, p. 40
(19) Ibid. p. 41
(20) Berger, p. 37
(21) Gilman & Xun, p. 124
(22) Walton, p. 39
(23) Gilman & Xun, p. 88
(24) Gilman & Xun, p. 15
(25) Corti, p. 19
(26) James Boswell, *Journal of the Tour of the Hebrides*, Koneman, 1785 (2000 edition); p. 9
(27) Berger, p. 45
(28) Berger, p. 44
(29) In Britain, the RSPCA was formed to campaign against cruelty to animals, famously predating the foundation of the NSPCC which aimed to do the same for children.
(30) 'Medical aspects of tobacco smoking and the anti-tobacco movement in Britain in the nineteenth century', R.B. Walker, *Medical History*, 1980, 24; p. 400
(31) Ian Tyrell, *Deadly Enemies*, UNSW, 1999; p. 9
(32) Walton, p. 66

(33) Ibid.
(34) Ibid.
(35) Ibid. p. 65
(36) Meta Lander, *The Tobacco Problem*, 1882; p. 48
(37) Ibid. p.86
(38) Ibid. p. 11
(39) Matthew Hilton, *Smoking in British Popular Culture*, Manchester University Press, 2000; p. 64
(40) Gilman & Xun, p. 25
(41) 'The Moral Statistician', Mark Twain, Originally published in *Sketches, Old and New*, 1893

2. 'A smokeless America by 1925'

(1) Robert F. Durden, *The Dukes of Durham 1865-1929*, Duke Uni. Press, 1987; p. 110
(2) 'James Buchanan Duke, tobacco king, 68, dies of pneumonia', *New York Times*, 11/10/25
(3) Gilda Berger, *Smoking not allowed*, Impact books, 1987; p. 52
(4) *The New York Times*, 29/1/1884
(5) Edward Behr, *Prohibition*, 1996 p.38
(6) Cassandra Tate, *Cigarette Wars*, OUP, 1999; p. 30
(7) Tate, p. 31
(8) Tate, p. 31
(9) Behr, p. 41
(10) 'Lost Cause: A portrait of Lucy Page Gaston', Frances Warfield, *Outlook and Independent*, 1930; 154:p. 244-247, 275-276.
(11) Herbert Asbury, *Carry Nation*, 1929
(12) Behr, p. 41
(13) Meta Lander, *The Tobacco Problem*, 1882; p.26
(14) *New York Times*, 12/12/1894
(15) Lander, p.63
(16) Ibid.
(17) James Walton (ed), *The Faber book of smoking*, Faber, 2000; p. 79
(18) Behr, p. 41
(19) Walton (ed), p. 80
(20) *New York Times*, 8/8/1907
(21) *Harpers Weekly*, 17/9/1910
(22) Matthew Hilton, *Smoking in British Popular Culture*, Manchester University Press, 2000, p. 74
(23) Ibid. p. 168
(24) *New York Times*, 15/6/1893
(25) *New York Times*, 19/4/1905; p. 10
(26) *Outlook*, 11/3/1905; p. 611
(27) Letter to the *New York Times*, 10/11/1911
(28) *Harpers Weekly*, 17/9/1910
(29) *New York Times*, 8/7/11
(30) 'Workers assail Dr Pease', *New York Times*, 10/8/08
(31) 'Smokers demand a place on cars', *New York Times*, 24/10/2008
(32) Berger, p. 42
(33) Walton, p. 40
(34) Ibid.
(35) Tate, p. 74
(36) Daniel A. Poling, *Huts in Hell*, Boston, 1918; p. 54-55
(37) Richard Kluger, *Ashes to Ashes*, Knopf, New York, 1996, p. 63
(38) Tate, p. 84
(39) *The Lancet*, 3/10/1914
(40) Hilton, p. 120

3. 'Your body belongs to the Fuhrer'

(1) Cassandra Tate, *Cigarette Wars*, OUP, 1999, p. 121
(2) Ibid. p. 122
(3) Ibid. p. 121
(4) Ibid. p. 127
(5) 'War is declared on 'demon' tobacco', *New York Times*, 2/9/23
(6) Cited in Milton Friedman, *'An Economist's Protest: Columns in political economy'*, Thomas Horton, New Jersey, 1972, p.160
(7) Tate, p. 122
(8) 'Anti-cigarette league and Miss Gaston part', *New York Times*, 27/8/21
(9) Tate, p. 114
(10) Ibid.
(11) Ibid.p. 115
(12) Ibid, p. 5
(13) Ibid, p. 100
(14) Ibid. p. 113
(15) Cited in Troyer & Markle, *'Cigarettes: The battle over smoking'*, The State University Press, 1983; p. 267
(16) Ibid.
(17) Count Corti, *A History of Smoking*, New York, 1931; p. 265
(18) Kluger, *Ashes to Ashes*, p. 105
(19) *Journal of American Medical Association*, 1948
(20) 'Tobacco and the individual', A.A. Brill, *International Journal of Psychoanalysis*, 1922
(21) Robert Proctor, *The Nazi War on Cancer*, Princeton University Press, 1999; p. 196
(22) Ibid. p. 184
(23) Ibid. p. 209
(24) Lickint's epic book, for example, was commissioned and funded by the Reich Committee for the Struggle Against Addictive Drugs and the German Anti-Tobacco League.
(25) Proctor. p. 204
(26) Ibid.
(27) 'The Nazis' campaign against tobacco: Science in a totalitarian state' in *Medicine and medical ethics in Nazi Germany* (ed. F. Nicosia & J. Huerer), Berghahn books, 2001
(28) 'Why does smoking so often produce dependence? A somewhat different view', John R. Hughes, *Tobacco Control*, 2001; 10 p. 62-64
(29) Meta Lander, *The Tobacco Problem*, 1882
(30) David Krogh, *The Artifical Passion*, W.H. Freeman & Co. 1991, pp. 51-52
(31) W. L. Dunn, *Smoking behaviour; Motives & Incentives*, Washington, V. H. Winston & Sons, 1973, p. 197-207
(32) Corti, p. 257
(33) James Boswell, *Journal of the tour of the Hebrides*, London, 1785, p.9
(34) Shown in experiments by Werbes & Warburton (1983) and Knott (1985)
(35) 'Smoking, obesity, and their co-occurence in the United States: Cross sectional analysis', Healton et al. *British Medical Journal*, Vol. 333:1/7/06
(36) Shown by Williams (1980) and Frankenhauser (1971)
(37) Whether smokers benefit from better concentration and performance levels overall is more debatable. Some studies have shown an overall superiority in ability, memory and learning when nonsmokers are given nicotine tablets but the evidence is neither strong nor consistent. Krogh believes that concentration levels are somewhat higher when nicotine is administered for certain tasks. He gives the example of the disproportionately large number of baseball players who chew tobacco as being suggestive that, in that sport at least, it can enhance performance and raise alertness. (Krogh, p. 64)
(38) 'The big draw', Daisy Garnett, *Vogue*, September 2006; p. 160
(39) Lander, p. 3
(40) Krogh. p. 65
(41) Shown by Knott & Venables (1978)
(42) Shown by Perkins (1989)
(43) Leo Tolstoy, *Why do men stupefy themselves? and other writings*, Hankins, New York Strength Books, 1975; pp. 55-56
(44) See Remington et al (1985), Green (1979), Kozlowski (1979), Hughes (1986), Glassman (1988). Krogh, p. 103

4. 'Some women would prefer having smaller babies'

(1) 'How to stop smoking', *Time* magazine, 15/09/52
(2) Lennox Johnston, *The Disease of Tobacco Smoking and its Cure*, London, Christopher Johnston, 1957, p. 76 & p. 96
(3) Ibid. p. 54
(4) Kluger, *Ashes to Ashes*; p. 169
(5) Ibid.
(6) *The Lancet*, 11/10/1952
(7) James Walton (ed), *The Faber Book of Smoking*, Faber; p. 96
(8) 'A Frank Statement to Cigarette Smokers', TIRC, 1953
(9) There were questions then, as there are questions now, about what protection, if any, was offered by filter tips. Richard Kluger, in *Ashes to Ashes*, describes them as 'placebos' but he still seems to accept that cellulose acetate filters block tarry materials.

Clinical trials have shown filters to be much more than placebos. Experiments on beagles carried out by Hammond and Auerbach in 1970 showed that 72% of the dogs exposed to normal cigarettes developed tumours; this fell to 33% for those exposed to filtered cigarettes. In Australia, the Commonwealth Department of Health investigated the issue and found "evidence that some protection was afforded by cigarette holders and efficient types of filters" and a comprehensive study in 2004 showed that filtered cigarettes are around 25% less harmful than their unfiltered cousins. ('Cigarette tar yields in relation to mortality from lung cancer in the cancer prevention study II prospective cohort, 1982-8', Jeffrey E Harris et al. *British Medical Journal*, 10/1/2004; 328:72)
(10) Maryland Medicaid Lawsuit, 1/5/96
(11) Kluger, p. 240
(12) Stanton Glantz et al., *The Cigarette Papers*, University of California Press, 1998; p. 109
(13) Ibid. p. 211
(14) Johnston, p. 19-20
(15) Ibid. p.21
(16) Ibid. p. 79
(17) *British Medical Journal*, letters, 15/12/79, p.1584
(18) Johnston, p. 77
(19) 'Smoking revenue outweighed risk, Macmillan told Cabinet', *Daily Telegraph*, 30/5/08, p. 12
(20) Hilton, pp. 205-213
(21) J. Walton (ed), p. 99
(22) Ibid.
(23) Internal Brown & Williamson memo from Addison Yeaman, July 17 1963. It is interesting to note that, if this memo is any indication, the tobacco industry believed that the 'smoking theory' might be disproved and, if not, that cigarettes could be made safe.
(24) Ian Tyrell, *Deadly Enemies*, UNSW Press, 1999; p. 178
(25) Tara Parker-Pope, *Cigarettes: Anatomy of an industry*, The New Press, New York, 2001, p.93
(26) 'How Banzhaf's Successful Antismoking Crusade Began' Frank Tursi, Susan E. White and Steve McQuilkin; *Winston-Salem Journal*, 11/18/99. Available at www.ash.org
(27) *Readers Digest*, March 1971
(28) Kluger, p. 306
(29) Parker-Pope, p.93
(30) Troyer & Markle, *Cigarettes: The battle over smoking*, The State Uni. Press, 1983; p. 114
(31) Ibid. p. 112
(32) Ibid. p. 112
(33) Ibid. p. 82
(34) Kluger, p. 358

5. 'Smokers should be eliminated'

(1) 'Science, Politics, and Ideology in the Campaign Against Environmental Tobacco Smoke' Ronald Bayer & James Colgrove, *American Journal of Public Health*. 2002 June; 92(6): pp. 949–954
(2) Jacob Sullum, *For Your Own Good*, Free Press, 1998, p. 114
(3) 'The Power of One: Agent of change: more than "a nuisance to the tobacco industry"', Simon Chapman, *Medical Journal of Australia*, 2002 177 (11/12); pp. 661-633

Notes

(4) 'BUGA UP (Smoking history), Australian Broadcasting Company, George Nexus Tonight, 22/11/04
(5) 'Social Movements as Catalysts', Constance A. Nathanson, *Journal of Health Politics, Policy and Law*, 24 (3), 06/03/99; pp. 421-488
(6) Steve Allen & Bill Adler, *The Passionate Nonsmokers Bill of Rights*, Bill Adler books, 1989; p. 61
(7) 'Mandarin branded anti-smoking group "militant"', David Turner & Ben Sherwood, *Financial Times*, 4/1/05
(8) Virginia Berridge, *Marketing Health*, Oxford, OUP, 2007, p. 167.

      The UK version of GASP was formed in 1979 and embarked on what its leader described as "wild and witty demonstrations," perhaps the best known being the submission of a painting of a lung cancer victim to the John Player-sponsored Portrait Award competition. (C. Farren, 'GASP: Picking off the pack of lies', *Tobacco Control*, 2004:13; p.100-101)

(9) Berridge, p. 182, 185, 187
(10) Troyer & Markle, *Cigarettes: The battle over smoking*, Rutgers, 1986; p. 104
(11) Memo from Fred Panzer to Horace Kornegay, 1/5/1972 www.tobaccodocuments.org
(12) Kluger, p. 445
(13) 'Mortality in relation to tar yield of cigarettes: a prospective study of four cohorts', J. Tang et al, *British Medical Journal*, 1995; 311: pp. 1530-1533
(14) 'Cigarette tar yields in relation to mortality from lung cancer in the cancer prevention study II prospective cohort, 1982-8', Jeffrey E Harris et al., *British Medical Journal*, 10/1/2004; pp. 328:72
(15) 'Out of the Ashes: The Life, Death, and Rebirth of the "Safer" Cigarette in the United States', Amy Fairchild and James Colgrove, *American Journal of Public Health*, February 2004; 94(2): pp. 192–204.
(16) 'Re-inventing the cigarette: Innovation in the cigarette industry', John Slade, *Priorities*, Summer 1990; pp. 5-9
(17) Gio Gori, Fred G. Bock (ed.), '*Banbury report: A safe cigarette?*', Cold Spring Harbour Laboratory, 1980; p. 43
(18) US Congress, 'Reviewing Progress Made Toward the Development and Marketing of a Less Hazardous Cigarette', in Hearings, 90th Congress, First Session, August 23, 24, and 25, 1967 (Washington, DC: Government Printing Office, 1968), p. 153.
(19) *The Health Consequences of Smoking*, Surgeon General's report, 1972, p. v
(20) Kluger. p. 460
(21) Ibid. p. 451
(22) 'The lawyers did it: The cigarette manufacturers' policy toward smoking and health' Martha Derthick, *Legality and Community*, ed. Kagan et al, Rowan & Littlefield, 2002; pp. 281-295
(23) Sullum, p. 71

6. 'Nonsmokers arise!'

(1) Richard Kluger, *Ashes to Ashes*, 1996 p. 375
(2) Ibid.
(3) Virginia Berridge, *Marketing Health*, p. 220
(4) 'Please put your cigarette out; the smoke is killing me!', John Banzhaf III, *Today's Health*, April 1972, pp.38-40
(5) "Nonsmokers arise!" Max Wiener, *Readers Digest*, Nov. 1972, pp 249-254
(6) 'A study of public attitudes towards cigarette smoking and the tobacco industry in 1978', The Roper Organisation (Tobacco Institute), May 1978
(7) 'Passive smoking: How great a hazard?' Gary Huber et al. *Consumers' Research*, July 1991, Vol. 74, No. 7, p. 13
(8) Kluger, p.553
(9) Roy J. Shephard, *Carbon Monoxide: The Silent Killer*, 1983. p. 117
(10) Roy J. Shephard, *The Risks of Passive Smoking*, 1982, pp. 38-39
(11) Ibid. pp.123-124
(12) Shephard, *Carbon Monoxide*, p. 166
(13) Jacob Sullum, *For Your Own Good*, 1998. p.176
(14) Shephard, p. 71
(15) Ibid. p. 82
(16) 'Indoor air pollution, tobacco smoke, and public health', J.C. Repace & A.H. Lowrey, *Science*, 208; 2/5/80, pp. 464-472
(17) 'Passive smoking: How great a hazard?' Gary Huber et al. *Consumers' Research*, July 1991, Vol. 74, No. 7; p. 13
(18) Quoted in Don Oakley, *Slow burn*, Eyrie Press, 1999; p. 234,
(19) Researchers in England have since shown that nonsmokers living and working with nonsmokers are exposed to the equivalent of six cigarettes per *year*, or one sixtieth of a cigarette per day (*The Daily Telegraph*, 'Passive smokers inhale six cigarettes a year', 16/8/98)
(20) Kluger, p. 497
(21) E. Wynder, *Workshop on guidelines to the epidemiology of weak associations*, 1987, pp.139-41

(22) 'Epidemiology faces its limits', *Science*, 14/7/95
(23) 'Non-smoking wives of heavy smokers have a higher risk of lung cancer: a study from Japan', Takeshi Hirayama, *British Medical Journal*, Vol. 282 17 Jan 1981; pp. 183-185
(24) 'A case-control study of lung cancer and environmental tobacco smoke among nonsmoking women living in Shanghai, China', Zhong et al., *Cancer Causes and Control*, 10:1999; pp. 607-616. See also Koo (1988)
(25) Zhong et al. 1999
(26) 'Misclassification rates for current smokers misclassified as nonsmokers', Wells et al., *American Journal of Public Health*, Oct. 1998; pp.1503-09
(27) 'Lung cancer and passive smoking', D. Trichopoulos, *International Journal of Cancer*, 1981: 27; pp.1-4
(28) 'A national dilemma: Cigarette smoking or the health of Americans', N.C.S.P.P Report 1978, New York; p. 71
(29) Berridge, p. 182
(30) Matthew Hilton, *Smoking in British Popular Culture*, p. 188
(31) James Le Fanu, *The Rise and Fall of Modern Medicine*, Abacus, London, 1999
(32) Michael Fitzpatrick, *The Tyranny of Health*, Routledge, 2001; p. 79
(33) Ibid. See also Theodore MacDonald's *Rethinking Health Promotion: A Global Approach*, Routledge, 1998
(34) Sir Douglas Black, *Inequalities of Health* report of a research working group, London, Pelican, 1981. Also known as the Black Report.
(35) Kluger, p. 537
(36) Troyer & Markle, p. 126
(37) Stanton A. Glantz's CV, http://tobaccodocuments.org/pm/2021181600-1616.html
(38) Jacob Sullum, *For Your Own Good*, 1996, p. 147
(39) *Washington Star*, 15/4/80, p. D1

7. 'A smoke-free America by 2000'

(1) Proceedings of the 5th World Conference on Smoking and Health, Canadian Council on Smoking & Health, 1983; pp. 479-481
(2) Ibid. p. 287
(3) Ibid. p. 191
(4) Ibid. p. 213
(5) 'Fifth World Conference on Smoking & Health - Winnipeg', Hans Verkerk, 1983; http://tobaccodocuments.org/pm/2501021564-1587.html
(6) Proceedings of the 5th World Conference on Smoking and Health, Canadian Council on Smoking & Health, 1983, p. 815
(7) Ibid.
(8) Ibid. p. 41
(9) San Francisco Smoking Pollution Control Ordinance, Section 1001, 1983
(10) 'If It's Good for Philip Morris, Can It Also Be Good for Public Health?', Joe Nocera, *New York Times*, 18/06/06
(11) 'Lung cancer in non-smokers in Hong Kong', Chan & Fung, Cancer Campaign, Vol. 6, *Cancer Epidemiology* (E. Grundmann (ed)), 1982 pp. 199-202
(12) 'Passive smoking and lung cancer,' Correa et al, *The Lancet*, 10/9/83; 2:8350; pp.595-597
(13) 'Time trends in lung cancer mortality among nonsmokers and a note on passive smoking', L. Garfinkel, *Journal of the National Cancer Institute*, 1981: 66; pp. 1061-1066
(14) Ibid.
(15) 'Relationship of passive smoking to risk of lung cancer and other smoking-associated diseases', P.N. Lee, British Journal of Cancer, July 1986; 54(1): pp. 97-105.
(16) Kluger, p. 502
(17) C. Evertt Koop, 'The health consequences of involuntary smoking', Surgeon General's Report 1986, Washington DC
(18) Ibid.
(19) Kluger, p. 540
(20) Ibid, p. 505
(21) Ibid. p. 763, pp. 503-504 (Kluger holds no brief for the tobacco industry. He has described it as a "slayer of an incubus that has defied all reason, thrived on greed and folly, and driven poor mortals to grasp onto it for succour in a fashion their Maker never designed their bodies to long endure." *Ashes to Ashes*,1996; p. 763)
(22) 'Achieving a smoke-free society', S. Glantz, *Circulation*, 76:4, Oct. 1987, pp. 746-752
(23) Troyer & Markle, p. 126

(24) 'Consummate consumer; pressing charges - students fight discriminatory fees', *Washington Post*, 29/6/80

(25) James Repace advises complaining to the pilot "if it gets stuffy". He says that he does so regularly and is always rewarded with the ventilation being increased. ('Rendez-Vous with James Repace', *Phillippe Boucher, Rendez-Vous*, no. 64; 26/4/2000)

(26) 'The man who would stamp out smoking', James F. McCarty, *Tristate* magazine, 5/1/86, pp.4-7

(27) 'Unhealthy haze spoils game', *USA Today*, June 12 1991,

(28) Glantz, 'Achieving a smoke-free society', pp. 746-752

(29) 'A disease model of cigarette use', John D. Slade, *New York State Journal of Medicine*, July 1985; pp.297

(30) Source: *Lung Cancer Alliance*

(31) Sullum, p. 135

(32) 'Tobacco Prevention', *Mammoth Lakes Weekly*, 18/2/93, p. 53

(33) 'Health groups squabble for tobacco tax funds', Ken Hoover, United Press International, 31/7/89

(34) According to the *Los Angeles Daily News*, much of this money was spent "collecting information on groups and individuals that the foundation believes are secretly working for Big Tobacco." *LA Daily News*, 6/12/99

(35) Spoken at 'Revolt against tobacco' conference, Los Angeles, 2/10/92. Transcript, p. 14. At the same conference, ANR spokesman Glenn Barr explained that the movement's aim was to "force [smokers] to do the right thing for themselves."

(36) 'The effect of environmental tobacco smoke in two urban communities in the west of Scotland', Gillis et al., *European Journal of Respiratory Disease*, 1984; p. 121-126

(37) 'Passive smoking and cardiorespiratory health in a general population in the west of Scotland', Hole et al., *British Medical Journal*, 12/8/89, 299: (6696); pp. 423-427

(38) 'Lung cancer in nonsmoking women: a multi-center case-control study', Fontham et al, *Cancer Epidemiology, Biomarkers and Prevention*, Vol. 1, Nov/Dec 1991; pp. 35-43

(39) 'Environmental tobacco smoke and lung cancer in nonsmoking women', Stockwell et al., *Journal of National Cancer Institute* 84, 1992; p. 1412-1422

(40) M. Perske, 'Cooking the Books: A Restaurant Study' 12/5/95

(41) Kluger, pp. 694-696

(42) 'Lung cancer and exposure to tobacco smoke in the household', Janerich. D.T, *New England Journal of Medicine* 6/9/90; pp. 632-636

(43) Ibid.

(44) Kluger, p. 693

(45) 'Wide peril is seen in passive smoking', *New York Times*, Philip J. Hilts, 10/5/90

(46) ABC TV, May 9, 1990. Daynard appeared on NBC's 'The Today Show', May 10, 1990

(47) *Phillippe Boucher's Rendez Vous: James Repace*, 20/4/00: http://www.tobacco.org/resources/rendezvous/repace.html (The full quote reads: "In 1986, EPA created an Indoor Air Staff, (which later became a Division), and I joined it. Based on these two reports, we were able to convince EPA top management *to initiate a request a research office staff to* produce the now-famous 1992 EPA risk assessment on passive smoking, to put the Agency as a whole on the record." The highlighted passage makes no sense and I assume is a typo. I have changed the second 'a' to 'for')

(48) Milloy, p. 158

(49) EPA report, 1993; p. A-136

(50) EPA, *Respiratory Health Effects of Passive Smoking*; pp. 5-2

(51) Kluger p. 739

(52) Opinion written by Judge William L. Osteen US District Judge, 4 F. Supp. 2nd 435;1998 US District LEXIS 10986

(53) Ibid.

(54) John Brignell, *The Epidemiologists*, Brignell Associates, 2004

8. 'This is a crusade, not a lawsuit'

(1) Proceedings of the 5th World Conference on Smoking and Health, Canadian Council on Smoking & Health; p. 481

(2) Hillary Rodham Clinton, *Living History*, Headline, London, 2003

(3) Ibid.

(4) Kluger, *Ashes to Ashes*, p. 437

(5) Sullum, *For Your Own Good*, p. 133

(6) Ibid. p. 133

(7) 'Tobacco costs more than you think', WHO 1995, World No-Tobacco Day advisory kit. Tobacco Alert, special issue.

(8) Sullum. p. 203-204
(9) 'Death in the West', Thames TV, 1976; Interview with presenter Peter Taylor and PM spokesman Helmut Wakeham
(10) 'Out of the Ashes: The Life, Death, and Rebirth of the "Safer" Cigarette in the United States', *American Journal of Public Health*. Amy Fairchild and James Colgrove, February 2004; 94(2): pp.192–204.
(11) 'Junking Science to Promote Tobacco', Derek Yach, *American Journal of Public Health*, Nov. 2001, Vol. 91, No. 11, pp.1745-48
(12) ASH Daily News, 24/10/06 www.ash.org.uk
(13) 'The safer cigarette: what the tobacco industry could do (...and why it hasn't done it)', ASH UK Press release, 3/3/99, available at www.ash.org.uk
(14) Tara Parker-Pope, '*Cigarettes: Anatomy of an Industry*', The New Press, New York, 2001, p.129
(15) 'Anti-Smoking Zealots' speech to RJ Reynolds employees, Herbert Osmon, 1991 http://tobaccodocuments.org/landman/511384849-4877.html
(16) 'Out of the Ashes: The Life, Death, and Rebirth of the "Safer" Cigarette in the United States', Amy Fairchild and James Colgrove, *American Journal of Public Health*, February 2004; 94(2); pp.192–204.
(17) 'Antismoking climate inspires suits by the dying', *New York Times*, David Margolick, 15/3/85
(18) RJ Reynolds Tobacco Co. v. Colluci, 8.2 TPLR 2.225 (n.C. Super. Ct. 1993)
(19) *New York Times*, 6/3/95
(20) Iain Gately, *La Diva Nicotina*, Simon & Schuster, 2001; p. 324
(21) Sullum, p. 253
(22) 'Blowing Smoke', *The Economist*, 20/12/97
(23) *Journal of the American Medical Association*, 12/7/95
(24) Sullum, p. 186
(25) Ibid. p. 202
(26) 'What deal? We got suckered', Stanton Glantz, *Los Angeles Times*, 23/6/97, p. B5
(27) Sullum, p. 205
(28) 'The case for smoker-free workplaces', Nigel Gray, *Tobacco Control* 2005; 14, p.143-144
(29) Kathleen E. Scheg, ASH, Senate Judiciary Hearings, 30/7/97
(30) Tara Parker-Pope, *Cigarettes: An Anatomy of an Industry*, The New Press, New York, 2001, p.27

9. 'I have a comic book mentality'

(1) 'Environmental tobacco smoke and lung cancer in nonsmoking women', Stockwell et al. *Journal of National Cancer Institute* 84: 1992; pp. 1412-1422
(2) Stanton Glantz, *Tobacco War*, Uni. of California Press, Berkeley, 2000; p.212
(3) Ibid. p. 226
(4) Ibid. p. 3
(5) The branding was considered too harrowing for broadcast and when the commercial was filmed, the tobacco cowboy merely rounds up some children, locks them up and takes them off in his cart.
(6) 'Cattle' and 'Nicotine Soundbites', TV advertisements, September/October, California
(7) C. W. Crocker Communications Inc. 'Save a Waitress' Script for radio advertisement. Sacremento, April 1996
(8) 'Show Me the Documents', Robert A. Levy, *Reason*, April, 2000
(9) Glantz, '*Tobacco War*', p. 243
(10) They were particularly bitter because the CMA had been ambivalent about Prop 99 until it was made law because the CMA expected it to be rejected by the electorate.
(11) Glantz, p. 117
(12) 'Suit questions use of state fund', Greg Lucas, *San Francisco Chronicle*, 24/3/94 p. A19
(13) *New York Times*, 3/4/97, p. A18
(14) Sullum, p. 5
(15) Ibid. p. xii
(16) Glantz et al. *The Cigarette Papers*, University of California Press, 1998; p. 180-181.
   Sullum's article was originally published in *The Wall Street Journal* as 'Smoke & Mirrors: EPA Wages War on Cigarettes'
(17) 'Show Me the Documents', Robert A. Levy, *Reason*, April 2000
(18) M. Perske, 'Cooking the Books: A Restaurant Study', 1995
(19) 'Junking Science to Promote Tobacco', Derek Yach, *American Journal of Public Health*, Nov. 2001, Vol. 91, No. 11, pp.1745-48

Notes

(20) Michael Siegel, The Rest of the Story blog; 20/7/05, http://tobaccoanalysis.blogspot.com/2005/07/challenging-dogma-post-2-anyone-who.html
(21) Ibid.
(22) 'Foundation gives cash to raise tobacco taxes', John Schmeltzer, *Salt Lake Tribune*, 16/8/94, p. D5
(23) Robert Wood Johnson Foundation 2005 Annual Report
(24) Ibid.
(25) 'Anti-smoking groups look to drug companies for funding', *Edmonton Journal*, 22/1/07
(26) 'The workplace: Haziness about tobacco', Thomas Fuller, *International Herald Tribune*, 8/6/05

10. 'Do not let them fool you'

(1) 'Cancer Facts and Figures 2006', American Cancer Society. US cigarette consumption peaked in 1963 at 4,345 per capita.
(2) Centers for Disease Control; National Youth Risk Behaviour Survey
(3) W. Kip Viscusi, *Smoking: Making the risky decision*, OUP, Oxford, 1992. p. 121
(4) Ibid. pp. 61-86
(5) Michael Fitzpatrick, *The Tyranny of Health*, Routledge, p. 15
(6) 'Long-Term Decline In Smoking in U.S. Is Apparently Over', *New York Times*, May 20, 1994, Philip J. Hilts
(7) Mark Lender, 'A new prohibition?' in '*Smoking: Who has the right?* Schaler & Schaler (ed.), Prometheus books, 1998; pp. 89-93
(8) Simon Chapman, *The Lancet*, 20/4/85, 1(8434):918-920
(9) 'It is time to abandon tobacco access programmes', Ling, Landman & Glantz, *Tobacco Control*; 11, p.3-6
(10) 'Is ban on underage smoking working?', Deborah Hirsch, *Charlotte Observer*, 17/9/2006
(11) 'Compete with the tobacco industry', Stanton Glantz, *Tobacco Control*, 2000; 9; p.241
(12) *The Lancet*, 17/10/98, Vol. 352, p. 1288
(13) *The Lancet*, 'Tobacco's industry efforts subverting International agency for Research on Cancer's second-hand smoke study"; Vol. 355, 8/4/00, p. 1255
(14) 'Multicenter Case-Control Study of Exposure to Environmental Tobacco Smoke and Lung Cancer in Europe', Paolo Boffetta et al., *Journal of the National Cancer Institute*, Vol. 90, No. 19, October 7, 1998, pp. 140-150
(15) ASH letter to PCC, 'Re: Sunday Telegraph reports on passive smoking - ref. 980522', Clive Bates, 29/5/98
(16) 'Passive smoking and lung cancer risk; What is the story now?', *Journal of the National Cancer Institute*, Vol. 90, No. 19, 7/10/98. p. 1416
(17) 'Resisting smoke and spin', *The Lancet*, Vol. 355, 8/4/00, p. 1197
(18) 'Smoking as "independent" risk factor for suicide: illustration of an artifact from observational epidemiology?', Smith et al, *The Lancet*, 1992, 340; pp. 709-712
(19) 'Truths and Myths: the cancer report (part two)', Peter Silveron, *The Guardian*, 15/10/00
(20) E-mail from Stanton Glantz (14/5/06); J. Enstrom, 20/9/06, Defending Legitimate Epidemiologic Research http://www.spiked-online.com/Articles/0000000CAA11.htm
(21) 'Tobacco's industry efforts subverting International agency for Research on Cancer's second-hand smoke study", *The Lancet*, vol. 355, 8/4/00. p. 1255
(22) 'Study flawed from outset' (letter), *British Medical Journal*, 2003; 327: 501, 30/8/03
(23) Thun also told the press that the ACS database had never been intended to study the ETS issue and that Enstrom and Kabat's use of it was therefore inappropriate. This objection had not prevented the ACS from allowing Enstrom to use the database in the first place, nor from them handing it to Lawrence Garfinkel for his 1981 report into passive smoking. Garfinkel, too, found no statistically significant relationship between secondhand smoke and lung cancer.
(24) *BMJ*, 'Study flawed from outset', 2003
(25) *BMJ*.com message board, 'BMJ turns tabloid' (comment), May 20 2004
(26) *BMJ*, 30/8/03, letters
(27) 'Defending Legitimate Epidemiologic Research', J. Enstrom, 20/9/06, http://www.spiked-online.com/Articles/0000000CAA11.htm
(28) *Sacramento Bee*, 16 May 2003
(29) 'A case-control study of lung cancer and environmental tobacco smoke among nonsmoking women living in Shanghai, China', Zhong et al., *Cancer causes and control*, 10:1999, pp. 607-616. Also, Kreuzer et al (2001) and Jockel GSF (1997)
(30) 'Mortality from cancer and other causes among airline cabin attendants in Germany 1960-1997', Blettner et al., *American Journal of Epidemiology* 2002; 156: pp. 556-565.

'Mortality among pilots and cabin crew in Greece 1960-1997', Paridou et al., *International Journal of Epidemiology*, 2003,; 32: pp. 244-247

'Mortality from cancer and other causes among male airline cockpit crew in Europe', Blettner et al., *International Journal of Cancer*, Oct 2003: 106(6); pp. 946-52

(31) 'Reiteration of existing OSHA policy on Indoor Air Quality: Office Temperature/Humidity and Environmental Tobacco Smoke', Richard Fairfax, 24/3/03; *Regulation* 29 CFK 1910.1000; www.osha.org

(32) 'Public smoking ban slashes heart attacks', *New Scientist*, 1/4/03

(33) Americans for Nonsmokers' Rights press release, 9/12/03

(34) 'Economic Losses Due to Smoking Bans in California and Other States' Kuneman, D.W., McFadden, M.J., Smoker's Club, 2005

(35) 'Heart disease & stroke statistics', 2005 Update, American Heart Association

(36) *USA Today*, 10/7/96

(37) 'The case for smoker-free workplaces', Nigel Gray, *Tobacco Control* 2005;14, p.143-144

(38) 'US laws that protect tobacco users from employment discrimination', J. Slade, *Tobacco Control*, 1993;2, pp. 132-138

(39) Berger, p.p. 13-14

(40) Kluger, p. 680

(41) 'Revolt against tobacco' conference, Los Angeles, 2/10/92. Transcript.

(42) Sullum, p. 271

(43) *Daily Telegraph*, 27/8/97

(44) *Daily Telegraph*, 28/8/98

(45) Martin Bell, *Smoking: The New Apartheid*, FOREST, 1999, pp. 7-9

(46) BBC.co.uk/news, 23/12/05

(47) 'From Eric Blair to Tony Blair', Mark Mason, *The Spectator*, 5/6/99

(48) 'Changing FDR's image', Caldwell & Titsworth, *Tobacco Control*, 1996: 5: pp. 312-315

(49) 'Smoking ban swayed jury's decisions, appeal argues', Tom Sheehan Sunday, *The Columbus Dispatch*, 6/8/2006

(50) 'The Anti-Anti-Smoking Rally', *The Village Voice*, Tricia Romano, 4/8/03

(51) By Linda Stasi at the *New York Post*

(52) 'The economic impact of the New York State Smoking ban on New York's bars', Ridgewood Economic Associates, May 2004

(53) 'Can displacement ventilation control secondhand ETS?', James L. Repace and Kenneth C. Johnson, *IAQ Applications*, Vol. 7, No. 4, 2006

(54) 'Pubs' takings fear on smoke ban', BBC.co.uk/news, 12.04.05

(55) 'Smoke-free ban in Ireland: A runaway success', F. Howell, *Tobacco Control* 2005:14; pp. 73-74

(56) Katherine Robinson, *Clear the Air - Coping with Smokers*; Government Printing Office, Wellington, 1987, pp. 38-39

(57) New Zealand tops the table for number of SIDS death at 1.5 per 1,000 live births, despite being one of the world leaders in tobacco control. Many of the countries with a large population of smokers have the fewest SIDS deaths, including Slovakia and Hong Kong. The latter has a death ratio of just 0.1 per 1,000 live births (Source: SIDS International) .

Epidemiologists have gone into overdrive in their efforts to explain the rise in asthma. In recent years all of the following have been "linked to" asthma: low vitamin E, paracetamol, autumn births, cat allergies, antibiotics, stress during pregnancy, mould, thunderstorms, air fresheners, eczema, obesity, chlorine, ear infections, pesticides, low birth weights, depression, swimming pool use, autism, diet, aspirin, gas heaters, nuts, plastic, emotive words, flu does, PVC flooring, margarine, breast-feeding and painkillers. Similar lists can be compiled for cot death, allergies and autism.

(58) Letter from Phipps Y. Cohe of SIDSA to John Banzhaf III, Dec. 4 1996

(59) *Breast Cancer Research and Treatment*, Volume 75, Number 2, September 2002, pp. 181-184

(60) 'Alcohol, tobacco and breast cancer', *British Journal of Cancer*, 2002, 87, pp. 1234-1245. See also 'Cigarette smoking and breast cancer', Field et al. *International Journal of Epidemiology* 1992; 21: 842–848.

(61) 'Active Smoking, Household Passive Smoking, and Breast Cancer: Evidence From the California Teachers Study', Reynolds et al, *Journal of the National Cancer Institute*, Volume 96, Number 1, 7 January 2004, pp. 29-37(9)

In 2008, a large study of 224,917 nonsmokers found no link whatsoever between passive smoke and breast cancer and concluded that: "The aggregate findings from the retrospective studies may have been distorted by some women becoming more likely to report past exposures because they knew that they had breast cancer." ('Passive smoking and breast cancer in never smokers: prospective study and meta-analysis', Pirie, Peto et al., *International Journal of Epidemiology*, 10/6/08, 37: pp. 1069-1079

(62) ASH press release, 2005 www.ash.org

(63) 'Lecture ties secondhand smoke to breast cancer', Michael Coburn, *The Dartmouth News*, 7.3.08

(64) 'Tobacco interests are now quoting ACS to discredit CalEPA', Stanton Glantz, UCSF message board, 18/2/06.

Notes

(65) Skin cancer publicised by ACS, 5/1/01. Lower back pain claim made in *BMJ* 8/5/93. Hair loss claim made in *LA Times* 21/4/03.

(66) 'Long-term tobacco smoking and colorectal cancer in a prospective cohort study', *International Journal of Cancer*, Terry et al, 2001 Feb 15;91(4):585-7

(67) 'Nuns, prostitutes, witches and toads', CJ Snowdon, www.velvetgloveironfist.com

(68) 'Secondhand smoke can 'increase the risk of dementia'', Kate Devlin, *Daily Telegraph*, 13.02.09

(69) David Krogh, *The Artificial Passion*, 1991; *'Tobacco-Related Health Problems & Older persons'*, Center for Social Gerontology, www.tcsg.org/tobacco/health.htm. (The impotence study in question was produced by Henry Feldman of the New England Research Institute, 2000.)

(70) 'Is smoking tobacco an independent risk factor for HIV infection and progression to AIDS? A systemic review', A. Furber et al. *Sexually Transmitted Infections*, 2006; 0:1-6

(71) UK Survey. The Survey Shop, www.tobacco.org. The survey found smoking prevalence was 41%, rising to 60% for the 25-34 age group.

(72) 'Elevated risk of lung cancer among people with AIDS', Chaturvedi et al, *AIDS*, 21, 2007; pp. 207-213

(73) ASH press release; 11/7/00

(74) *Addiction*, December 2006, Vol. 101

(75) 'Smoking as "independent" risk factor for suicide: illustration of an artifact from observational epidemiology?', Smith et al, *The Lancet*, 1992;340:709-712

(76) Letters, *American Journal of Epidemiology*, Smith & Phillips, Vol. 153, 2001, p. 307

ii. 'How do you sleep at night Mr Blair?'

(1) 'Smokers get militant over ban', BBC.co.uk/news; 9/9/98

(2) 'Government denies smoking ban press reports', BBC.co.uk/news; 20/6/2005

(3) One correspondent was Terence Gerace who, in 1999, had proposed the 'Toxic Tobacco Law' in America. This would have involved making the plainest cigarettes for twenty years prior to outlawing the product absolutely. Koop and the FDA's David Kessler had publicly supported the idea and, by allowing him to state his case for a twenty year amnesty, *The Lancet* editorial gave Gerace a rare opportunity to present himself as a moderate.

(4) 'The Hippocratic Wars', *New York Times Magazine*, 28/6/98.

(5) Ibid.

(6) Glantz et al, *The Cigarette Papers*, p. 430

(7) BBC.co.uk/news, 23/2/04

(8) 'Toward a comprehensive long term nicotine policy' N. Gray et al, *Tobacco Control* 2005;14 pp.161-165

(9) 'Passive smoke risk 'even greater'', BBC.co.uk/news 29/6/04

(10) 'Smoke screen', Tim Luckhurst, *The Independent* (Review), 16/11/04

(11) Steve Milloy, *Junk Science Judo*, p. 104

(12) 'Yet Another Anti-Abortion Scare Tactic: False Claims of Breast Cancer Risk', Center for Reproductive Rights Press Release, April 2004

(13) 'Analysis of 23 Studies Suggests Abortion Can Slightly Raise the Risk of Breast Cancer', Jane E. Brody, *New York Times* ; 12/10/96

(14) 'Breast cancer and alcohol consumption: A study in weak associations', R.E. Harris and E.L. Wynder, *JAMA*: Vol. 259 No. 19, May 20, 1988

(15) 'US laws that protect tobacco users from employment discrimination', J. Slade, *Tobacco Control*, 1993, 2; pp. 132-138

(16) 'Evaluation of the Potential Carcinogenicity of Electromagnetic Fields', U.S. Environmental Protection Agency. Review Draft, October 1990, p. 6-2.

(17) 'Much ado about mobile phones', Kelly Morris, *The Lancet Oncology*, Vol 2, March 2001, p. 124

(18) 'Safety doubt for more painkillers', BBC.co.uk/news; 10/6/05

(19) Ibid.

(20) 'Milk linked to Parkinson's risk', BBC.co.uk/news; 07/4/05

(21) 'Epidemiology faces its limits', *Science*, 14/7/95

(22) BBC.co.uk/news, 14/2/05

(23) BBC.co.uk/news, 5/8/05

(24) BBC.co.uk/news, 13/1/05

(25) 'Rural pubs will suffer from smoking ban', D. Lister, *The Times*, 27/2/07

(26) Ibid.

(27) In addition, a European Union ruling banned the tobacco industry from describing its brands as 'light' or 'mild', thereby creating a bizarre situation whereby millions of smokers successfully conducted transactions in shops asking for, and receiving, products which did not technically exist.

The debate about filtered and low yield cigarettes, like the passive smoking debate, was by now considered closed. The American Medical Association announced that "It is imperative that physicians realise that there will never be a 'less hazardous' cigarette." The ACS's Michael Thun co-authored a paper, published in the *BMJ*, which announced that all cigarettes were equally harmful. Only those who read the paper in full would have seen that the study showed those who smoked high-tar cigarettes had the highest rate of lung cancer and co-author Jeffrey Harris later told the press that filters clearly did reduce risk.

(28) 'UK stops short of outright smoking ban in enclosed public places', Kaye McIntosh, *BMJ*, 25 June 2008; 330: p. 1468

(29) BBC.co.uk/news, 27/7/06

(30) Ibid.

(31) Sullum, p. 179

(32) 'Choosing Health', UK Dept. of Health, 2004

(33) *BMJ*; 5/2/05; p.265

(34) 'Environmental tobacco smoke and risk of respiratory cancer and chronic obstructive pulmonary disease in former smokers and never smokers in the EPIC prospective study', P. Vineis, *BMJ*; 5/2/05, pp.277-280

(35) 'Slaying myths about passive smoking', K. Jamrozik, *Tobacco Control* 2005:14;p.294-295. See also 'Policy priorities for tobacco control', K. Jamrozik, *British Medical Journal*, Vol. 328, 24/4/04 p. 1007

(36) As the Vineis study had shown just a few weeks earlier in the same journal, even light smokers have a reading of 138 ng/ml.

(37) 'Cigarette Smoking and Stroke in a Cohort of U.S. Male Physicians', Robbins et al., *Annals of internal medicine*, 15/3/94, Volume 120 Issue 6, Pages 458-462

(38) 'Mortality in relation to smoking: 50 years' observations on male British doctors mortality in relation to smoking: 50 years', Doll, Peto et al, *British Medical Journal*; 22/6/04; No. 328

(39) 'Estimate of deaths attributable to passive smoking among UK adults: database analysis', K. Jamrozik, *BMJ*; 9/4/05; pp. 812-815. Realising the hospitality industry has an unusually high turnover of staff and that few people work in bars all their lives, he estimated that 20% chose bar-work as their "chief lifetime occupation" and so divided his figures by five. This, he admitted, was nothing more than a guess since the real figure "is not known."

(40) Ibid.

(41) 'Passive smoking killing thousands', BBC.co.uk/news; 3/2/05

(42) 'Controlling Tobacco Smoke Pollution', James Repace, *American Society of Heating, Refrigerating and Air-Conditioning Engineers*, 2005

(43) 'James Repace thinks of a number', CJ Snowdon, 2008, www.velvetgloveironfist.com

(44) 'Blowing smoke: British American Tobacco's air filtration scheme'; Rae et al., *BMJ* ,28/1/06, pp. 227-229

(45) ASH financial accounts 2006-07, Charities Commission

(46) 'Government denies smoking ban aim', BBC.co.uk/news; 19/6/05.

(47) 'Smoke and mirrors', D. Arnott and I. Willmore, *The Guardian*, 19/7/06

(48) 'Prisoners are sentenced to nicotine patch for their days in the dock', Richard Ford, *The Times*, 6/4/07 p. 25

(49) *The Daily Telegraph*, editorial, 15/2/06

(50) 'Mixed reaction to ban on smoking', BBC.co.uk/news, 14/02/06.

(51) Ibid.

(52) Ibid.

(53) Ibid.

(54) 'Arctic Monkeys draw heat over smoking album cover', *The Herald*, 2/3/06. (The band said that the criticism was "a bit rich coming from a country that eats fried Mars Bars for a living.")

(55) 'US laws that protect tobacco users from employment discrimination', J. Slade, *Tobacco Control*, 1993;2, pp. 132-138

(56) 'Smoking ban leads to fall in drink sales', Shan Ross, *The Scotsman*, 24/8/06

(57) BBC.co.uk/news, 17/5/06

(58) 'Bingo profits plunge 62% on smoke ban', *The Scotsman*, Claire Smith, 30/4/07

(59) 'Ban has led to drop in takings', BBC.co.uk/news, 23/8/06,

(60) 'Smoking ban leads to fall in drink sales', Shan Ross, *The Scotsman*, 24/8/06

(61) BBC.co.uk/news, 27/7/06

(62) 'Pub crisis: 27 close each week', *Morning Advertiser*, Ewan Turney, 05/03/2008 (Statistics from the British Beer and Pub Association); 'Pubs closing at rate of 39 per week', Matt Eley, *The Publican*, 19.01.09

(63) 'Over 1,000 pubs shut since smoking ban', London *Metro*, 1/7/08; 'Smoking ban has 'devastated licensed trade', *Lancashire Telegraph*, 27/2/08; 'Public smoking ban hits pubs' beer sales' *The Observer*, 6/7/08

(64) '20,000 Pubs in danger', M. Baker and T. Latchem, *Sunday People*, 29/6/08,

(65) 'The economic impact of the New York State Smoking ban on New York's bars', Ridgewood Economic Associates, May 2004

(66) 'Bad air', M. Moynihan, *Reason*, November 2007, Vol. 39, No. 6, p. 10

(67) *The New Paper* (Singapore); 6/4/06, p.2-3

(68) 'Cigarette butts and the building of socialism in East Germany', Young-sun Hong, *Central European History*, vol. 35, no.3, p. 341

(69) Ibid. p. 339

(70) 'Germany 's highest court rules against smoking ban', Reuters, 30.07.08

(71) 'Dutch tobacco smoke means cafe smokers can only light up cannabis cigarettes', Lucy Cockcroft, *The Daily Telegraph*, 1/7/08

12. 'Developed societies are paternalistic'

(1) 'No signs posted on eve of outdoor smoking ban', Charlie Goodyear, *San Francisco Chronicle*, 25/6/05

(2) 'Safe rooms for smokers', Kylie Hansen, *Herald Sun*, 09/10/02

(3) City of Calabasas Ordinance 2006-217

(4) 'Belmont considers nation's toughest smoking ban', *CBS News*, 15/11/06

(5) 'Belmont, Oakland ponder smoking laws', *San Francisco Chronicle*, 13/6/07, B1

(6) 'Belmont to be first US City to ban smoking', Dana Yates, *The Daily Journal*, 11/6/07

(7) James Repace, 'Measurements of outdoor air pollution for second hand smoke on the UMBC campus'; 1/6/05

(8) ASH Press Release, 'Majority Favors Outdoor Smoking Bans' 4/11/06

(9) 'Researchers Light Up for Nicotine, the Wonder Drug', Marty Graham, *Wired* magazine, 06/20/07

(10) Robert Wood Johnson Foundation, 2005 Annual Report

(11) New Survey Extinguishes 'Smoking is Sexy' Myth', GlaxoSmithKline Consumer Healthcare press release: 29/3/05

(12) 'Glaxo pays for Chantix woes', Lisa LaMota, *Forbes*, 26.06.08 ; 'Can Chantix make a comeback?', Matthew Harper, *Forbes*, 12.09.08

(13) 'Toward a comprehensive long term nicotine policy', N Gray et al, *Tobacco Control*, 2005;14: pp.161-165

(14) Supreme Court of the United States, 'Food and Drug Administration et al. v. Brown & Williamson tobacco corp. et al' No. 98-1152.

The Supreme Court's report emphasised that the FDA had never claimed such authority until relatively recently and expressed a degree of weariness with the interminable requests from tobacco's opponents begging them to change their mind. Recognising the prohibitionist intent that lay behind these pleas, and mindful of the crime and misery that invariably accompanies prohibition, the Supreme Court noted that "banning [tobacco products] would cause a greater harm to public health than leaving them on the market."

Canada's attempts to emulate the US were given a lift when their own Supreme Court ruled that a recent effort by British Columbia to sue the tobacco industry was lawful. The province had passed a Florida-inspired bill to relieve the prosecution of the obligation to provide proof in cases against Big Tobacco. The industry appealed and the Supreme Court allowed British Columbia to proceed with their $8.6 billion (US) action, albeit asking them to provide some evidence to give it legal credibility. As in America, the Canadians demanded that the tobacco industry reimburse the state for the cost of treating smoking related diseases even though, by this time, taxes on cigarettes were so high that the Canadian government was making $9 billion a year from them.

(15) Glantz, p. 379

(16) www.smokefreemovies.ucsf.edu/problem/new_smokers.html

(17) 'Film rating board to consider smoking as a factor', MPAA press release, 10/5/07

(18) www.nyclash.com

(19) D. Simpson in *Tobacco Control*, 2003

(20) 'Party for the right to smoke', R. Kerbaj, *The Australian*, 16/1/06, p.5

(21) 'Smoke ban rebel fined again', BBC.co.uk/news, 26/3/08 ; 'Nick Hogan to appeal against smoking fine', *The Bolton News*, Jane Lavender, 29/1/08; '£12,000 blow for smoke ban rebel Tony', *The Publican*, Matt Eley; 7/3/08

(22) 'Survey shows smoking up since 2002', Patrick Logue, *Irish Times*, 29/4/08

(23) 'The big draw', Daisy Garnett, *Vogue*, September 2006; p. 158

(24) Ibid.

(25) University of Alberta Express News, 25/5/06, www.expressnews.ualberta.ca

(26) 'Agent of change: more than "a nuisance to the tobacco industry"', Simon Chapman, *Medical Journal of Australia*, 2002, 177 (11/12): pp. 661-633

(27) 'No butts about it', Susan Alexander, *San Francisco Chronicle*, 29/1/07

(28) BBC forum, 4/12/06

(29) 'Smokers turning to pub crawls' (reader comment), *The Scotsman* website, posted 11/5/07

(30) www.justrage.com, posted 2/6/06

(31) Ibid. posted 4/6/06

(32) 'Seventh Futures Forum on Unpopular Decisions in Public Health', A. Arnaudova, WHO (Europe), 2005
(33) 'Reasons for banning smoking in certain public outdoor places', ASH, www.ash.org
(34) WHO, 'Seventh Futures', 2005
(35) 'Choosing Health: Making healthy choices easier - Executive Summary', Department of Health, 16 November 2004
(36) 'Choosing health? First choose your philosophy', *The Lancet*, 365; 29/1/05 p. 369
(37) John Stuart Mill, *On Liberty*, Penguin, London, 1974 (first published 1859)
(38) '3,000 new criminal offences since Tony Blair came to power', Kirsty Walker, *The Daily Mail*, 16/8/06
(39) 'Health inequalities under the UK presidency', Liam Donaldson, *Eurohealth*, No. 11, Vol. 4, 2005, p.1
(40) Mill, p. 166
(41) Mill, p. 166
(42) Mill, p. 170
(43) Mill, p. 172
(44) 'Councils push to stamp out outdoor smoking', *Sydney Morning Herald*, Sunanda Creagh, 14/9/2007
(45) Mill, p.69
(46) As far back as 1980, Margaret Thatcher's junior health minister explicitly challenged Mill's principle, saying:

"The traditional role of politicians has been to prevent an individual causing harm to others, but to allow him to do harm to himself. However, as modern society has made us all more interdependent, this attitude is now changing."

It was questionable whether people were really more "interdependent" than in their grandmother's day, but the point was nonetheless made that established principles of personal liberty were not relevant to contemporary society. (Quoted in Heather Ashton and Rob Stepney, *Smoking: Psychology and Pharmacology*, Tavistock Publications, London, 1983, p. 144)
(47) Mill, p. 7, Introduction by Gertrude Himmelfarb. Hayek made the same observation when he noted that the word liberty is "used as freely in totalitarian states as elsewhere." (*The Road to Serfdom*, p. 162)
(48) 'Am I guilty of oldthink or is this sensefree?', Mick Hume, *The Times*, 27/6/07
(49) George Orwell, *The Complete Novels* (*1984*), 1983, Penguin, p. 865
(50) WHO, Youth Tobacco Assessment and Response Guide, 2002, Chapter 6.
(51) '£10 government permit plan to deter smokers', *The Guardian*, John Carvel, 15/2/08; BBC.co.uk/news, £10 licence to smoke proposed, 15/2/08
(52) 'Framing Tobacco Control efforts within an ethical context', B. J. Fox, *Tobacco Control* 2005;(Supp. II)ii38-ii44
(53) 'Social movements and human rights rhetoric in tobacco control', Jacobson & Banjeree, *Tobacco Control*, Supp II, ii45-49
(54) Ibid.
(55) 'Individual rights advocacy in tobacco control policies: an assessment and recommendation', J. E. Katz, *Tobacco Control*, 2005;14 (Supp. 2):pp. ii31-ii37
(56) Ibid.
(57) Ibid.

13. 'The next logical step'

(1) *Portland Oregonian*, 11/12/19
(2) 'War is declared on 'demon' tobacco', *New York Times* 2/9/23
(3) Richard Kluger, *Ashes to Ashes*, Knopf, New York, p. 463
(4) 'California Activists' Success Ignites a Not-So-Slow-Burn', John Schwartz, *Washington Post*, 30/5/94, p. 1
(5) (India) 'How have the disadvantaged fared in India? An analysis of poverty and inequality in the 1990s', J.V.Meenakshi & Ranjan Ray, 2002; (UK) New Policy Institute, The Poverty Site, www.npi.org.uk
(6) Le Fanu, p. 376
(7) Fitzpatrick, p. 7
(8) 'Male manual workers 'live longer', BBC.co.uk/news, 9/11/07. 'William Hill slashes odds on living to 100 'Miles Brignall and Patrick Collinson, *The Guardian*, 28/04/07
(9) 'Life expectancy in Great Britain rises—but later years are still spent in poor health', Karen Hébert; *BMJ*, 31/07/2004; 329:p. 250
(10) *BMJ*, News, 329: 250 (31/7/04)
(11) BBC.co.uk/news, 30/9/05
(12) 'Smoker population, smoking deaths, prognoses', WHO/Tobacco Free Initiative
(13) 'Junk food ad ban attacked from both sides', O. Gibson & R. Smithers, *The Guardian*, 18/11/06, p. 6

(14) BBC.co.uk/news, 'Junk food advert code launched'; 15/3/08

(15) 'CDC study overstated obesity as a cause of death', *The Wall Street Journal*, Betsy McKay, 23/11/04
Criticism of the anti-fat movement came from an unexpected quarter. The CDC's estimate of 400,000 deaths per annum was all too close to their oft-cited figure of 435,000 tobacco deaths, and the worsening nature of the obesity 'crisis' suggested that it would soon overtake tobacco as public health enemy number one. Concerned that they were about to be eclipsed, some of the biggest names in tobacco control came out to pour water on the findings. Senator Henry Waxman requested a government investigation into how the CDC had come to such a figure and Stanton Glantz wrote to *JAMA* to disparage the report and sent a flurry of e-mails to his followers urging them to ignore it entirely. With the threat of money being redirected towards the bright young things of the anti-fat movement, Glantz wrote: "I don't think that anyone should rely on the CDC paper for anything, especially policy making and *resource allocation*." (my emphasis)
The CDC backtracked. They suddenly admitted to serious errors in their calculations and declared that the true annual body count was in fact 365,000 which, as the media quickly appreciated, equated to 1,000 deaths a day. The following year, a new study gave an estimate of just 25,814 obesity deaths per annum and confusion reigned until the CDC finally settled on a figure of 112,000 - less than a third of its original estimate. Tobacco was reinstated as the country's most infamous killer and anti-smoking activists continued to receive the lion's share of public health funding. Obesity, on the other hand, was apparently now killing far fewer people than it had a decade earlier.

(16) 'Half of Britons will be obese by 2050', Daniel Martin, *The Daily Mail*, 17/10/07

(17) 'Obesity? This is a job for Supernanny', Minette Marrin, *The Sunday Times*, 27/8/06

(18) 'Larger-size clothes should come with warning to lose weight, say experts', *The Times*, 15/15/06

(19) Centers for Disease Control statistic, 2005; 'Obesity: The "Big" Picture', Stan Reents, www.atheleteinme.com, 6/5/07

(20) 'Study claims poor diets are costing NHS £6bn per year', Lyndsay Moss, *Edinburgh Evening News*, 15/11/05

(21) 'We need a heavy tax on chocolate to fight obesity, says doctor', Lyndsay Moss, *The Scotsman*, 5/3/09

(22) 'Are we turning our children into fat junkies?' Ellen Ruppel Shell, *The Guardian*, 12/10/03

(23) www.banzhaf.net/obesitylinks.html

(24) 'Who should pay for obesity?', John Banzhaf III, *San Francisco Daily Journal*, 4/2/02

(25) 'Obesity crisis to cost £45 billion a year', Denis Campbell, *The Observer*, 14/10/07

(26) 'Tackling obesity: Future choices', October 2007, Department of Innovation Universities and Skills.

(27) 'Obesity "not individual's fault"', BBC.co.uk/news, 17/10/07

(28) 'Lunchtime lock-in may be used in schools to beat obesity', Frank Urquhart, *The Scotsman*, 15/11/07

(29) 'Burgers and Coke criticised as Games sponsors', *The Daily Telegraph*, Sally Pook, 16/06/2006

(30) 'Federal fascists uber alles', Walter Williams, *Human Events*, 22/10/99, Vol. 55;39. p. 14

(31) *Newark Star-Ledger*, 30/4/02

(32) Glantz, *Tobacco War*, p. 379

(33) '"Direct link" between cancer and obesity', *The Independent*, 31/10/07

(34) '"Ban bacon" say cancer experts', Emily Garnham, *Daily Express*, 31/10/07; 'Bacon Butty Ban to Beat Cancer', *Daily Mirror*, 31/10/07,

(35) 'Fatties' axe on chip shop', *The Sun*, 9/6/07

(36) 'New York City bans use of trans-fats in restaurants', Lisa Pickoff-White, *The National Academies*, 12/12/06

(37) 'Three drink limit urged in Scottish bars', Marc Horne, *The Sunday Times*, 11/12/05

(38) Ibid.

(39) BBC.co.uk/news, 18/10/05

(40) 'The normalisation of binge-drinking?', Virginia Berridge, Centre for History in Public Health, 2007, p. 32-33

(41) Fitzpatrick, p. 47

(42) 'How 'safe drinking' experts let a bottle or two go to their heads', *The Times*, Andrew Norfolk, 20/10/07

(43) 'British drinking: a suitable case for treatment?', *British Medical Journal*, 10/9/05; 331: 527-528

(44) 'Alcohol abuse "becoming epidemic"', BBC.co.uk/news, 2/11/06

(45) British Crime Survey (June 2006)

(46) British Beer and Pub Association

(47) Ibid.

(48) BBPA and HM Revenue and Customs, BBPA Statistical Handbook 2007

(49) Crime in England and Wales 2005/06, Alison Walker, Chris Kershaw and Sian Nicholas, ONS, July 2006. See also 'Violent crime, disorder and criminal damage since the introduction of the Licensing Act 2003', Penny Babb, Home Office, July 2007

(50) 'Violence down amid pub law change', 10/2/06; www.ias.org.uk
Violent crime fell 17% in York, 24% in Selby, 8% in South Tyneside, 11% in Leamington Spa. Merseyside, Norwich and Cumbria constabularies both reported a drop in assaults since the ban and Sussex police recorded a 1.1% drop in violent crime that fell to 10.3% when 'violence not resulting in injury' was excluded. The Institute of Alcohol Studies is primarily funded by the prohibitionist Alcohol Health Alliance (formerly known as

the UK Alliance for the Suppression of the Traffic in all Intoxicating Liquors) whose aim is "to spread the principles of total abstinence from alcoholic drinks."

(51) 'Impact of the new UK licensing law on emergency hospital attendances: a cohort study', Alastair Newton, *Emergency Medicine Journal* 2007; 24, pp. 532-534

(52) 'Time for a sober look at 'epidemic' nonsense', *The Daily Telegraph*, Charles Moore, 32/2/08

(53) 'Time called on happy hours as drinking costs the NHS £2.7 billion', Joanna Sugden, *The Times*, 22.07.08.
    Refusing to be outflanked, ASH responded three months later with a press release that stated: "The annual cost of smoking to the NHS in England has soared from £1.7 billion a year in 1998 to £2.7 billion this year." ('Smoking Costing NHS £2.7 billion a year', ASH press release, 07.10.08)

(54) 'For middle class read guzzle class', Sarah Jarvis, *The Sunday Times*, News Review, p. 7

(55) 'Campaigners want alcohol tax rise', BBC.co.uk/news, 13/11/07

(56) 'Europe to crack down on 'passive drinking', says leaked report', Bruno Waterfield, *Spiked Online*, 26/5/06

(57) Ibid.

(58) www.actionagainstobesity.com. The group have since launched a campaign to boycott cookies sold by Girl Guides. Roth calls this "using young girls as a front to push millions of cookies." ('Girl Scout cookies boycott called for by National Action Against Obesity' NAAO press release 19/2/07)

(59) 'Smoke-free legislation linked to drop in gambling', Smokefree Coalition press release, 25/1/06

(60) 'Gambling Ads should have warnings', *The Argus Lite*, 14/8/06, p. 3

(61) 'A very big bet: Why doctors say the new casino culture is bad for you', Sophie Goodchild and Ian Griggs; *Independent on Sunday*, 14/1/07

(62) 'Gambling with the nation's health?', *British Medical Journal*, 26/8/1995; 311: pp. 521-522

(63) Ibid.

(64) 'Gambling with the nation's health', Middleton and Latif, *British Medical Journal*, 21/4/07;334:828-829

(65) 'Doctors attack gambling policies', BBC.co.uk/news, 19 April 2007

(66) 'DDT: A case of scientific fraud', J. Gordon Edwards, *Journal of American Physicians and Surgeons*, Vol 9, number 3, Fall 2004, pp. 83-88

(67) Rachel Carson, *Silent Spring*, 1994, Boston/New York: Houghton Mifflin (introduction by Al Gore)

(68) 'DDT and its derivatives', World Health Organization: Environmental health criteria 9: WHO, Geneva, 194 pp (1979).

(69) 'Study of the potential carcinogenicity of DDT in the Syrian Golden Hamster', Agthe, C., H. Garcia, P. Shubik, L. Tomatis, & E.Wenyon: *Proc.Soc.Exp.Biol.*134, 113 (1970). 'DDT and its metabolites in body fat and liver of albino mice'. Banerjee, B. D : *J.com. Dis* (1982). 'Lack of carcinogenicity of DDT in hamsters'. Cabral, J.R.P., L.Rossie, S.A. Bronczyk and P. Shubik :*Tumori* 68, 11 (1982). 'No effect caused by DDT on birds or their egg shells', Edwards, J.G : *Chemical and Engineering News*. Aug. 16. (1971). 'Effects of DDT on reproduction in multiple generations of Beagle dog's. Ottoboni, A., G. D. Bissel, and A.C Hexter : *Arch. Environ.Contam. Toxicol.* 6, 83 (1977). 'Other pollutants may cause thin egg shells' Tucker, R.K, *Utah Science*, pp 47-49, (June 1971). 'DDT and its derivatives', World Health Organization : *Environmental health criteria* 9; WHO, Geneva, 194 pp (1979).

(70) 'A Case of the DDTs: The war against the war against malaria', Roger Bate, *National Review*, Inc, May 14, 2001, Vol. LIII, No. 9

(71) WHO Framework Convention on Tobacco Control, WHO, Geneva, 2003

(72) 'WHO gives indoor use of DDT a clean bill of health for controlling malaria', WHO press release, 15/9/07

14. 'The scene is set for the final curtain'

(1) 'The Smell Test', Colin Nickerson, *The Boston Globe*, 5/26/2000, p. A01

(2) Steve Allen and Bill Adler Jr, *The Passionate Nonsmokers' Bill of Rights*; Bill Adler books, 1989, p. 199

(3) *Rome News Tribune*, 30/1/03

(4) 'As the smoking ban looms, far fewer are kicking the habit', Jonathan Owen, *The Independent*, 27/5/07

(5) *Yes, Prime Minster*, 'Power to the people', Anthony Jay & Johnathan Lynn, BBC Television, 1988

(6) '£10 cigs', *The People*, 9/3/08

(7) Ibid.

(8) 'Now drivers face ban on smoking at the wheel', Juliette Jowit & Denis Campbell, *The Observer*, 13/5/07

(9) 'City tries to ban drinkers from standing at the bar', Alan Hamilton, *The Times*, 2/8/06,

(10) 'Alcohol should carry graphic warning pictures say doctors', Rebecca Smith, *The Daily Telegraph*, 21/7/08

(11) 'Call for alcohol ban in supermarkets', Rebecca Smith and Toby Helm, *The Daily Telegraph*, 26/2/08. 'Alcohol on TV prompts drinking', BBC.co.uk/news, 4.03.09

(12) 'Health warnings for holiday ads', BBC.co.uk/news, 5/4/07

(13) 'Laws prohibit smoking around children', Emily Bazar, *USA Today*, 28/11/06

(14) 'Melbourne, Florida, may ban off-the-job smoking by employees', ASH PR, 09/02/06

(15) 'The case for smoker-free workplaces', Nigel Gray, *Tobacco Control* 2005; 14, p.143-144

(16) 'US laws that protect tobacco users from employment discrimination', J. Slade, *Tobacco Control*, 1993;2, pp. 132-138

(17) 'Get healthy or get fired', Tim Jones, *Baltimore Sun*, 26/9/07

(18) 'Myth: Secondhand smoke is a killer', *ABC News*, 12/5/06

(19) 'New Surgeon General's report expands list of diseases caused by smoking', US Dept of Health & Human Services, Press release, 27/5/2004

(20) Richard Carmona, 'Remarks at press conference to launch "Health consequences of involuntary exposure to tobacco smoke: A report from the Surgeon General'; Washington DC, 27/6/06,

(21) 'US Details Dangers of secondhand smoking', Marc Kaufman, *Washington Post*, 29/6/06

(22) 'Smoking out bad science', Lorraine Mooney, *Wall Street Journal* (European edition), 12/3/98

(23) Ibid.

(24) 'And now, a subsidy to attract smokers the city drove away', Craig Westover, *St. Paul Pioneer Press*, 11/10/06

(25) 'Senate votes to ban smoking in cars carrying young kids', *Mercury News*, 31/8/06

(26) British Columbia Minsitry of Health, Tobacco Prevention Series no. 30c, August 2005. This particular myth is assessed in 'Secondhand News' by CJ Snowdon, 2008; www.velvetgloveironfist.com

(27) 'Anti-smoking campaigner Carr is diagnosed with lung cancer', Sophie Kirkham, *The Sunday Times*, 30/7/06; (Carr himself never made such a claim.)

(28) 'WHO denounces health benefits of alcohol', N. Craft, *British Medical Journal* 1994; 309: p. 1249 (12 November)

(29) 'Households contaminated by environmental tobacco smoke: sources of infant exposures', G.E.Matt et al, *Tobacco Control*, 2004, Vol. 13, pp. 29-37

(30) '"Smoking outside "is still a risk to babies"', Adrian Radnedge, London *Metro*, 8/8/06, p. 1.

(31) 'Smoker's breath is harmful to health', ASH press release, 22/6/08

(32) www.blackpooltoday.co.uk, 14/9/06

(33) 'The dangers of secondhand smoke', Elizabeth Bartholomew, Baptist Memorial Health Care Corporation, 19/9/06

(34) 'Do smoking bans cause a 27% to 40% drop in admissions for myocardial infarction in hospitals?', Kuneman & McFadden, 29/11/2005

(35) See 'New Study Concludes that Bowling Green Smoking Ban Reduced Heart Disease Admissions by 47%; Unfortunately, Science is Weak and Conclusions Unjustified', Michal Siegel, Rest of The Story blog; http://tobaccoanalysis.blogspot.com/2007/05/new-study-concludes-that-bowling-green.html

(36) 'The impact of a smoking ban on hospital admissions for coronary heart disease', Khuder et al., *Preventive Medicine*, July 2007;45(1): pp. 3-8.

(37) 'Beliefs about the health effects of 'thirdhand' smoke and home smoking bans', Winickoff et al., Pediatrics, Vol. 123, No. 1, January 2009; e74-e79

(38) 'Don't mangle the facts, even in a good cause', *New Scientist*; 10/5/07

(39) 'Warning: Anti-tobacco activism may be hazardous to epidemiologic science', Carl V. Phillips, *Epidemiologic Perspectives & Innovations;* 2007:4: p. 13

(40) 'Outdoor smoking bans are seldom justifiable', Simon Chapman, *Tobacco Control*, 2000:9, p. 95-97

(41) 'What should be done about smoking in movies?', *Tobacco Control* e-letters, Simon Chapman, 27.11.08

(42) 'Surgeon General's report blows smoke', Elizabeth Whelan, ACSH Press release, 14/7/06

(43) PR Watch (8) Fourth quarter 1998, Vol 5 No. 4 (9)

Whelan's heresy provoked an angry reaction from her erstwhile comrades. Despite having devoted years of her life to the cause, she was accused, effectively, of faking it. Since it was plainly ludicrous to pretend that Whelan was in the pay of the tobacco industry, she was accused instead of being in the pay of 'industry' in general, and the chemical industry in particular.

ACSH had defended various products that the environmental lobby wanted banning - such as dioxin, Alar and DDT - and so her detractors accused her of using the smoking issue to, as Michael Jacobson, director of the Center for Science in the Public Interest, put it "deflect criticism that it always defends industry." Whelan had heard it all before. It was the exactly the same line of attack the tobacco industry had used against ACSH in the early 1990s when they, too, tried to rubbish the organisation.

(44) Phillippe Boucher's Rendez-Vouz with Alan Blum 30/12/99, www.tobacco.org/News/rendezvouz/blum1.html

(45) Interview with the author, March 2009

(46) M. Siegel, *Rest of the Story* blog, http://tobaccoanalysis.blogspot.com; 4/5/06

(47) 'Phase out cigarette sales in 10 years', ASH NZ, Smokefree Coalition and Te Reo Marama PR; 5/9/2007,

(48) Ibid.

(49) 'Scents and Senselessness', Michael Fumento, *The American Spectator*, April 2000

(50) 'Halifax hysteria. Non-scents in Nova Scotia', Leah McLaren, *The Globe and Mail*, 29/4/00

(51) Ibid.

(52) 'First they came for the smokers...', Kevin Steel, *Alberta Report*, 18/5/98, Vol. 25, Issue 22, p. 17

(53) 'MCS: Mis-concern serious', Dr Stephen Barrett, *Priorities* Vol 11, no. 1, 1/1/99

(54) 'Are some people sensitive to mobile phone signals?', G.J. Rubin, *British Medical Journal*; doi:10.1136/bmj. 38765.519850.55; 6/3/06

(55) 'Phone mast allergy "in the mind"', BBC.co.uk/news, 25/7/07

(56) 'The smell test, Halifax stirs emotions with ban on scents', Colin Nickerson, *Bolston Globe*, 5/26/2000

(57) 'Evil genes and antifreeze: TV gurus' toxic talk put under the microscope', Alok Jha, *The Guardian*, 3/1/08,

(58) 'Halifax Hysteria, Non-scents in Nova Scotia', Leah McLaren, *The Globe and Mail*, 29/4/2000

(59) Senior Programs Tri-Center Newsletter, August, 2006, Volume 40, Number 8, City of Berkeley

(60) 'Scents and Senselessness', Michael Fumento, *The American Spectator*, April 2000

(61) Jacob Sullum, *For Your Own Good*, 1996, p. 147

(62) 'The Anti-Fragrance Movement has its nose out of joint – and sweet-smelling Canada is leading the way', Michael Fumento, *The American Spectator*, April 2000

(63) 'Avoid Valentines Day headaches - don't buy your lover perfume', WWF press release, 11 February 2005

(64) 'DJ wins $10m over rival's scent that made her sick', *The Times*, Chris Ayres, 27/5/05

(65) 'Radio DJ wins $10.6 million in stink over perfume', David Shepardson, *The Detroit News*, 24/5/2005,

(66) 'The Smell Test', Colin Nickerson, *The Boston Globe*, 5/26/2000, p. A01

(67) 'Spraying Yourself With Toxic Chemicals is Not Sexy', Wendy Priesnitz, *Natural Life* no. 87; Sept/Oct 2002

(68) 'But the fire is not delightful', Julie Mellum, *Minneapolis-St Paul Star Tribune*, 04.12.07

(69) Senior Programs Tri-Center Newsletter, August, 2006, Volume 40, Number 8, City of Berkeley

(70) 'Spraying Yourself With Toxic Chemicals is Not Sexy', Wendy Priesnitz, *Natural Life* no. 87; Sept/Oct 2002

(71) Michael McFadden, *Dissecting Antismokers Brains*, Aethna press, 2003; p. 65

(72) 'Use sun cream all year round to stop skin damage - doctor', Sarah-Kate Templeton, *The Sunday Times*, 5/8/06

(73) Ibid.

(74) 'Phones CAN make you ill', *The Daily Mail*, Fiona McRae, 12/9/05

(75) 'Experts put a health warning on 'electrical allergy' advice', *The Daily Telegraph*, Nic Fleming, 4/11/05

(76) 'The classroom 'cancer risk' of wi-fi internet', *The Daily Mail*, Daniel Martin, 21/5/07

(77) 'Pupils 'are wi-fi guinea pigs', BBC.co.uk/news, 1/8/07

(78) Rob Cunningham, *Smoke and Mirrors: The Canadian Tobacco War*, International Development Centre, Ottowa, 1996 pp. 278-279. (The phrase 'shower-adjusters' was probably borrowed from the US tobacco industry spokesman William F. Dwyer; Kluger p. 468)

(79) 'Reasons for banning smoking in certain outdoor places', ASH, www.ash.org

(80) Ibid.

(81) Harvard Medical School Office of Public Affairs, 'Obesity Spreads through social networks ', 23/7/07

(82) Ibid.

(83) Ibid.

(84) Walton, p. 66

(85) Fitzpatrick, p. 70

(86) Claire Fox of the Institute of Ideas, quoted in 'Huffing & Puffing', *The Daily Telegraph*, Adam Edwards, 27/6/07

(87) 'Reasons for banning smoking in certain outdoor places', ASH, www.ash.org

(88) Ibid.

(89) 'Framing Tobacco Control efforts within an ethical context', B. J. Fox, *Tobacco Control*, 2005; (Supp. II), pp. ii38-ii44

(90) Egon Corti, 'A History of Smoking', 1931, p. 267

(91) Ibid.

Selected bibliography

Allen, Steve & Adler, Bill, *A Passionate Nonsmokers Bill of Rights*, Bill Adler Books, 1989

American Tobacco Company, *Sold American! The first fifty years*, 1954

Basham et al., *Diet Nation*, The Social Affairs Unit, London, 2006

Bate, Roger (ed.), *What Risk?*, Butterworth Heineman, Oxford, 1997

Behr, Edward, *Prohibition*, Arcade Publishing, New York, 1996

Berger, Gilda, *Smoking Not Allowed: The Debate*, Franklin Watts, New York, 1987

Berridge, Virginia, *Marketing Health: Smoking & the Discourse of Public Health in Britain, 1945-2000*, OUP, Oxford, *2007*

Booker & North, *Scared to Death*, Continuum, London, 2007

Brignell, John, *The Epidemiologists*, Brignell Associates, 2004

Corti, Egon (translated by Paul England), *A History of Smoking*, Bracken Books, London, 1931

Cunningham, Rob, *Smoke and Mirrors: The Canadian Tobacco War*, International Development Centre, Ottowa, 1996

Davis, Devra, *The Secret History of the War on Cancer*, Basic Books, New York, 2007

Department of Health, Education & Welfare, *A History of Cancer Control in the United States*, 1977

Feldman & Marks (ed.), *Panic Nation!*, John Blake, London, 2007

Fitzpatrick, Michael, *The Tyranny of Health*, Routledge, London, 2001

Ford, Barry, *Smokescreen*, Halcyon Press, Perth, 1994

Gately, Iain, *La Diva Nicotina*, Simon & Schuster, 2001

Gilman & Xun (ed.), *Smoke: A Global History of Smoking*, Reaktion Books, London, 2004

Glantz, Stanton et al. *The Cigarette Papers*, University of California Press, Berkeley, 1996

Glantz & Balbach, *Tobacco War*, University of California Press, Berkeley, 2000

Goodman, Jordan, *Tobacco in History: The Culture of Dependance*, Routledge, London, 1993

Goodman, Jordan, *Tobacco in History and Culture: An Encyclopaedia*, Charles Scribener's Sons, New York, *2004*

Harsanyi, David, *Nanny State*, Broadway Books, New York, 2007

Hayek, F.A., *The Road to Serfdom*, Routledge, New York, 1943

Hilton, Matthew, *Smoking in British Popular Culture 1800-2000*, Manchester University Press, 2000

Johnston, Lennox, *The Disease of Tobacco Smoking and Its Cure*, Christopher Johnson, 1957

Kerr, K. Austin, *Organised for Prohibition*, Yale University Press, New Haven, 1985

Kierman, V.G, *Tobacco: A History*, Hutchinson Radius, London, 1991

Kluger, Richard, *Ashes to Ashes*, Knopf, New York, 1996

Krough, David, *The Artificial Passion*, W. H. Freeman, New York, 1991

Le Fanu, James, *The Rise and Fall of Modern Medicine*, Abacus, London, 2000

McFadden, Michael, *Dissecting Antismokers' Brains*, Aethna, 2003

Milloy, Steven, *Junk Science Judo*, Cato, Washington, 2001

Oakley, Don, *Slow Burn*, Eyrie Press, 1999

Parker-Pope, Tara, *Cigarettes: Anatomy of an industry,* The New Press, New York, 2001

Pollock, David, *Denial and Delay*, Action on Smoking and Health, London, 1999

Proctor, Robert, *The Nazi War on Cancer*, Princeton University Press, 1999

Rabinoff, Michael, *Ending the Tobacco Holocaust*, Elite Books, Santa Rose, 2006

Reeves, Richard, *John Stuart Mill: Victorian Firebrand*, Atlantic Books, London, 2007

Schaler & Schaler (ed.), *Smoking: Who Has the Right?*, Prometheus Books, New York, 1998

Shephard, Roy, *The Risks of Passive Smoking*, Croom Helm, London, 1982

Sullum, Jacob, *For Your Own Good*, The Free Press, New York, 1998

Tate, Cassandra, *Cigarette Wars: The Triumph of the Little White Slaver*, OUP, New York, 1999

Taverne, Dick, *The March of Unreason*, OUP, Oxford, 2006

Tollinson, Robert, *Smoking and Society*, Lexington, Massachusetts, 1986

Troyer & Markle, *Cigarettes: The Battle over Smoking*, The State Univeristy, 1983

Tyrell, Ian, *Deadly Enemies*, UNSW Press, New South Wales, 1999

Viscusi, W. Kip, *Smoking: Making the Risky Decision*, OUP, New York, 1992

Walker, Robin, *Under Fire*, Melbourne University Press, Melbourne, 1984

Walton, James (ed), *Faber Book of Smoking*, Faber & Faber, London, 2000

Wootton, David, *Bad Medicine*, OUP, Oxford, 2006

Index

CPSIA information can be obtained at www.ICGtesting.com
Printed in the USA
BVOW11s0959250715

410135BV00009B/90/P